SYSTEMIC SCLEROSIS – AN UPDATE ON THE ABERRANT IMMUNE SYSTEM AND CLINICAL FEATURES

Edited by **Timothy Radstake**

Systemic Sclerosis – An Update on the Aberrant Immune System and Clinical Features
Edited by Timothy Radstake

Published by InTech
Janeza Trdine 9, 51000 Rijeka, Croatia

Publishing Process Manager Ivona Lovric

Technical Editor Teodora Smiljanic

Cover Designer InTech Design Team

Additional hard copies can be obtained from orders@intechopen.com

Systemic Sclerosis – An Update on the Aberrant Immune System and Clinical Features,
Edited by Timothy Radstake
p. cm.
ISBN 978-953-307-869-4

Meet the editor

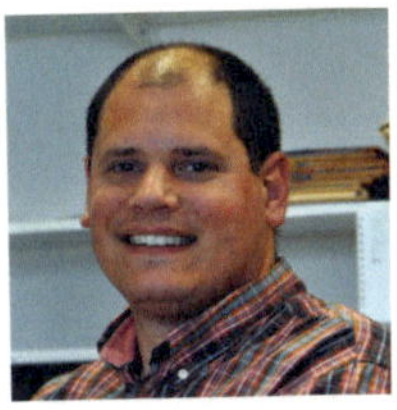

Dr Timothy Radstake, MD, PhD, attended medical school at the Radboud University in Nijmegen, the Netherlands, where he graduated in 2000 with the judicium Cum Laude. In 2003, he obtained his PhD (Cum Laude) on the genetic factors that determine the susceptibility to Rheumatoid arthritis, and the role of dendritic cells in this condition. He then started with his trainee ship rheumatology at the department of Rheumatology of the Radboud University Nijmegen Medical Centre. He became a staff rheumatologist in July 2011. From 2007 – 2008, he performed a post-doctoral fellowship at the Scleroderma center of the Boston University School of Medicine in Boston, MA, USA. Since then, he holds a faculty position, and together, with Prof. R. Lafyatis and Prof. M. Trojanowska, runs the immunology research line at this center. Currently, he is principal investigator of the research group translational immunology at the Nijmegen Center of Molecular Life Sciences (NCMLS) and Nijmegen Institute of Infection, Inflammation and Immunity (N4i).

Contents

Preface

Scleroderma, or systemic sclerosis (Ssc), means "tight skin" and is caused by the fibrosis of skin and disappearance of subcutaneous fat. There is much more involved, however. Although the fibrosis of the skin is a disabling and often painful sign of SSc, the involvement of the kidneys (see chapter on renal failure), lungs, and heart mostly lead to severe co-morbidity and premature death. The exact cause of SSc is unknown but there is accumulating evidence that the immune systems drives the three hallmarks that are observed in SSc patients: endothelial cell dysfunction, presence of autoantibodies, and fibroblast activation. In order to update the readers in the multiple facets of Ssc, this book covers two issues. In the first eight chapters, multiple key authors will provide better insights into the role of endothelial damage (chapter 1), platelets (chapter 2), and the observations that came forth from proteomic studies so far (chapter 3). T lymphocytes (chapter 4) and IL-17; a cytokine more recently shown to be increased in the circulation, and T cells isolated from SSc patients (chapter 5) are then discussed. In chapter 6, Broen and colleagues dive deeper into the potential role of the telomere and its dysfunction in SSc. Chapter 7 and 8 will deal with fibroblasts and thrombin as a potential therapeutic target of this clinical syndrome.

Besides the immunopathology of this disease, various clinical issues will be dealt with in the next issues. As such, novel issues with regard to diagnosis and pathogenesis will be discussed (chapter 9), as well as the potential role of capillary nail fold lesions in the diagnosis and follow-up (chapter 10). Scleroderma renal crisis is a feared complication of SSc and will be further discussed in chapter 11. Finally, the hurdles and pitfalls with regard pregnancy in a patient with SSc is widely discussed.

Altogether, although significant advances have occurred in our understanding SSc, the exact cause and most optimal way of treatment remains a medical conundrum. This book is meant to provide an up-to-date in SSc pathogenesis and clinical features. We believe that this book will be able to provide both researchers and clinicians dealing with SSc with the most modern information that will aid them in their work. However, the research into its cause and most efficient treatment is rapidly expanding, hopefully resulting in highly needed updates in the not to distant future.

Dr Timothy Radstake, MD, PhD
Department of Rheumatology, Radboud University Medical Center, Nijmegen, The Netherlands
The Scleroderma Center, Boston University School of Medicine, Massachusetts, U.S.A.

Part 1

The Immune System in SSc

1

Pathogenesis of the Endothelial Damage and Related Factors

Paola Cipriani, Vasiliki Liakouli, Alessandra Marrelli,
Roberto Perricone and Roberto Giacomelli
University of L'Aquila
Italy

1. Introduction

Systemic sclerosis (SSc) is an autoimmune connective tissue disorder characterized by a widespread microangiopathy, autoimmunity and fibrosis of the skin and of various internal organs. Vascular damage occurs early in the course of the disease as showed by the presence of Raynaud's phenomenon (RP) that can precede the fibrotic process of months or years. A complex interaction between endothelial cells (ECs), smooth muscle cells (SMCs), pericytes, extracellular matrix (ECM), and intravascular circulating factors is now recognized to contribute to the vascular reactivity, remodeling, and occlusive disease of SSc (Gabrielli et al., 2009). Chronic platelet activation and enhanced coagulation with reduced fibrinolysis, secondary to EC activation that leads to fibrin deposits and contribute to the intimal proliferation and luminal narrowing are also found. The identity of the initial trigger of EC damage remains unknown. Current hypotheses suggest a possible infectious or chemical trigger(s) that activates both cellular and humoral immunity. Products of immune activation may lead to vascular injury possibly through the production of autoantibodies and the release of products of activated T cells that can directly damage the endothelium (Kahaleh, 2008). Microangiopathy is characterized by a reduced capillary density and an irregular chaotic architecture that leads to chronic tissue hypoxia and organ dysfunction with eventual organ failure. Vascular complications, including pulmonary arterial hypertension (PAH) and scleroderma renal crisis (SRC) have emerged as leading causes of disability and mortality in SSc (Guiducci et al., 2007). Despite the hypoxic conditions, there is no evidence for a sufficient compensative angiogenesis in SSc (Distler O et al., 2002). Furthermore, vasculogenesis, the *de novo* formation of blood vessels, is also impaired. An imbalance between angiogenic and angiostatic factors as well as functional alterations of the cellular players, involved in the angiogenic and vasculogenic program, might explain the pathogenetic mechanisms of SSc vasculopathy (Liakouli, 2011; Cipriani, 2011). Either angiogenic or vasculogenic mechanisms may potentially become in the future the target of novel therapeutic strategies to promote vascular regeneration in SSc.

2. Vascular endothelial cell damage

Microvascular endothelial cell (MVEC) injury and apoptosis is an early and central event in the pathogenesis of SSc vasculopathy that leads to microcirculatory dysfunction and loss of capillaries with consequent vascular desertification, tissue chronic ischemia and eventual organ failure. The initiating factors or cause of the vascular insult in scleroderma remain unknown. Current hypotheses in SSc vascular disease pathogenesis suggest a possible infectious or chemical trigger(s) that activates both cellular and humoral immunity. Products of immune activation may lead to vascular injury possibly through the production of autoantibodies and the release of products of activated T cells that can directly damage the endothelium. In particular, primary activation of ECs in SSc include autoantibodies showing cross-reactivity between Cytomegalovirus (CMV) epitopes and specific surface molecules of ECs, inducing apoptosis. However, this is unlikely to be the only aetiological factor, since CMV is ubiquitous in the normal population (Lunardi et al., 2000). Anti-endothelial cells antibodies (AECAs) present in the SSc sera are reported to activate EC and, induce EC apoptosis *in vivo* independent of the Fas–Fas ligand pathway. This is clearly shown in the chicken model of SSc (UCD-200), where serum transfer into normal chicken embryos results in binding of antibodies to the microvasculature in the chorioallantoic membrane in association with endothelial apoptosis (Worda et al., 2003). The exact identity of the endothelial antigen is not known; (Worda M et al., 2003). Moreover, SSc sera containing distinct AECA subsets (ACAs for limited cutaneous SSc or anti-topoisomerase I antibodies for diffuse cutaneous SSc) can induce EC apoptosis in association with increased gene expression of caspase 3 and the reexpression of EC SSc autoantigen fibrillin 1 (Ahmed et al., 2006). Anti-endothelial cells antibodies (AECAs) are present in 40–50% of the SSc sera and are mostly of the IgG1 isotype. The antibody titres correlate negatively with pulmonary diffusion capacity and positively with pulmonary hypertension and with digital ischemic ulcers, suggesting a pathological role in the development of the vascular disease. The only published proteomic analysis of endothelial antigen(s) recognized by AECA identified 53 proteins consisting of cytoskeleton proteins, proteins involved in cellular mobility, regulation of apoptosis and senescence as well as proteins implicated in clotting and antigen presentation (Bordron et al., 1998). Thus, vascular cell apoptosis could, in turn, expose autoantigens to immune surveillance, evoking an autoimmune response and perpetuating autoimmunity to blood vessels in SSc (Ahmed et al., 2006). However, AECAs are detected in a variety of vascular diseases and specific epitopes and mechanisms have not been clarified in SSc. High levels of reactive oxygen species and oxidative stress have been directly or indirectly implicated in scleroderma (Sambo et al., 2001, 1999; Servettazet al., 2007). The source of reactive oxygen species is the membrane NADPH oxidase system, which is stimulated in all cell types within or surrounding the vessel wall in response to injury (Lassegue, 2001; Sturroch, 2005; Holland, 1998). In scleroderma, the high levels of reactive oxygen species in mesenchymal cells (MSCs) are relatively independent of the inflammatory status; they persist *in vitro* in the absence of growth factors and cytokines, render cells sensitive to stress, and induce DNA damage (Svegliati et al., 2006). MSCs become progressively hypersensitive to cytokines induced by local reactive oxygen species (Sullivan et al., 2008). Cytokines activate mesenchymal precursor cells and lead to the transformation of fibroblasts to myofibroblasts with consequent abnormal collagen synthesis. Furthermore, free radicals contribute to the release of mediators implicated in fibrosis (Bellocq et al., 1999; Barcellos-Hoff et al., 1996). EC apoptosis may also activate the immune-inflammatory system by dendritic cells and macrophage presentation of self-antigen present in the apoptotic debris to CD8+ T cells, and by the direct activation of the alternate complement and coagulation cascades leading to microvascular thrombosis and further vessel compromise. MVEC apoptosis can result from their interaction with cytotoxic T cells either by Fas or granzymes/perforin-related mechanisms. For example, CD4+ T cells can mediate MVEC apoptosis by a Fas-related mechanism as seen in cytolytic T cells killing of vascular endothelium in the rejection reaction, whereas the granzyme/perforin system mediates apoptosis by the major cytotoxic cells, the CD8+ T cells, NK and LAK cells. Involvement of cytotoxic T cells in SSc is suggested by the presence of a 60 kDa protein in SSc sera that was described as an endothelial cytotoxic factor. This factor was characterized as the granular enzyme, and was detected in the perivascular spaces in SSc skin biopsies. Cytotoxic T lymphocytes (in particular CD8+ T cells, NK cells, LAK cells) granule-specific products such as granzyme B and perforin are able to induce apoptosis in cultured ECs. Granzymes gain access to the cells following cellular membrane damage by perforin (Kahaleh, 1997). The majority of autoantigens targeted in SSc can be cleaved by granzyme B and are recognized preferentially by patients antibodies (Schachna et al., 2002). Furthermore, the activation of cytotoxic cell-mediated pathways is plausible and may be involved in early vascular injury thus initiating and propagating the autoimmune response in SSc. Antibody-dependent cellular cytotoxicity of vascular endothelium is reported in up to 40% of the SSc patients. The effector cells express Fc receptors and are both non-T cells and non adherent T lymphocytes, while the antibody is an IgG with MVEC specificity that mediate MVEC cytotoxicity via the Fas pathway (Sgonc et al., 2000). EC apoptosis may also confer a state of resistance to apoptosis by the surrounding fibroblasts that may lead to myofibroblast differentiation and tissue fibrotic changes that follow (Laplante et al., 2005). However, EC damage and apoptosis is an early event in the course of the disease with progressive loss of capillaries, responsible on one hand of the typical clinical manifestations of vasculopathy and on the other hand the chronic tissue ischemia that leads to organ dysfunction and eventual organ failure.

3. Vascular endothelial cell alterations and fibroproliferative vasculopathy

Vascular disease in scleroderma patients is both functional and structural with reversible vasospasm as well as a reduction in the capillary density followed by obliterative vasculopathy. These vascular changes involving capillaries, arterioles and small arteries may be observed by nail-fold capillaroscopy.

Important features of the tissue lesions in various stages of scleroderma are early microvascular damage, mononuclear-cell infiltrates, and slowly developing fibrosis. In later stages of scleroderma, the main findings are very densely packed collagen in the dermis, loss of cells, and atrophy. In particular, in the early phase of the disease, endothelial damage is characterized by collapse of vimentin's filaments in the perinuclear region, vacuolization, granular degeneration of the nucleus, cellular necrosis, gaps between endothelial cells, reduplication of basal membranes, followed by vascular lumen obstruction, altered permeability of vessel wall that induce increased passage of both plasma and mononuclear cells with perivascular infiltrates formation in which T lymphocytes and monocytes bearing macrophage markers predominate (Fleischmajer, 1980, 1977; Ishikawa, 1992) with more CD4+ than CD8+ cells (Roumm, 1984). In fact, T cells in skin lesions are predominantly CD4+ cells, display markers of activation, exhibit oligoclonal expansion (Sakkas et al., 2002) and are predominantly type 2 helper T (Th2) cells (Mavalia et al., 1997). Moreover, an increase in the Vdelta1 + T cells subset that express both adhesion molecules and activation markers suggests a selective V gene subset expansion (Giacomelli et al., 1998). In advanced phases, intimal thickening, delamination, vessel narrowing or obliteration and perivascular fibrosis are present (Rodnan et al., 1980).

At the cellular level, the changes that characterized the early lesions are: loss of endothelial cells, proliferating pericytes and vascular smooth muscle cells, and immune cells in the perivascular space. Endothelial cells are the only mesenchymal cell type that undergo apoptosis in the early phase of scleroderma, whereas vascular smooth-muscle cells and pericytes proliferate vigorously thus leading to the characteristic fibroproliferative SSc vasculopathy. The activation of vascular smooth muscle leads to migration of these cells into the intimal layer of the vessel where they differentiate into a myofibroblast. Fibroblasts and pericytes may also transform into myofibroblasts in scleroderma disease (Rajkumar et al., 2005). It is also suggested that, following vascular injury, bone marrow-derived circulating mesenchymal progenitor cells (e.g., fibrocytes), and epithelial cells via epithelial to mesenchymal transition (EMT) can become myofibroblasts. Recently, a study provided evidence that abnormal fibrillin-1 expression and chronic oxidative stress mediate endothelial-mesenchymal transition (EndoMT) in the tight skin murine model of SSc (Xu et al, 2010) and more recently evidence indicates that the c-Abl tyrosine kinase and the protein kinase C δ (PKC-δ), are crucial for TGFβ induction of EndoMT *in vitro*, and that imatinib mesylate and rottlerin, or similar kinase inhibitor molecules, may be effective therapeutic agents for SSc and other fibroproliferative vasculopathies in which EndoMT is involved (Li & Jimenez, 2011). The exact mediator of cell activation in scleroderma is unknown, but speculation includes the release of mediators from the activated endothelium (e.g., endothelin- 1 (ET-1)) and platelets (e.g., thromboxane or platelet derived growth factor. In fact, endothelial damage cause an imbalance in endothelial vascular signals with increased endothelin production and impaired nitric oxide and prostacyclin release that mediates the vasospasm and contribute to intimal proliferation and vascular fibrosis and stiffness of the vessel wall. Recently, Interleukin 33 (IL-33), a novel member of the IL1 family that promotes Th2 responses and inflammation through the ST2 receptor, was found to be abnormally expressed in the SSc tissue and sera. In particular, in the early phase of the disease, upon EC activation/damage IL-33 may be mobilised from ECs into the circulation to signal through ST2 in key profibrotic players such as inflammatory/immune cells and fibroblasts/myofibroblasts. (Manetti, 2010, 2011). This step probably corresponds to the first symptom of scleroderma. Recurrent Raynaud's phenomenon could be the direct consequence of the structural changes of the vessel and the perturbed control of vascular tone due to an imbalance between vasodilatory and vasoconstrictive mediators. At this stage, the patient may have early signs of skin and visceral fibrosis. Platelet activation and enhanced coagulation with reduced fibrinolysis lead to fibrin deposits and contribute to the intimal proliferation and luminal narrowing.

Besides the skin, fibroproliferative vasculopathy is present in the lungs, kidneys and other organs (Dorfmuller et al., 2007; Nagai et al., 2007; Guiducci et al., 2007). However, the mechanisms underlying the pathological vascular changes in SSc still remain unclear.

4. Impaired angiogenesis and vasculogenesis in SSc

In the adult mammalian organism, the vasculature is normally quiescent and the ECs have an extremely low turn-over rate with the exception of the reproductive cycle (ovulation, implanation, pregnancy) and wound healing or tissue regeneration (Carmeliet, 2003).

However, after endothelial cell injury, and in response to appropriate stimuli, mature and progenitor ECs they can form new blood vessels through a combination of two separate processes: angiogenesis and vasculogenesis. The term angiogenesis describes the formation of new capillaries and larger vessels by sprouting of differentiated EC from pre-existing vessels. Angiogenesis is a highly complex and requires a dynamic, temporally and spatially interaction among ECs, ECM molecules, adhesion molecules, proteolytic enzymes and the subtle balance between proangiogenic and angiostatic factors (Distler et al., 2003). In particular, proangiogenic stimuli activate EC, which degrade the basal membrane and the perivascular extracellular matrix, proliferate and migrate into the site of new vessel formation. Stabilisation of vessel wall by pericytes is the final process of sprouting angiogenesis and leads to a functional network of new capillary. In contrast to angiogenesis, vasculogenesis describes the formation of new vessels by circulating EPC, independent from pre-existing vessels. Vasculogenesis was regarded to be restricted to embryogenesis but the discovery of EPC in adult bone marrow and peripheral blood has challenged this theory (Asahara et al., 1997; Shi et al., 1998). After birth, postnatal vasculogenesis contributes to vascular healing in response to endothelial injury through the processes of rapid reendothelialization of denuded vessels and collateral vessel formation in ischemic tissues. In particular, following tissue ischemia, EPC are mobilized from their bone marrow niches into the circulation in response to stress- and/or damage related signals, migrate through the bloodstream and home to the sites of vascular injury, where they contribute to the formation as well of neovessels as to the repair of damaged vessels, collaborating with pre-existing mature EC (Urbich et al., 2004). Several studies showed that EPCs promotes structural and functional repair in several organs such as the heart, liver, kidney or brain. However, as mentioned above, progenitor cells can migrate to sites of vascular injury and differentiate not only into an endothelial phenotype (vascular repair), but also into vascular smooth muscle cells contributing to neointimal hyperplasia and eventually fibroproliferative vasculopathy.

Both angiogenic and vasculogenic processes are impaired in SSc. The progressive loss of capillaries on one hand, and the vascular remodeling of arteriolar vessels on the other result in insufficient blood flow, causing severe and chronic hypoxia. Tissue hypoxia usually initiates the formation of new blood vessels from the pre-existing microvasculature leading to the expression of pro-angiogenic molecules, mainly of Vascular Endothelial Growth Factor (VEGF), which triggers the angiogenic process. Despite the hypoxic conditions and the increased levels of VEGF in skin and serum of SSc patients, there is, paradoxically, no evidence for a sufficient angiogenesis, thus perpetuating the vicious circle leading to tissue ischemia (Distler JH et al., 2006; Distler O et al., 2004, 2002). Vasculogenesis, is also impaired in SSc patients with a decreased number and several functional defects of endothelial progenitor cells (EPCs) (Kuwana et al., 2004; Del Papa et al., 2006) and mesenchymal stem cells (MSCs), the latter deriving from the bone marrow population and the tissue resident cells, was observed in SSc patients (Cipriani et al., 2007).

5. Endothelial cells

The aetiological factors involved in the pathogenesis of SSc-associated vascular defects determine a complicate network of EC alterations which account for the lost ability of these cells to perform *in vitro* angiogenesis.

Angiogenic process is an invasive event in which proteolytic activities by EC are required. Specific proteases are needed for the degradation of the membrane basement, for cell migration and for creating space in the matrix, to allow the formation of new tubules. Besides their substrate specific properties, proteases exert more complex pro- or anti-angiogenic activities, including the activation and modification of growth factors, cytokines and receptors and the generation of matrix fragments which inhibit angiogenesis (Van Hinsberg et al., 2008). Evidence for a mechanism of dysregulated angiogenesis involving these proteases in SSc has emerged from recent experimental studies. A decreased urokinase plasminogen activator (uPA) dependent invasion, proliferation, and capillary morphogenesis, was showed in SSc EC. Urokinase plasminogen activator receptor (uPAR) undergoes truncation between domains 1 and 2, and this modification prevents EC from entering in an angiogenic program (D'Alessio et al., 2004). Furthermore, SSc MVECs produce large amounts of antiangiogenic molecules such as matrix metalloproteinase 12 (MMP-12), involved in the cleavage of the domain of the uPAR, and pentraxin 3 (PTX3). Silencing these two molecules in SSc-MVEC, restore their ability to produce capillaries in vitro (Margheri et al., 2010). Recent work has provided the evidence for the association between a uPAR gene variant, *UPAR* rs344781, and vascular complications, such as digital ulcerations, suggesting a role of this gene in the vascular pathophysiology of SSc (Manetti et al., 2011).

Endothelial cells are directly involved also in vasculogenic process, through the expression of SDF-1. In fact, SDF-1 is a pivotal molecule in the recruitment and retention of CXCR4+ EPC into neo-angiogenic niches (Petit et al., 2007). This molecule, expressed and presented by EC at the site of injury triggers cell arrest and emigration of circulating cells, facilitating the formation of stable vasculature and supporting organ repair (Yao et al., 2003). Additionally, SDF-1 has an angiogenic effect on endothelial cells by inducing cell proliferation, differentiation, sprouting and tube formation in vitro (Salvucci et al., 2002; Yamaguchi et al., 2011). It has been reported that SDF-1 and CXCR4 are clearly up-regulated in the skin and in microvascular endothelial cells during the early edematous phases of SSc. The production of these two molecules progressively decreased, with the lowest levels in the latest phases of the disease. These data strongly suggest that an impairment of EC ability to promote a sustained response to chronic ischemic stress through SDF-1 expression could compromise an adaptive angiogenesis and vasculogenesis in the disease, contributing to the disappearance of the vessels (Cipriani et al., 2006).

Finally, it has been demonstrated that in SSc skin, along with the loss of capillaries, there is a dramatic change in the endothelial phenotype of residual microvessels, characterized by loss of vascular endothelial cadherin (VEcadherin), supposed to be an universal endothelial marker required for tube formation, as well as the over-expression of the anti-angiogenic interferon-α (IFN-α) and over-expression of RGS5, a signaling molecule whose expression coincides with the end of new vessel formation during embryo development and tumour angiogenesis (Fleming et al., 2008).

5.1 Endothelial progenitors

5.1.1 Hematopoietic endothelial progenitor cells

Endothelial progenitor cells are known to be a key cellular effectors of vascular regeneration. Growing evidence shows that EPC play an important role in the homeostasis of physiologic vascular network and are involved both in new vessel formation after ischemic insult and in the repair mechanisms of existing vessels (Shi et al., 1998; Urbich et al., 2004; Zammaretti & Zisch, 2005; Adams et al., 2004). Endothelial progenitor cells have emerged as crucial regulators of cardiovascular integrity. Reduced numbers and altered

functions of these cells have been found to be involved in the pathogenesis of cardiovascular disease (Adams et al., 2004, Dimmeler et al., 2001; Hill et al., 2003).
At least two different types of circulating progenitors appear able to become mature endothelium (Smadja et al., 2007). One type of progenitor cells displays the markers CD133, CD34, and vascular endothelial growth factor receptor 2 (VEGFR2) (Hristov et al., 2004). These are harvested from late-outgrowth cultures, possess a high proliferation capacity and are sometimes referred as "true EPC "; most of studies focus on this population. A second type of progenitor population is a subset of CD14+ monocytes distinguishable from the conventional endothelial progenitor cells by the fact that they are CD34− (Hristov et al., 2004; Zhao et al., 2003), arise from short-term cultures and show little proliferative capacity. Both circulating progenitor cell types can differentiate into mature endothelium in culture. It has been precisely characterized using, genome-wide transcriptional study, the molecular fingerprint of two distinct EPCs, showing that early-outhgrowth EPC are haematopoietic cells with a molecular phenotype linked to monocytes; whereas late-outgrowth EPC exhibit commitment to the endothelial lineage (Medina et al., 2010). Interestingly both populations can form capillary tubes in vitro, mediate reendothelialization after injury and improve neovascularization (Urbich et al., 2004). It has been previously demonstrated that both subsets contribute to angiogenesis, but through different mechanisms, CD14+ EPC supporting vasculogenic process by paracrine production of growth factors, while late-outgrowth CD14- EPC directly incorporating into vessel wall (Sieveking et al., 2008; Mukai et al., 2008). Neovascularization and reendothelialization event are complex multistep processes, requiring EPC chemoattraction, adhesion, and finally differentiation into mature EC. Although the signaling cascades that regulate these steps are still incompletely understood, it is well known that VEGF and SDF-1, induced by hypoxia, play a pivotal role in the EPC mobilization from bone marrow, differentiation and attraction to site of ischemia. Recently several studies have demonstrated a role of EPC in the pathogenesis of SSc, suggesting that alteration in the vasculogenic process might contribute to the vasculopathy, distinctive features of the disease. Apparently conflicting results have raised on quantitative and functional characteristics of EPC from SSc patients, probably due to unclear distinctive markers of the several cell subsets belonging to the EPC population.
A lower number of circulating EPC, defined as CD34+CD133+VEGFR-2+ mononuclear cells in patients with SSc than in patients with RA or in healthy subjects was seen (Kuwana et al., 2006). In SSc patients, EPC counts did not correlate with the disease subset, the disease duration, or the modified Rodnan skin thickness score. However, the numbers of these cells were lower in SSc patients with pitting scars and active fingertip ulcers. Furthermore, EPC, obtained from the peripheral blood of SSc patients demonstrated an impaired differentiation capacity into mature EC, as shown by a reduced expression of the EC marker von Willebrand factor.
In contrast to these findings, in another study was found a significantly increase in the number of circulating EPC, identified via the same cell surface markers CD34+ CD133+VEGFR-2+, in SSc patients. Further subgroup analysis revealed a negative correlation between EPC count and disease duration (Del Papa et al., 2008). Based on this finding, the authors suggested that differences in disease duration might account for the discrepancy between their results and the findings reported by the other authors. Apart from disease duration, no correlations between EPC counts and clinical parameters, including digital ulcers, were observed. In this study bone marrow EPC were also evaluated. The number of bone marrow CD133+ cells was significantly decreased in SSc patients compared to healthy controls. Their ability to differentiate into EC *in vitro* was

found reduced in SSc patients. Finally, the number and the size of colonies were reduced, and cells from patients showed morphologic signs of cellular senescence.

Another study assessed EPC counts in the whole blood of patients with SSc, osteoarthritis (OA), and RA (Allanore et al., 2007). Circulating CD34+CD133+ cells were increased in patients with SSc as compared with patients with OA, but the same cells were lower than those in RA patients. The analysis of potential correlations with clinical parameters showed that CD34+CD133+ counts increased in parallel with the European League Against Rheumatism Scleroderma Trial and Research (EUSTAR) group disease activity score. Of note, the authors did not analyse the expression of VEGFR-2.

In another study, the same authors (Avouac et al., 2008) assessed EPC, evaluating VEGFR-2 and lineage (Lin) markers as additional markers, and using 7-aminoactinomycin D (7-AAD) as viability marker. Again, patients with SSc displayed higher numbers of circulating Lin-7AAD-CD34+CD133+VEGFR-2+ EPC than did healthy subjects. Lower EPC counts in SSc patients were associated with higher Medsger severity scores for SSc and with digital ulcers. A decreased CD34+CD133+VEGFR-2+ EPC counts was found in both limited and diffuse subsets of recent-onset, and late-stage SSc, as compared with healthy individuals. The authors showed an increased rate of apoptosis in freshly isolated EPC from SSc patients. Addition of sera from the same patients to cultured EPC from healthy volunteers was able to induce apoptosis of EPC. The proapoptotic effects of SSc sera were abolished by depletion of the IgG fraction, suggesting the presence of anti-EPC autoantibodies in the SSc patient sera (Zhu et al., 2008).

It has been also found a raise of circulating EPC in early stage SSc, in response to tissue ischemia, but they dropped with disease progression. EPC reduction was linked with endothelial dysfunction and capillary loss, as well as the development of severe cardiac involvement and pulmonary arterial hypertension (Nevsakaya et al., 2008).

Whether EPC counts are altered in the peripheral blood of SSc patients is still a matter of controversy. Apparent contradiction in EPC counts between the different studies might be explained by use of different combinations of surface markers, resulting in the analysis of different cell subsets, or by differences in the mean disease duration and severity. Nevertheless, functional defects of EPC in the peripheral blood as well as in the bone marrow have consistently been reported (Del papa et al., 2006; Kuwana et al., 2004) indicating a critical role of EPC in the pathogenesis of SSc. Further studies on the molecular mechanisms underlying these defects is needed in order to develop specific treatment options and restore functional vasculogenesis in patients with SSc.

Several lines of evidence indicate that EPC obtained by short term culture of peripheral blood mononuclear cells (PBMCs) in media favouring endothelial differentiation, are composed predominantly of endothelial-like cells derived from circulating monocytes (Rehman et al., 2003; Urbich et al., 2003). Moreover, it has been identified a monocyte-derived multipotent cells positive for CD14, CD45, CD34, which contain progenitors able to differentiate into several distinct mesenchymal cell types, including bone, cartilage, fat, and skeletal and cardiac muscle cells, as well as neurons (Kuwana et al., 2003; Kodama et al., 2005, 2006). It has been recently shown that this population of multipotent cells, is able to differentiate into endothelium of a mature phenotype with typical morphologic and functional characteristics (Kuwana et al., 2006). These findings indicate a potential developmental relationship between monocytes and endothelial cells and suggest that the monocyte population could be recruited for vasculogenesis and represent an endothelial precursor population.

A recent study demonstrated that circulating monocytic EPCs were increased in the peripheral blood of SSc patients. *In vitro* and *in vivo* functional analyses revealed that monocytic EPCs derived from SSc patients had an enhanced ability to promote blood vessel formation, when co-cultured with HUVEC. In contrast, the EPC ability to be incorporated into vessels and differentiate into mature endothelial cells was rather impaired in SSc patients. This characteristic was primarily attributable to an enhanced angiogenic property through production of angiogenic factors (Yamaguchi et al., 2010). Because EPCs may critically contribute to the homeostasis of the physiological vascular network, these progenitor cells might be considered interesting candidates for novel cell therapies for the treatment of various ischemic diseases.

5.1.2 Mesenchymal stem cells (MSCs)

Endothelial cells could also originate from non- hematopoietic stem cells of the bone marrow (Drake et al., 2003). Mesenchymal stem cells are multipotent cells that are present in the bone marrow and in some tissues as resident stem cells. They retain the capacity to differentiate into several cell lineages of mesenchymal tissues, i.e. bone, cartilage, muscle, tendon or adipose tissue and serve for the preservation and repair of tissues and organs (Tuan et al., 2003; Arnhold et al., 2007). Multipotent mesenchymal progenitor cells have been isolated from bone marrow. Under exposition to angiogenic factors, these cells differentiated to angioblasts *in vitro* (CD34-positive, flk-1- positive, vascular endothelial cadherin-positive) and finally to mature endothelial cells, expressing specific endothelial markers, showing characteristics endothelial functional features and participating in neovascularization of tumours or wound healing *in vitro* (Reyes et al., 2001, 2002). Transplanted MSCs were able to enhance angiogenesis and contribute to remodelling of the vasculature *in vitro* (Ladage et al., 2007; Choi et al., 2008; Copland et al., 2008). Taken together, these data suggest that human MSCs may be considered an alternative source of EPCs (Oswald et al., 2004).

There are several evidences that in SSc there is a complex impairment in the BM microenvironment, involving not only the endothelial compartment but also the MSC, thus hypothesizing that alteration in this cell population may also contribute to the defective vasculogenesis in SSc (Del Papa et al., 2006; Cipriani et al., 2007). In particular, it has been reported that the number of colonies formed by MSC obtained from bone marrow of SSc patients were reduced in comparison with healthy controls. The colonies were small and did not expand, and the cells rapidly showed aging and signs of stress (Del Papa et al., 2006). Furthermore, nother study provided evidence of a reduced differentiative ability *in vitro* toward an endothelial phenotype of bone marrow MSC from SSc patients. These cells displayed both an early senescence and decreased capacity to perform specific endothelial activities, such as capillary morphogenesis and chemoinvasion, after VEGF and SDF-1 stimulation (Cipriani et al., 2007). All above suggests that a functional impairment of this population of endothelial progenitors cells may affect endothelial repair machinery, contributing to the defective angiogenesis and vasculogenesis in the disease.

In the last few years bone marrow-derived MSCs have shown great promise for tissue repair. In experimental models of acute myocardial infarction, intramyocardial injection of mesenchymal stem cells restored cardiac function through the formation of a new vascular network and arteriogenesis (Torensma et al., 2004). Autologous implantation of bone marrow–derived mesenchymal stem cells into chronic nonhealing ulcers has been shown to accelerate the healing process and significantly improve clinical parameters (Martens et al.,

2006). Recently, it has been showed that in one patient with systemic sclerosis who have severe peripheral ischemia, intravenous infusion of expanded autologous mesenchymal stem cells may promote the recovery of the vascular network, restore blood flow, and reduce skin necrosis (Guiducci et al., 2010). Further studies on a larger number of patients with systemic sclerosis are needed to confirm the short- and long-term efficacy and safety of mesenchymal stem-cell infusion as treatment of severe digital ulcers and gangrene of the extremities that are resistant to conventional therapies.

6. Angiogenic factors

6.1 Vascular endothelial growth factor (VEGF)

VEGF, one of the strongest angiogenic factors known in biology, is involved in several steps of physiological and pathological angiogenesis. VEGF increases the vascular permeability, stimulates the migration and proliferation of ECs and induces tube formation. The biological effects of VEGF are extremely dose dependent. Loss of even a single allele results in lethal vascular defects in the embryo, and postnatal inhibition of VEGF leads to impaired organ development and growth arrest in mice. Application of VEGF as a recombinant protein or by gene transfer augmented perfusion and development of collateral vessels in animal models of hindlimb ischemia, thereby making VEGF an interesting target for therapeutic angiogenesis (Takeshita et al., 1994, 1996). During SSc, VEGF is strongly overexpressed in the skin and sera (Distle O et al., 2002) of these patients. VEGF exerts its biological functions by binding to 2 different tyrosine kinase receptors: VEGFR-1 and VEGFR-2, which are both upregulated in the affected skin of SSc patients (Distler O et al., 2004), although non compensative new vessel formation is observed. The serum levels of VEGF significantly correlate with the development of fingertip ulcers in these patients. Although elevated levels of VEGF are consistent with active angiogenesis, an uncontrolled chronic over-expression, as seen in SSc patients, throughout various disease stages, might contribute to disturbed vessel morphology and endothelial disturbances rather than to promote new vessel formation. On the other hand, a brief upregulation of VEGF results in instability of newly formed vessels ((Dor et al., 2002). The mechanisms that lead to an over-expression of VEGF in SSc are unclear. Isolated microvascular endothelial cells (MVECs) from SSc patients show an impaired response to VEGF and other growth factors in the Matrigel capillary morphogenesis assay, suggesting that VEGF receptor signaling might be impaired in these cells (D'Alessio et al., 2004). Hypoxia-induced expression of hypoxia inducible factor-1α (HIF1-α) does not appear to play a major role in the induction of VEGF in SSc (Distler O et al., 2004), whereas induction by cytokines such as platelet derived growth factor (PDGF) and transforming growth factor beta (TGF-β) appear to be more important. The function of TGF-β in angiogenesis is strongly context dependent. A weak TGF-β stimulation may cause induction of several angiogenic regulators such as VEGF and matrix proteins to promote angiogenesis, whereas at high TGF-β concentrations, growth-inhibitory effect dominate (Bobik et al., 2006). Functionally important gene polymorphisms that lead to an impairment in biological properties of VEGF have not still been shown in SSc patients (Allanore et al., 2007).

6.2 Transforming growth factor beta (TGF-β) and Endoglin (ENG)

The vascular effect of TGF-β in angiogenesis results in activation of ECs and vascular smooth muscle cells (VSMCs). It regulates the activation state of ECs, via 2 different types of I receptors, ALK-5, and ALK-1. The TGF-β/ALK-1 pathway stimulates ECs proliferation and migration, whereas the TGF-β/ALK-5 pathway inhibits these processes. ALK-5 deficiency not only impairs TGF-β/ALK-5 signaling but also reduces TGF-β/ALK-1 responses, suggesting that ALK-5 is essential for efficient ALK-1 activation and recruitment into a TGF-β/receptor complex (Bobik et al., 2006). These effects are mainly mediated by ENG (CD105), a coreceptor of TGF-β, predominantly expressed on cell surfaces of ECs. ENG plays a role in vascular integrity and endothelium functioning, whereas soluble ENG (sENG) acts as an antiangiogenic protein interfering with the binding of TGF-β to its receptors. Conflicting results have been reported in the available literature concerning the relationship between ENG and PAH. A previous paper reported an association between a 6-base insertion in intron 7 (6bINS) polymorphism of ENG gene and SSc-related PAH (Wipff et al., 2007). More recently, increased sENG levels were found in SSc patients, both with and without PAH, suggesting a role for ENG in SSc vasculopathy, independent of PAH presence (Coral-Alvarado et al., 2010). Furthermore, ENG might act on fibroblasts to modulate TGF-β signaling by acting as a molecular link regulating or reducing the total pool of TGF-β available for activating signal-transducing receptors.

6.3 Platelet derived growth factor (PDGF)

The PDGF family consists of four different PDGF strands (A-D), establishing functional homodimers (PDGF-AA, PDGF-BB, PDGF-CC, and PDGF-DD) or an heterodimer PDGF-AB. They exert their biological activities by activating 2 structurally related tyrosine kinase receptors, PDGFRα and PDGFRβ. Ligand-induced receptor homo- or hetero-dimerization leads to autophosphorylation of specific tyrosine residues within the cytoplasmic domain. PDGF-A activates PDGFRα exclusively, while PDGF-B is capable of activating PDGFRαα, PDGFRαβ and PDGFRββ. PDGF-AB and PDGF-C activate PDGFRαα and PDGFRαβ, whereas PDGF-D preferentially activates PDGFRββ. PDGF-B and the PDGFRβ are primarily required for the development of the vasculature both under physiological and pathological angiogenic conditions e.g. during myocardial infarction (Zymek et al., 2006) and tumor vascularization (Vrekoussis et al., 2007) while, they are almost undetectable in healthy tissues. PDGFBB/PDGFRβ signaling-axis is also involved in recruiting pericytes and smooth muscle cells thus contributing to the maturation of the vessel wall (Lindblom et al., 2003). PDGF plays an important role in the pathogenesis of scleroderma and elevated expression of PDGF and its receptors has been found in SSc skin and lung diseases. In particular, expression of PDGF-B was detected in endothelial cell lining of small capillaries and in the infiltrating cells (Gay et al., 1989; Klareskoog et al., 1990). Likewise, elevated levels of PDGF-A and PDGF-B were found in bronchoalveolar lavage (BAL) fluid obtained from SSc patients (Ludwicka et al., 1995). Moreover, elevated plasma levels of PDFG-BB were reported in patients with SSc (Hummers et al., 2009). Indeed, recent studies suggest that the reciprocal induction of pro-angiogenic factors could promote vascularization and improve vessel maturation compared with the release of a single factor, and the interplay between PDGF and VEGF-mediated signalling pathways is just emerging (Bianco et al., 2007; Reinmuth et al., 2007). In fact, activated platelets carry in their alpha granules a set of angiogenesis stimulators such as VEGF, PDGF and SDF-1. Moreover, EPCs trigger EC thus inducing a pro-angiogenic phenotype including the up-regulation of PDGFRβ, thereby turning the PDGFBB/PDGFRβ signaling-axis into a critical element of EPC-induced endothelial angiogenesis (Wyler von Ballmoos et al., 2010). This finding may be utilized to enhance EPC-based therapy of ischemic tissue in future. Furthermore, the recent discovery of novel agonistic antibodies targeting the PDGF receptor that represents a pathogenetic link between immune system and fibrosis might lead to perform intense investigations to clarify the possible role that PDGF might exert on the SSc vasculopathy (Baroni et al., 2006). Finally,

PDGF receptor antagonist STI571 (imatinib) reversed advanced pulmonary vascular disease in 2 animal models of pulmonary hypertension (Schermuly et al., 2005).

6.4 Stromal cell-derived factor 1 (SDF-1/CXCL12)

The CXC chemokine SDF-1, the most important chemokine induced by ischemia, and its receptor, CXCR4, regulates specific steps in new vessel formation (Salcedo et al., 2003). Experimental deficiency in *SDF-1* or *CXCR4* gene in the embryo results in a lethal phenotype characterised by defective development of cardiovascular system (Kucia et al., 2004). As already mentioned above, SDF-1 is a potent chemoattractant for mature ECs, hematopoietic stem cells (HSCs) and EPCs expressing CXCR4 on their surface, thus influencing both angiogenesis and vasculogenesis (De Falco et al., 2004). SDF-1–CXCR4 interaction further amplifies angiogenesis by increasing VEGF release by ECs. VEGF elevated levels, in turn, promote enhanced expression of CXCR4 on endothelial cells, which can then respond to SDF-1. SDF-1, also prevents the apoptosis of EPCs. Also, SDF-1 contributes to the stabilization of neo-vessel formation by recruiting CXCR4+PDGFR+cKit+ smooth muscle progenitor cells during recovery for vascular injury. In SSc, due to the transient nature of SDF-1 expression, its modulation could be considered a future therapeutic target for inducing new vessel formation in this disease (Cipriani et al., 2006). Finally, SDF-1 polymorphism may modulate SSc vascular phenotype, further arguing for a critical role of SDF-1/CXCR4 axis in the vascular component of SSc pathogenesis (Manetti et al., 2009).

6.5 Endothelin 1 (ET-1)

ET-1, a highly vasoconstrictor molecule produced from endothelial cells and mesodermal cells such as fibroblasts and smooth muscle cells, promotes leukocyte adhesion to the endothelium as well as vascular smooth muscle cell proliferation and fibroblast activation (Abraham & Distler, 2006). ET-1 expression levels are increased in blood vessels, lung, kidney and skin of patients with SSc. Plasma ET-1 levels are also increased in SSc patients in both early and late stage (Kahaleh, 1991; Kadono et al., 1995). ET-1 mediates its biological effects via the ETA and ETB receptors. ETA receptors are expressed by vascular smooth muscle cells and can mediate vasoconstriction, smooth muscle cell proliferation, fibrosis and inflammation. ETB receptors are predominantly expressed on endothelial cells mediating vasodilation via the release of nitric oxide or potassium channel activation, and removing ET-1 from the circulation. In SSc vasculopathy, ETB receptors are down regulated on endothelial cells which may diminish their vasodilatory role while are up-regulated on smooth muscle cells and can contribute to cell proliferation, hypertrophy, inflammation, fibrosis and vasoconstriction (Abraham et al., 1997; Bauer et al., 20029). ETA/B receptor antagonists including bosentan are now commonly used for the treatment of PAH (Channick et al., 2001; Rubin et al., 2002) and of the prevention of new digital ulcers related to SSc (Matucci-Cerinic et al., 2011). ET-1 represents a potent molecular target for intervention in the management of patients with SSc.

6.6 Angiopoietins

Angiopoietins are known to be involved in the development, remodeling and stability of blood vessels. Recently has been clarified as they might act alongside VEGF (Ashara et al., 1998). However, Ang-1 and -2 have opposing functions. Ang-1 under physiological conditions has vasoprotective and anti-inflammatory actions (Kim et al., 2001), mediates vessel maturation and maintains vessel integrity by the recruitment of periendothelial cells. On the contrary, Ang-2 acts as a vessel-destabilizing cytokine, playing an essential role in vascular remodeling. Recently, has been demonstrated that Ang-1 and -2 are differentially expressed in the sera of patients with SSc. Ang-1, was significantly decreased in SSc patients contributing to the development of SSc-related vasculopathy through promoting activation and apoptosis of ECs and destabilization of blood vessels. On the other hand, Ang-2, was significantly increased in SSc patients (Michalska et al., 2010)). Moreover, high Ang-2 levels are associated with greater severity and higher activity of the disease. Thus, the Ang-1/ Ang-2 imbalance might contribute to the development of the disease, and represent a new promising therapeutic target in SSc.

6.7 uPAR and kallikreins

As already mentioned above, MVECS can perform angiogenesis only when provided with a proper enzymatic machinery, enabling them to lyse the extracellular matrix and invade the surrounding tissue. In this regard, the serine protease urokinase- type plasminogen activator uPA-uPAR system is known to play a crucial role in angiogenesis by modulating the adhesive properties of ECs in their interactions with the extracellular matrix and in the degradation of matrix components (Van Hinsberg et al., 2008); D'Alessio et al., 2004; Margheri et al., 2006; Manetti et al., 2011).

Another angiogenesis-associated serine protease family, potentially involved in the angiogenic program of SSc are some members of kallikreins. Kallikreins hydrolyze kininogen to kinin. Kinins promote angiogenesis, since they play a role that leads to endothelial cell migration, proliferation and differentiation. Kallikreins 9, 11, and 12, which are associated with proangiogenesis, were downregulated in SSc patients, whereas anti-angiogenic kallikrein 3 was upregulated. Further experiments using healthy MVECs treated with antibodies against the relevant kallikreins revealed that while kallikreins 9, 11, and 12 induced cell growth, only kallikrein 12 regulated invasion and capillary morphogenesis. Buffering of kallikrein 12 with antibodies resulted in the acquisition of an SSc-like pattern by normal cells *in vitro* angiogenesis (Giusti et al., 2005).

6.8 Adhesion molecules

Another pro-angiogenic marker of SSc vasculopathy is the presence of adhesion proteins involved in cell-cell interaction and cell-extracellular matrix interactions that are found increased in SSc skin (Gruscwitz et al., 1992). In particular, increased expression of the adhesion proteins such as intercellular adhesion molecule 1 (ICAM-1), endothelial leukocyte adhesion molecule 1 (ELAM-1), vascular adhesion molecule (VCAM-1), E-selectin, P-selectin in endothelial cells in the skin of patients with a rapidly progressive systemic sclerosis was observed (Sollberg et al., 1992; Gruschwitz et al., 1995; Ihn et al., 1997; Kiener et al., 1994; Ihn et al., 1998). To evaluate the relationship between systemic manifestations and immunological markers of endothelial cell activation, soluble VCAM-1 (sVCAM-1), soluble E selectin (sE-selectin), VEGF, and ET-1 were determined. Interestingly, the injury to the pulmonary and renal vascular trees might have distinct pathogenic mechanisms (Stratton et al., 1998). In particular, in patients with SRC, the level of E-selectin, sVCAM-1, and soluble ICAM-1 (sICAM-1) were elevated, but they were not consistently elevated in patients with pulmonary hypertension.

7. Angiostatic factors

7.1 Endostatin and Angiostatin

Breakdown of the extracellular matrix by granzyme B and other proteases contained in T cell granule content, may contribute to defective wound healing and vascular repair in SSc patients. Among these extracellular matrix derived angiostatic growth factors, endostatin has been characterized as a potent inhibitor of VEGF-induced angiogenesis. Endostatin is a C-terminal, 20 kDa fragment of the basement protein collagen type XVIII that inhibits angiogenesis and tumor growth strongly by reducing endothelial cell proliferation and migration. Circulating endostatin concentrations are significantly increased in patients with SSc and this increase is associated with the presence of more severe clinical involvement (Distler O et al., 2002). Angiostatin is another antiangiogenic factor derived from the cleavage of the plasminogen and proangiogenic plasmin. Recent data suggest that there is a decreased presence and activity of proangiogenic plasmin, and increased production of antiangiogenic angiostatin in SSc plasma. This increase in angiostatin production may account for some of the vascular defects observed in patients with SSc (Mullighan-Kehoe et al., 2007). Finally, circulating thrombospondin-1 (TSP-1), a counteradhesive protein with angiostatic and apoptotic properties was found increased in patients with SSc (Macko et al., 2002).

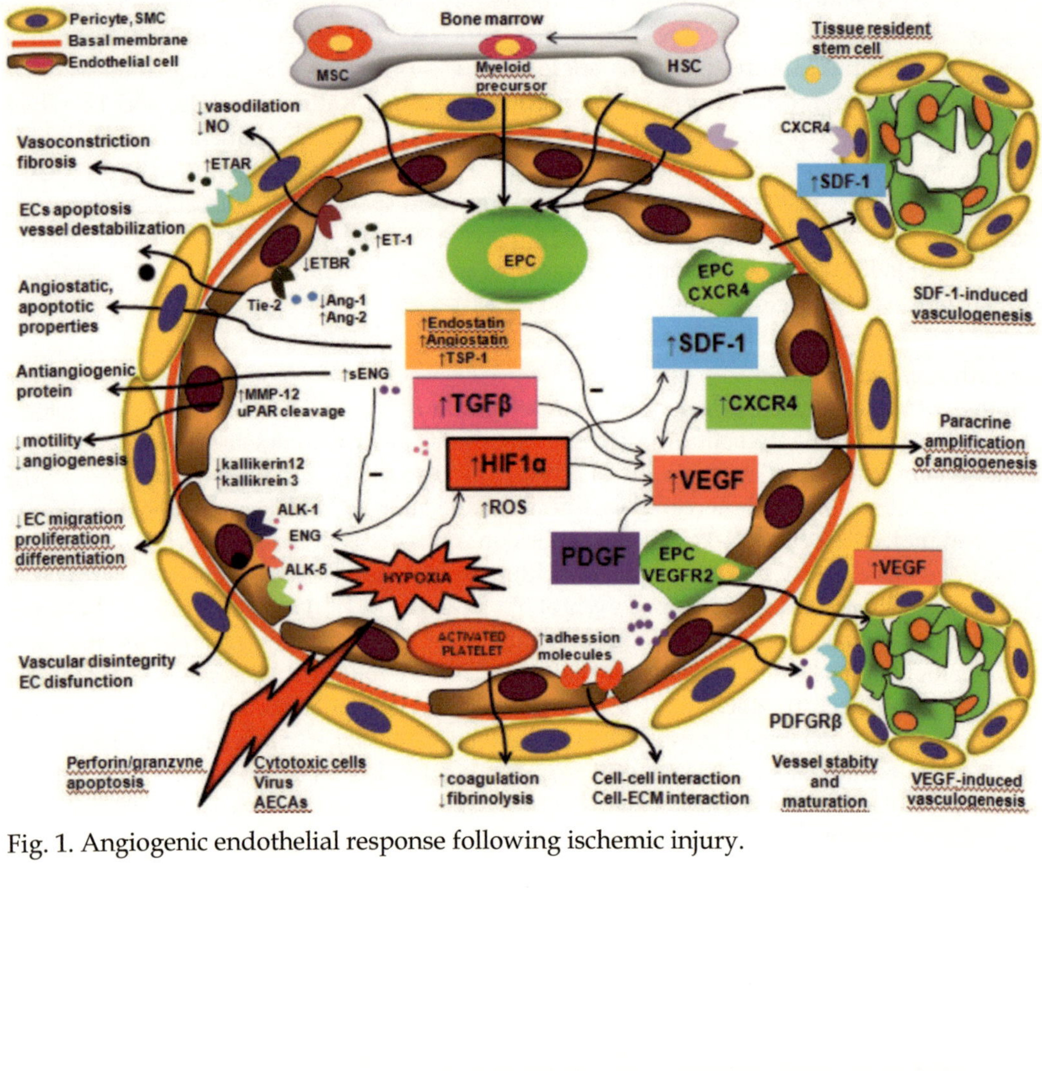

Fig. 1. Angiogenic endothelial response following ischemic injury.

For the specific function of involved molecules and cells see the text. EPC: circulating endothelial progenitors; MSC: mesenchymal stem cells; HSC: hematopoietic stem cells; ROS: reactive oxygen species; TGFβ: transforming growth factor beta; HIF1α: hypoxia inducible factor 1 alfa; PDGF: platelet derived factor; PDGFR: platelet derived factor receptor; VEGF: vascular endothelial growth factor; VEGFR: vascular endothelial growth factor receptor; SDF-1: stromal cell-derived factor 1; CXCR4: SDF-1 receptor; ENG: endoglin; sENG: soluble endoglin; ALK-1 and ALK-5: activin receptor-like kinase-1 and -5; Ang-1 and Ang-2: angiopoietin 1 and 2; Tie-2: tyrosine kinase receptor; ET1: endothelin-1; ETAR and ETBR: endothelin receptor A and B; MMP12: matrix metalloproteinase 12; uPAR: urokinase-type plasminogen activator.

8. Conclusions

Vascular endothelial cell damage is and early an probably initiating event in the pathogenesis of the SSc resulting in endothelial dysfunction and loss of capillaries. The dysregulation of the angiogenic homeostasis seen in SSc, leads to failure in replacing damaged vessels, thus contributing to the vascular desertification and the chronic ischemia characteristic of the disease. Vasculogenesis is also impaired in SSc. Failure of the angiogenic process in SSc largely depends on alteration in the balance between angiogenic and angiostatic factors. At present, data describing the process of dysregulation in angiogenic homeostasis are incomplete and need further research. On the other hand functional alterations of the cellular players involved in the angiogenic and vasculogenic program are also demonstared. The possibility of reversing this impairment opens new perspectives for regenerative cellular therapy for the vascular damage of this disease.

9. Acknowledgment

This work was supported in part by PRIN 2008:200884K784 and FIRA ONLUS 2009.

10. References

Abraham DJ, Vancheeswaran R, Dashwood MR, Rajkumar VS, Pantelides P, Xu SW & du Bois RM, Black CM.(1997). Increased levels of endothelin-1 and differential endothelin type A and B receptor expression in scleroderma-associated fibrotic lung disease. *Am J Pathol* Sep;151(3):831–41

Abraham D, Distler O. (2007). How does endothelial cell injury start? The role of endothelin in systemic sclerosis. *Arthritis Res Ther*. 2007; 9(Suppl 2): S2.

Adams V, Lenk K, Linke A, Lenz D, Erbs S, Sandri M, Tarnok A, Gielen S, Emmrich F, Schuler G & Hambrecht R. (2004). Increase of circulating endothelial progenitor cells in patients with coronary artery disease after exercise-induced ischemia. *Arterioscler Thromb Vasc Biol* 2004 Apr;24(4):684–90

Ahmed SS, Tan FK, Arnett FC, Jin L & Geng YJ. (2006). Induction of apoptosis and fibrillin 1 expression in human dermal endothelial cells by scleroderma sera containing antiendothelial cell antibodies. *Arthritis Rheum*. 2006;54(7):2250–62.

Allanore Y, Borderie D, Airo P, Guiducci S, Czirják L, Nasonov EL, Riemekasten G, Caramaschi P, Majdan M, Krasowska D, Friedl E, Lemarechal H, Ananieva LP, Nievskaya T, Ekindjian OG, Matucci-Cerinic M & Kahan A. (2007). Lack of association between 3 vascular endothelial growth factor gene polymorphisms and systemic sclerosis: results from a multicenter EUSTAR study of European Caucasian patients. *Ann Rheum Dis* 2007 Feb 66(2):257-259.

Arnhold S. J., Goletz I., Klein H., Stumpf G, Beluche L. A., Rohde C., Addicks K & Litzke LF .(2007). Isolation and characterization of bone marrow-derived equine mesenchymal stem cells. *Am. J. Vet. Res.* 2007 Oct 68(10):1095–1105

Asahara T, Murohara T, Sullivan A, Silver M, van der Zee R, Li T, Witzenbichler B, Schatteman G & Isner JM. (1997). Isolation of putative progenitor endothelial cells for angiogenesis. *Science* 1997 Feb 14; 275(5302):964-7.26, 27

Asahara T, Chen D, Takahashi T, Fujikawa K, Kearney M, Magner M, Yancopoulos GD & Isner JM. (1998). Tie2 receptor ligands, angiopoietin-1 and angiopoietin-2, modulate VEGF induced postnatal neovascularization. *Circ Res* 1998 Aug 10;83(3): 233-40

Avouac J, Juin F, Wipff J, Couraud P, Chiocchia G, Kahan A, Boileau C, Uzan G & Allanore Y. (2008). Circulating endothelial progenitor cells in systemic sclerosis: association with disease severity. *Ann Rheum Dis* 2008 Oct;67(10):1455–60.

Barcellos-Hoff MH, & Dix TA. (1996). Redoxmediated activation of latent transforming growth factor-beta 1. *Mol Endocrinol.* 1996 Sep;10(9):1077-83.

Baroni SS, Santillo M, Bevilacqua F, Luchetti M, Spadoni T, Mancini M, Fraticelli P, Sambo P, Funaro A, Kazlauskas A, Avvedimento EV & Gabrielli A. (2006). Stimulatory autoantibodies to the PDGF receptor in systemic sclerosis. *N Engl J Med.* 2006 Jun *22;* 354(25):2667-76

Bauer M, Wilkens H, Langer F, Schneider SO, Lausberg H & Schäfers HJ. (2002). Selective upregulation of endothelin B receptor gene expression in severe pulmonary hypertension. *Circulation* 2002 March 5; 105(9):1034–6

Bellini A & Mattoli S. (2007). The role of the fibrocyte, a bone marrow-derived mesenchymal progenitor, in reactive and reparative fibroses. *Lab Invest* 2007 Sep;87(9):858-70. Epub 2007 Jul 2. Review.

Bellocq A, Azoulay E, Marullo S, Flahault A, Fouqueray B, Philippe C, Cadranel J & Baud L. (1999). Reactive oxygen species and nitrogen intermediates increase transforming growth factor-beta1 release from human epithelial alveolar cells through two different mechanisms. *Am J Respir Cell Mol Biol.* 1999 Jul 21(1):128-36

Bianco A, Poukkula M, Cliffe A, Mathieu J, Luque CM, Fulga TA & Rørth P. (2007). Two distinct modes of guidance signalling during collective migration of border cells. *Nature* 2007 Jul 19;448(7151):362–365.

Bobik A. Transforming growth factor-betas and vascular disorders. (2006). *Arterioscler Thromb Vasc Biol* 2006 Aug 26(8):1712–20 Epub 2006 May 4.

Bordron A, Dueymes M, Levy Y, Jamin C, Leroy JP, Piette JC, Shoenfeld Y & Youinou PY. (1998). The binding of some human antiendothelial cell antibodies induces endothelial cell apoptosis. *J Clin Invest* 1998 May 15;101(10):2029–35.

Carmeliet P. (2003). Angiogenesis in health and disease. *Nat Med,* 9(6), (Jun 2003), 653-60. Review.

Channick RN, Simonneau G, Sitbon O, Robbins IM, Frost A, Tapson VF, Badesch DB, Roux S, Rainisio M, Bodin F & Rubin LJ. (2001). Effects of the dual endothelin-receptor antagonist bosentan in patients with pulmonary hypertension: a randomised placebo-controlled study. *Lancet* 358(9288), Oct 2001, 1119–1123

Choi SC, Shim WJ & Lim DS. (2008). Specific monitoring of cardiomyogenic and endothelial differentiation by dual promoter-driven reporter systems in bone marrow mesenchymal stem cells. *Biotechnol Lett.* 30(5), May 2008, 835-43 Epub 2008 Jan 4.

Cipriani P, Milia AF, Liakouli V, Pacini A, Manetti M, Marrelli A, Toscano A, Pingiotti E, Fulminis A, Guiducci S, Perricone R, Kahaleh B, Matucci-Cerinic M, Ibba-Manneschi L & Giacomelli R. (2006). Differential expression of stromal cell-derived factor 1 and its receptor CXCR4 in the skin and endothelial cells of systemic sclerosis patients: pathogenetic implications. *Arthritis Rheum* 54 Sep 2006, 3022-33

Cipriani, P.; Guiducci, S.; Miniati, I.; Cinelli, M.; Urbani, S.; Marrelli, A.; Dolo, V.; Pavan, A., Saccardi, R.; Tyndall, A.; Giacomelli, R. & Cerinic MM. (2007). Impairment of endothelial cell differentiation from bone marrow-derived mesenchymal stem cells: new insight into the pathogenesis of systemic sclerosis. *Arthritis Rheum.* 56(6), Jun 2007, 1994-2004

Cipriani P, Marrelli A, Liakouli V, Di Benedetto P & Giacomelli R. (2011). Cellular players in angiogenesis during the course of systemic sclerosis. *Autoimmun Rev.* Apr 22 2011 [Epub ahead of print]

Copland I, Sharma K, Lejeune L, Eliopoulos N, Stewart D, Liu P, Lachapelle K & Galipeau J. (2008). CD34 expression on murine marrow-derived mesenchymal stromal cells: impact on neovascularization. *Exp Hematol.* 36(1), Jan 2008, 93-103, Epub 2007 Nov 26.

Coral-Alvarado PX, Garces MF, Caminos JE, Iglesias-Gamarra A, Restrepo JF & Quintana G. (2010). Serum endoglin levels in patients suffering from systemic sclerosis and elevated systolic pulmonary arterial pressure. *Int J Rheumatol.*2010. pii: 969383. Epub 2010 Aug 24

D'Alessio S, Fibbi G, Cinelli M, Guiducci S, Del Rosso A, Margheri F Serratì S, Pucci M, Kahaleh B, Fan P, Annunziato F, Cosmi L, Liotta F, Matucci-Cerinic M & Del Rosso M. (2004). Matrix metalloproteinase 12-dependent cleavage of urokinase receptor in systemic sclerosis microvascular endothelial cells results in impaired angiogenesis. *Arthritis Rheum,* 50(10), Oct 2010, 3275-85

De Falco E, Porcelli D, Torella AR, Straino S, Iachininoto MG, Orlandi A, Truffa S, Biglioli P, Napolitano M, Capogrossi MC & Pesce M. (2004). SDF-1 involvement in endothelial phenotype and ischemia-induced recruitment of bone marrow progenitor cells. *Blood,* 104(12), Dec 1 2004, 3472-82 Epub 2004 Jul 29.

Del Papa N, Quirici N, Soligo D, Scavullo C, Cortiana M, Borsotti C, Maglione W, Comina DP, Vitali C, Fraticelli P, Gabrielli A, Cortelezzi A & Lambertenghi-Deliliers G. (2006). Bone marrow endothelial progenitors are defective in systemic sclerosis. Arthritis Rheum, 54(8), (Aug 6 2008), 2605-15.

Del Papa N, Cortiana M, Vitali C, Silvestris I, Maglione W, Comina DP, Lucchi T & Cortelezzi A. (2008). Simvastatin reduces endothelial activation and damage but is partially ineffective in inducing endothelial repair in systemic sclerosis. *J Rheumatol* 35(7), (Jul 2008), 1323–8.

Dimmeler S, Aicher A, Vasa M, Mildner-Rihm C, Adler K, Tiemann M, Rütten H, Fichtlscherer S, Martin H & Zeiher AM. (2001). HMG-CoA reductase inhibitors (statins) increase endothelial progenitor cells via the PI 3-kinase/Akt pathway. *J Clin Invest,* 108(3), (Aug 2008), 391–7

Distler, O.; Del Rosso, A.; Giacomelli, R.; Cipriani, P.; Conforti, ML.; Guiducci, S.; Gay, RE.; Michel, BA.; Brühlmann, P.; Müller-Ladner, U.; Gay, S. & Matucci-Cerinic, M.

(2002). Angiogenic and angiostatic factors in systemic sclerosis: increased levels of vascular endothelial growth factor are a feature of the earliest disease stages and are associated with the absence of fingertip ulcers. *Arthritis Res.* 4(6):R11. Epub 2002 Aug 30.

Distler, O.; Distler, JH.; Scheid, A.; Acker, T.; Hirth, A.; Rethage, J.; Michel, BA.; Gay, RE.; Müller-Ladner, U.; Matucci-Cerinic, M.; Plate, KH.; Gassmann, M. & Gay, S. (2004). Uncontrolled expression of vascular endothelial growth factor and its receptors leads to insufficient skin angiogenesis in patients with systemic sclerosis. *Circ Res.*

Distler J, Hirth A, Kurowska-Stolarska M, Gay RE, Gay S & Distler O. (2003). Angiogenic and angiostatic factors in the molecular control of angiogenesis. *Q J Nucl Med* 47(3), (Sep 2003), 149–61.

Distler JH, Gay S & Distler O. (2006). Angiogenesis and vasculogenesis in systemic sclerosis. *Rheumatology (Oxford)* 2006 Oct;45 Suppl 3:iii26-7. Review. Erratum in: Rheumatology (Oxford). 2008 Feb;47(2):234-5.

Dor Y, Djonov V, Abramovitch R, Itin A, Fishman GI, Carmeliet P, Goelman G & Keshet E. (2002). Conditional switching of VEGF provides new insights into adult neovascularization and proangiogenic therapy. *EMBO J* 21(8), (Apr 2002), 1939–47.

Dorfmuller, P, Humbert M, Perros F, Sanchez O, Simonneau G, Müller KM & Capron F. (2007). Fibrous remodeling of the pulmonary venous system in pulmonary arterial hypertension associated with connective tissue diseases. *Hum. Pathol.* 2007 Jun;38(6):893-902. Epub 2007 Mar 21. 8, 893–902

Drake C. J. (2003). Embryonic and adult vasculogenesis. Birth Defects Res. *C Embryo Today* 2003 Feb;69(1):73-82

Fleischmajer R, Perlish JS & Reeves JR. (1977). *Cellular infiltrates in scleroderma skin. Arthritis Rheum.* 20(4):975-84.

Fleischmajer R & Perlish JS. (1980). Capillary alterations in scleroderma. *J Am Acad Dermatol.* 2(2):161-70

Fleming JN, Nash RA, McLeod DO, Fiorentino DF, Shulman HM, Connolly MK Molitor JA, Henstorf G, Lafyatis R, Pritchard DK, Adams LD, Furst DE & Schwartz SM. (2008). Capillary regeneration in scleroderma: stem cell therapy reverses phenotype? *PLoS ONE* 3: e1452 31 Erratum in: PLoS ONE. 2008;3(8). doi: 10.1371/annotation/6b021f46-17bd-4ffe-a378-a1b8d24a1398.

Gabrielli A, Avvedimento EV & Krieg T. (2009). Scleroderma. *N Engl J Med.* 360(19):1989-2003. Review.

Gay S, Jones RE Jr, Huang GQ & Gay RE. (1989). Immunohistologic demonstration of platelet-derived growth factor (PDGF) and sis-oncogene expression in scleroderma. *J Invest Dermatol* 92:301–3.

Giacomelli R, Cipriani P, Lattanzio R, Di Franco M, Locanto M, Parzanese I, Passacantando A, Ciocci A & Tonietti G. (1997). Circulating levels of soluble CD30 are increased in patients with systemic sclerosis (SSc) and correlate with serological and clinical features of the disease. *Clin Exp Immunol.* 108(1):42-6.

Giacomelli R, Matucci-Cerinic M, Cipriani P, Ghersetich I, Lattanzio R, Pavan A, Pignone A, Cagnoni ML, Lotti T & Tonietti G. (1998). Circulating Vdelta1+ T cells are activated and accumulate in the skin of systemic sclerosis patients. *Arthritis Rheum.* 41(2):327-34. Review

Giusti B, Serrati S, Margheri F, Papucci L, Rossi L, Poggi F, Magi A, Del Rosso A, Cinelli M, Guiducci S, Kahaleh B, Matucci-Cerinic M, Abbate R, Fibbi G, Del Rosso M.et al. (2005). The antiangiogenic tissue kallikrein pattern of endothelial cells in systemic sclerosis. *Arthritis Rheum* 52:3618-3628

Gruschwitz M, von den DP, Kellner I, Hornstein OP & Sterry W. (1992). Expression of adhesion proteins involved in cell–cell and cell–matrix interactions in the skin of patients with progressive systemic sclerosis. *J Am Acad Dermatol* 27:169–177

Gruschwitz MS, Hornstein OP & von Den DP. (1995). Correlation of soluble adhesion molecules in the peripheral blood of scleroderma patients with their in situ expression and with disease activity. *Arthritis Rheum* 38:184–1899

Guiducci, S.; Giacomelli, R. & Cerinic MM. (2007). Vascular complications of scleroderma. *Autoimmun Rev*. 6(8):520-3. Epub 2007 Jan 12. Review.

Guiducci S, Porta F, Saccardi R, Guidi S, Ibba-Manneschi L, Manetti M, Mazzanti B, Dal Pozzo S, Milia AF, Bellando-Randone S, Miniati I, Fiori G, Fontana R, Amanzi L, Braschi F, Bosi A & Matucci-Cerinic M. (2010). Autologous mesenchymal stem cells foster revascularization of ischemic limbs in systemic sclerosis: a case report. *Ann Intern Med.* 153(10):650

Helmbold P, Fiedler E, Fischer M & Marsch WC (2004). Hyperplasia of dermal microvascular pericytes in scleroderma. J Cutan Pathol 31:431-40.

Hill JM, Zalos G, Halcox JP, Schenke WH, Waclawiw MA, Quyyumi AA & Finkel T. (2003). Circulating endothelial progenitor cells, vascular function, and cardiovascular risk. N Engl J Med (2003) 348: 593–600

Holland JA, Meyer JW, Chang MM, O'Donnell RW, Johnson DK & Ziegler LM. Thrombin stimulated reactive oxygen species production in cultured endothelial cells. Endothelium 1998;6:113-21.

Hristov M, & Weber C. (2004). Endothelial progenitor cells: characterization, pathophysiology, and possible clinical relevance. *J Cell Mol Med* 8:498–508.

Hummers LK, Hall A, Wigley FM & Simons M. (2009). Abnormalities in the regulators of angiogenesis in patients with scleroderma. *J Rheumatol*. 36(3):576-82. Epub 2009 Feb 17

Ihn H, Sato S, Fujimoto M, Kikuchi K, Kadono T, Tamaki K & Takehara K. (1997). Circulating intercellular adhesion molecule-1 in the sera of patients with systemic sclerosis: enhancement by inflammatory cytokines. *Br J Rheumatol* 36:1270–1275

Ihn H, Sato S, Fujimoto M, Takehara K & Tamaki K. (1998). Increased serum levels of soluble vascular cell adhesion molecule-1 and E-selectin in patients with systemic sclerosis. *Br J Rheumatol* 37:1188–1192

Ishikawa O & Ishikawa H. (1992). Macrophage infiltration in the skin of patients with systemic sclerosis. *J Rheumatol*. 19(8):1202-6.

Kadono T, Kikuchi K, Sato S, Soma Y, Tamaki K & Takehara K. (1995). Elevated plasma endothelin levels in systemic sclerosis. *Arch Dermatol Res* 287:439–442

Kahaleh MB. (1991). Endothelin, an endothelial-dependent vasoconstrictor in scleroderma. Enhanced production and profibrotic action. *Arthritis Rheum* 34:978–983,

Kahaleh MB & Fan PS (1997) Mechanism of serum-mediated endothelial injury in scleroderma: identification of a granular enzyme in scleroderma skin and sera. *Clin Immunol Immunopathol* 83:32–40

Kahaleh B. (2004). Progress in research into systemic sclerosis. Lancet. 364: 561-2.

Kahaleh B. (2008). The microvascular endothelium in scleroderma.. Rheumatology (Oxford). 47 Suppl 5:v14-5. Review.

Kalluri R & Neilson EG (2003). Epithelial-mesenchymal transition and its implications for fibrosis. J Clin Invest. 2003 Dec;112(12):1776-84. Review.

Kiener H, Graninger W, Machold K, Aringer M & Graninger WB. (1994). Increased levels of circulating intercellular adhesion molecule-1 in patients with systemic sclerosis. *Clin Exp Rheumatol* 12:483–487

Kim I, Moon SO, Park SK, Chae SW & Koh GY. (2001). Angiopoietin-1 reduces VEGF-stimulated leukocyte adhesion to endothelial cells by reducing ICAM-1, VCAM-1, and E-selectin expression. *Circ Res* 89:477-9

Klareskog L, Gustafsson R, Scheynius A & Hallgren R. (1990). Increased expression of platelet-derived growth factor type B receptors in the skin of patients with systemic sclerosis. Arthritis Rheum 33:1534–41

Kodama H, Inoue T, Watanabe R, Yasuoka H, Kawakami Y, Ogawa S, Ikeda Y, Mikoshiba K & Kuwana M. (2005). Cardiomyogenic potential of mesenchymal progenitors derived from human circulating CD14+ monocytes. Stem Cell Dev 14:676–686.

Kodama H, Inoue T, Watanabe R, Yasutomi D, Kawakami Y, Ogawa S, Mikoshiba K, Ikeda Y & Kuwana M. (2006). Neurogenic potential of progenitors derived from human circulating CD14+ monocytes. Immunol Cell Biol 84:209 –217

Kucia M, Jankowski K, Reca R, Wysoczynski M, Bandura L, Allendorf DJ, Zhang J, Ratajczak J & Ratajczak MZ. (2004). CXCR4–SDF-1 signalling, locomotion, chemotaxis and adhesion. J Mol Histol 35:233-45.

Kuwana M, Okazaki Y, Kodama H, Izumi K, Yasuoka H, Ogawa Y, Kawakami Y & Ikeda Y. (2003). Human circulating CD14+ monocytes as a source of progenitors that exhibit mesenchymal cell differentiation. J Leukoc Biol 74:833– 845

Kuwana, M.; Okazaki, Y.; Yasuoka, H.; Kawakami, Y. & Ikeda Y. (2004). Defective vasculogenesis in systemic sclerosis. *Lancet*. 14-20;364(9434):603-10.

Kuwana M, Okazaki Y, Kodama H, Satoh T, Kawakami Y & Ikeda Y. (2006). Endothelial differentiation potential of human monocyte derived multipotential cells. *Stem Cells* 24:2733–43.

Ladage D, Brixius K, Steingen C, Mehlhorn U, Schwinger RH, Bloch W & Schwinger RH. (2007). Mesenchymal stem cells induce endothelial activation via paracine mechanisms. *Endothelium*. 14(2):53-63

Laplante P, Raymond MA, Gagnon G, Vigneault N, Sasseville AM, Langelier Y, Bernard M, Raymond Y & Hébert MJ. (2005). Novel fibrogenic pathways are activated in response to endothelial apoptosis: implications in the pathophysiology of systemic sclerosis. *J Immunol*. 174(9):5740-9.

Lassegue B, Sorescu D, Szocs K, Yin Q, Akers M, Zhang Y, Grant SL, Lambeth JD & Griendling KK. (2001). Novel gp91 (phox) homologues in vascular smooth muscle cells: nox1 mediates angiotensin II-induced superoxide formation and redox-sensitive signaling pathways. *Circ Res*. 88:888-94.

Li Z, Jimenez SA (2011). Protein kinase C δ and the c-Abl kinase are required for transforming growth factor-β induction of endothelial-mesenchymal transition in vitro. *Arthritis Rheum*. 2011 [Epub ahead of print]

Liakouli V, Cipriani P, Marrelli A, Alvaro S, Ruscitti P & Giacomelli R. (2011). Angiogenic cytokines and growth factors in systemic sclerosis. *Autoimmun Rev.* [Epub ahead of print]

Lindblom P, Gerhardt H, Liebner S, Abramsson A, Enge M, Hellstrom M, Backstrom G, Fredriksson S, Landegren U, Nystrom HC, Bergstrom G, Dejana E, Ostman A, Lindahl P & Betsholtz C. (2003). Endothelial PDGF-B retention is required for proper investment of pericytes in the microvessel wall. *Genes Dev.* 17(15):1835-40.

Ludwicka A, Ohba T, Trojanowska M, Yamakage A, Strange C, Smith EA, Leroy EC, Sutherland S & Silver RM. (1995). Elevated levels of platelet derived growth factor and transforming growth factor-beta 1 in bronchoalveolar lavage fluid from patients with scleroderma. *J Rheumatol* 22:1876–83.

Lunardi C, Bason C, Navone R, Millo E, Damonte G, Corrocher R & Puccetti A. (2000). Systemic sclerosis immunoglobulin G autoantibodies bind the human cytomegalovirus late protein UL94 and induce apoptosis in human endothelial cells. *Nat Med.* 6(10):1183-6.

Macko RF, Gelber AC, Young BA, Lowitt MH, White B, Wigley FM & Goldblum SE. (2002). Increased circulating concentrations of the counteradhesive proteins SPARC and thrombospondin-1 in systemic sclerosis (scleroderma). Relationship to platelet and endothelial cell activation. *J Rheumatol* 29(12):2565-70

Manetti M, Liakouli V, Fatini C, Cipriani P, Bonino C, Vettori S, Guiducci S, Montecucco C, Abbate R, Valentini G, Matucci-Cerinic M, Giacomelli R & Ibba-Manneschi L. (2009). Association between a stromal cell-derived factor 1 (SDF-1/CXCL12) gene polymorphism and microvascular disease in systemic sclerosis. *Ann Rheum Dis.* 68(3):408-11. Epub 2008 Oct 17

Manetti M, Ibba-Manneschi L, Liakouli V, Guiducci S, Milia AF, Benelli G, Marrelli A, Conforti ML, Romano E, Giacomelli R, Matucci-Cerinic M & Cipriani P. (2010). The IL1-like cytokine IL33 and its receptor ST2 are abnormally expressed in the affected skin and visceral organs of patients with systemic sclerosis. *Ann Rheum Dis.* 69(3):598-605. Epub 2009 Sep 23.

Manetti M, Guiducci S, Ceccarelli C, Romano E, Bellando-Randone S, Conforti ML, Ibba-Manneschi L & Matucci-Cerinic M (2011). Increased circulating levels of interleukin 33 in systemic sclerosis correlate with early disease stage and microvascular involvement. *Ann Rheum Dis.* [Epub ahead of print]

Manetti M, Allanore Y, Revillod L, Fatini C, Guiducci S, Cuomo G, Bonino C, Riccieri V, Bazzichi L, Liakouli V, Cipriani P, Giacomelli R, Abbate R, Bombardieri S, Valesini G, Montecucco C, Valentini G, Ibba-Manneschi L, Matucci-Cerinic M. (2011). A genetic variation located in the promoter region of the UPAR (CD87) gene is associated with the vascular complications of systemic sclerosis. *Arthritis Rheum* 63(1):247-56. doi: 10.1002/art.30101.

Mantovani A, Allavena P, Sica A & Balkwill F. (2008). Cancer-related inflammation. *Nature.* 454:436-44.

Margheri F, Manetti M, Serratì S, Nosi D, Pucci M, Matucci-Cerinic M, Kahaleh B, Bazzichi L, Fibbi G, Ibba-Manneschi L, Del Rosso M. (2006). Domain 1 of the urokinase-type plasminogen activator receptor is required for its morphologic and functional, β2 integrin-mediated connection with actin cytoskeleton in human microvascular endothelial cells: failure of association in systemic sclerosis endothelial cells. *Arthritis Rheum.* 54(12):3926-38.

Margheri F, Serratì S, Lapucci A, Chillà A, Bazzichi L, Bombardieri S, Kahaleh B, Calorini L, Bianchini F, Fibbi G & Del Rosso M. (2010). Modulation of the angiogenic phenotype of normal and systemic sclerosis endothelial cells by gain-loss of function of pentraxin 3 and matrix metalloproteinase 12. *Arthritis Rheum.* 62(8):2488-98

Martens TP, See F, Schuster MD, Sondermeijer HP, Hefti MM, Zannettino A, Gronthos S, Seki T, Itescu S. (2006). Mesenchymal lineage precursor cells induce vascular network formation in ischemic myocardium. *Nat Clin Pract Cardiovasc Med.* 3 Suppl 1:S18-22

Matucci-Cerinic M, Denton CP, Furst DE, Mayes MD, Hsu VM, Carpentier P, Wigley FM, Black CM, Fessler BJ, Merkel PA, Pope JE, Sweiss NJ, Doyle MK, Hellmich B, Medsger TA Jr, Morganti A, Kramer F, Korn JH, Seibold JR. (2011). Bosentan treatment of digital ulcers related to systemic sclerosis: results from the RAPIDS-2 randomised, double-blind, placebo-contro lled trial. *Ann Rheum Dis* 70(1):32-8. Epub 2010 Aug 30

Mavalia C, Scaletti C, Romagnani P, Carossino AM, Pignone A, Emmi L, Pupilli C, Pizzolo G, Maggi E, Romagnani S. (1997). Type 2 helper T-cell predominance and high CD30 expression in systemic sclerosis. *Am J Pathol* 151:1751-8.

Medina RJ, O'Neill CL, Sweeney M, Guduric-Fuchs J, Gardiner TA, Simpson DA & Stitt AW. (2010). Molecular analysis of endothelial progenitor cell (EPC) subtypes reveals two distinct cell populations with different identities. *BMC Med Genomics.* 13;3:18

Michalska-Jakubus M, Kowal-Bielecka O, Chodorowska G, Bielecki M & Krasowska D. (2010). Angiopoietins-1 and -2 are differentially expressed in the sera of patients with systemic sclerosis: high angiopoietin-2 levels are associated with greater severity and higher activity of the disease. *Rheumatology (Oxford)* 2010 [Epub ahead of print]

Morgan-Rowe L, Nikitorowitcz J, Shiwen X, Leask A, Tsui J, Abraham D & Stratton R. (2011). Thrombospondin-1 in hypoxia conditioned media blocks the growth of human microvascular endothelial cells and is increased in systemic sclerosis tissues. *Fibrogenesis Tissue Repair.* 2;4(1):13. [Epub ahead of print]

Mukai N, Akahori T, Komaki M, Li Q, Kanayasu-Toyoda T, Ishii-Watabe A, Kobayashi A, Yamaguchi T, Abe M, Amagasa T, Morita I. (2008). A comparison of the tube forming potentials of early and late endothelial progenitor cells. *Exp Cell Res* 314(3):430-440

Mulligan-Kehoe MJ, Drinane MC, Mollmark J, Casciola-Rosen L, Hummers LK, Hall A, Rosen A, Wigley FM & Simons M. (2007). Antiangiogenic plasma activity in patients with systemic sclerosis. *Arthritis Rheum.* 56(10):3448-58

Murrell GAC, Francis MJ & Bromley L. (1990). Modulation of fibroblast proliferation by oxygen free radicals. *Biochem J.* 265: 659-65.

Nagai, Y, Yamanaka M, Hashimoto C, Nakano A, Hasegawa A, Tanaka Y, Yokoo H, Nakazato Y & Ishikawa O. (2007) Autopsy case of systemic sclerosis with severe pulmonary hypertension. *J. Dermatol.* 34, 769–772 (2007).

Nevskaya T, Bykovskaia S, Lyssuk E, Shakhov I, Zaprjagaeva M, Mach E, Ananieva L, Guseva N & Nassonov E. (2008). Circulating endothelial progenitor cells in systemic sclerosis: relation to impaired angiogenesis and cardiovascular manifestations. *Clin Exp Rheumatol.* 26: 421-9

Oswald J, Boxberger S, Jorgensen B, Feldmann S, Ehninger G, Bornhauser M & Werner C. (2004). Mesenchymal stem cells can be differentiated into endothelial cells in vitro. *Stem Cells* 22:377–84

Petit I, Jin D & Rafii S. (2007). The SDF-1-CXCR4 signaling pathway: a molecular hub modulating neo-angiogenesis. *Trends Immunol.* 28(7):299-307

Rajkumar VS, Howell K, Csiszar K, Denton CP, Black CM & Abraham DJ. (2005). Shared expression of phenotypic markers in systemic sclerosis indicates a convergence of pericytes and fibroblasts to a myofibroblast lineage in fibrosis. *Arthritis Res Ther* 7:R1113-R1123.

Reinmuth N, Rensinghoff S, Raedel M, Fehrmann N, Schwoppe C, Kessler T, Bisping G, Hilberg F, Roth GJ, Berdel W, Thomas M & Mesters RM. (2007). Paracrine interactions of vascular endothelial growth factor and platelet-derived growth factor in endothelial and lung cancer cells. *Int J Oncol* 31:621–626.

Reyes M, Lund T, Lenvik T, Aguiar D, Koodie L & Verfaillie CM. (2001). Purification and ex vivo expansion of postnatal human marrow mesodermal progenitor cells. *Blood.* 98(9):2615-25

Reyes M., Dudek A., Jahagirdar B., Koodie L., Marker P. H & Verfaillie C. M. (2002). Origin of endothelial progenitors in human postnatal bone marrow. *J. Clin. Invest.* 109, 337–346. 2002

Rodnan GP, Myerowitz RL & Justh GO. (1980). Morphologic changes in the digital arteries of patients with progressive systemic sclerosis (scleroderma) and Raynaud phenomenon. Medicine (Baltimore). 59(6):393-408.

Roumm AD, Whiteside TL, Medsger TA Jr, & Rodnan GP. (1984). Lymphocytes in the skin of patients with progressive systemic sclerosis. Quantification, subtyping, and clinical correlations. *Arthritis Rheum.* 27(6):645-53.

Rubin LJ, Badesch DB, Barst RJ, Galie N, Black CM, Keogh A, Pulido T, Frost A, Roux S, Leconte I, Landzberg M, Simonneau G. (2002). Bosentan therapy for pulmonary arterial hypertension. *N Engl J Med* 346:896–903

Sakkas LI, Xu B, Artlett CM, Lu S, Jiminez SA & Platsoucas CD.(2002). Oligoclonal T cell expansion in the skin of patients with systemic sclerosis. *J Immunol* 168: 3649-59.

Salcedo R & Oppenheim JJ. (2003). Role of chemokines in angiogenesis: CXCL12/SDF-1 and CXCR4 interaction, a key regulator of endothelial cell responses. *Microcirculation* 10:359-70

Salvucci O, Yao L, Villalba S, Sajewicz A, Pittaluga S & Tosato G. (2002). Regulation of endothelial cell branching morphogenesis by endogenous chemokine stromal-derived factor-1. *Blood* 99(8):2703-11

Sambo P, Jannino L, Candela M, Salvi A, Donini M, Dusi S, Luchetti MM & Gabrielli A. (1999). Monocytes of patients with systemic sclerosis (scleroderma) spontaneously release in vitro increased amounts of superoxide anion. *J Invest Dermatol.* 112:78-84.

Sambo P, Baroni SS, Luchetti M, Paroncini P, Dusi S, Orlandini G & Gabrielli A. (2001). Oxidative stress in scleroderma: maintenance of scleroderma fibroblast phenotype by the constitutive up-regulation of reactive oxygen species generation through the NADPH oxidase complex pathway. *Arthritis Rheum* 44:2653-64.

Schachna L, Wigley FM, Morris S, Gelber AC, Rosen A & Casciola-Rosen L. (2002). Recognition of Granzyme B-generated autoantigen fragments in scleroderma patients with ischemic digital loss. Arthritis Rheum. 46(7):1873-84

Schermuly RT, Dony E, Ghofrani HA, Pullamsetti S, Savai R, Roth M, Sydykov A, Lai YJ, Weissmann N, Seeger W & Grimminger F. (2005). Reversal of experimental pulmonary hypertension by PDGF inhibition. *J Clin Invest* 115(10):2811-21.

Servettaz A, Guilpain P, Goulvestre C, Chéreau C, Hercend C, Nicco C, Guillevin L, Weill B, Mouthon L & Batteux F. (2007). Radical oxygen species production induced by advanced oxidation protein products predicts clinical evolution and response to treatment in systemic sclerosis. *Ann Rheum Dis.* 66:1202-9.

Sgonc R, Gruschwitz MS, Boeck G, Sepp N, Gruber J & Wick G. (2000). Endothelial cell apoptosis in systemic sclerosis is induced by antibody-dependent cell-mediated cytotoxicity via CD95. *Arthritis Rheum.* 43(11):2550-62.

Shi Q, Rafii S, Wu MH, Wijelath ES, Yu C, Ishida A, Fujita Y, Kothari S, Mohle R, Sauvage LR, Moore MA, Storb RF, Hammond WP. (1998). Evidence for circulating bone marrow-derived endothelial cells. *Blood* 92: 362-7.

Sieveking DP, Buckle A, Celermajer DS & Ng MK. (2008). Strikingly different angiogenic properties of endothelial progenitor cell subpopulations: insights from a novel human angiogenesis assay. *J Am Coll Cardiol* 51(6):660-668.

Smadja DM, Cornet A, Emmerich J, Aiach M & Gaussem P. (2007). Endothelial progenitor cells: characterization, in vitro expansion, and prospects for autologous cell therapy. *Cell Biol Toxicol* 23:223–239

Sollberg S, Peltonen J, Uitto J & Jimenez SA. (1992). Elevated expression of beta 1 and beta 2 integrins, intercellular adhesion molecule 1, and endothelial leukocyte adhesion molecule 1 in the skin of patients with systemic sclerosis of recent onset. *Arthritis Rheum* 35:290–298

Sondergaard K, Stengaard-Pedersen K, Zachariae H, Heickendorff L, Deleuran M & Deleuran B. (1998). Soluble intercellular adhesion molecule-1 (sICAM-1) and soluble interleukin- 2 receptors (sIL-2R) in scleroderma skin. *Br J Rheumatol* 37:304-10

Stratton RJ, Coghlan JG, Pearson JD, Burns A, Sweny P, Abraham DJ & Black CM. (1998). Different patterns of endothelial cell activation in renal and pulmonary vascular disease in scleroderma. *QJM* 91:561–566.

Sturrock A, Cahill B, Norman K, Huecksteadt TP, Hill K, Sanders K, Karwande SV, Stringham JC, Bull DA, Gleich M, Kennedy TP & Hoidal JR. (2005). Transforming growth factor-beta1 induces Nox4 NAD(P)H oxidase and reactive oxygen species-dependent proliferation in human pulmonary artery smooth muscle cells. *Am J Physiol Lung Cell Mol Physiol.* 290:L661-L673.

Sullivan DE, Ferris M, Pociask D & Brody AR. (2008). The latent form of TGFbeta(1) is induced by TNFalpha through an ERK specific pathway and is activated by asbestos-deived reactive oxygen species in vitro and in vivo. *J Immunotoxicol.* 5:145-9.

Svegliati S, Cancello R, Sambo P, Luchetti M, Paroncini P, Orlandini G, Discepoli G, Paterno R, Santillo M, Cuozzo C, Cassano S, Avvedimento EV, Gabrielli A. (2005). Platelet-derived growth factor and reactive oxygen species (ROS) regulate Ras protein levels in primary human fibroblasts via ERK1/2:amplification of ROS and Ras in systemic sclerosis fibroblasts. *J Biol Chem.* 280:36474-82

Takeshita S, Zheng LP, Brogi E, Kearney M, Pu LQ, Bunting S, Ferrara N, Symes JF & Isner JM. (1994). Therapeutic angiogenesis. A single intraarterial bolus of vascular endothelial growth factor augments revascularization in a rabbit ischemic hind limb model. *J Clin Invest* 93:662-670.

Takeshita S, Tsurumi Y, Couffinahl T, Asahara T, Bauters C, Symes J, Ferrara N & Isner JM. (1996). Gene transfer of naked DNA encoding for three isoforms of vascular endothelial growth factor stimulates collateral development in vivo. *Lab Invest* 75:487-501.

Torensma R & Figdor CG. (2004). Differentiating stem cells mask their origins. *Stem Cells* 22:250–23

Tuan R. S., Boland G & Tuli R. (2003). Adult mesenchymal stem cells and cell-based tissue engineering. *Arthritis Res. Ther*. 5, 32–45

Urbich C & Dimmeler S. (2004). Endothelial progenitor cells: characterization and role in vascular biology. *Circ Res*. 95: 343-53

Van Hinsbergh VW & Koolwijk P. Endothelial sprouting and angiogenesis: matrix metalloproteinases in the lead. Cardiovasc Res. (2008) May 1;78(2):203-12

Vrekoussis T, Stathopoulos EN, Kafousi M, Navrozoglou I & Zoras O. (2007). Expression of endothelial PDGF receptors alpha and beta in breast cancer: up-regulation of endothelial PDGF receptor beta. *Oncol Rep* 17:1115–1119.

Xu H, Zaidi M, Struve J, Jones DW, Krolikowski JG, Nandedkar S, Lohr NL, Gadicherla A, Pagel PS, Csuka ME, Pritchard KA & Weihrauch (2011). Abnormal fibrillin-1 expression and chronic oxidative stress mediate endothelial mesenchymal transition in a murine model of systemic sclerosis. *Am J Physiol Cell Physiol.* 300(3):C550-6. Epub 2010 Dec 15.

Yamaguchi J, Kusano KF, Masuo O, Kawamoto A, Silver M, Murasawa S, Bosch-Marce M, Masuda H, Losordo DW, Isner JM, Asahara T. (2003). Stromal cell-derived factor-1 effects on ex vivo expanded endothelial progenitor cell recruitment for ischemic neovascularization. *Circulation.* 107(9):1322-8 –30

Yamaguchi Y, Okazaki Y, Seta N, Satoh T, Takahashi K, Ikezawa Z & Kuwana M. (2010). M Enhanced angiogenic potency of monocytic endothelial progenitor cells in patients with systemic sclerosis. *Arthritis Res Ther*. Nov 4;12(6):R205.

Yao L, Salvucci O, Cardones AR, Hwang ST, Aoki Y, De La Luz Sierra M, Sajewicz A, Pittaluga S, Yarchoan R & Tosato G. (2003). Selective expression of stromal-derived factor-1 in the capillary vascular endothelium plays a role in Kaposi sarcoma pathogenesis. *Blood*. 102(12):3900-5

Zammaretti P & Zisch AH (2005). Adult 'endothelial progenitor cells': renewing vasculature. *Int J Biochem Cell Biol* 37:493–503.

Zhao Y, Glesne D, Huberman E. (2003). A human peripheral blood monocyte-derived subset acts as pluripotent stem cells. *Proc Natl Acad Sci USA* 100:2426–2431.

Zhu S, Evans S, Yan B, Povsic TJ, Tapson V, Goldschmidt- Clermont PJ, & Dong C. (2008). Transcriptional regulation of Bim by FOXO3a and Akt mediates scleroderma serum-induced apoptosis in endothelial progenitor cells. *Circulation* 118:2156–65

Zymek P, Bujak M, Chatila K, Cieslak A, Thakker G, Entman ML & Frangogiannis NG. (2006). The role of platelet-derived growth factor signaling in healing myocardial infarcts. *J Am Coll Cardiol* 48:2315–2323.

Wipff J, Kahan A, Hachulla E, Sibilia J, Cabane J, Meyer O, Mouthon L, Guillevin L, Junien C, Boileau C & Allanore Y. (2007). Association between an endoglin gene polymorphism and systemic sclerosis related pulmonary arterial hypertension. *Rheumatology* 46:622

Worda M, Sgonc R, Dietrich H, Niederegger H, Sundick RS, Gershwin ME & Wick G. (2003). In vivo analysis of the apoptosis-inducing effect of anti endothelial cell antibodies in systemic sclerosis by the chorionallantoic membrane assay. *Arthritis Rheum.* 48:2605–14.

Wyler von Ballmoos M, Yang Z, Völzmann J, Baumgartner I, Kalka C & Di Santo S. (2010). Endothelial progenitor cells induce a phenotype shift in differentiated endothelial cells towards PDGF/PDGFRβ axis-mediated angiogenesis. *PLoS One.* 5(11):e14107.

2

Blood Platelets and Systemic Sclerosis

Sébastien Lepreux[1], Anne Solanilla[1], Julien Villeneuve[2], Joël Constans[3], Alexis Desmoulière[4] and Jean Ripoche[1]
[1]*INSERM U 1026 and Université de Bordeaux, Bordeaux*
[2]*CRG, Barcelona*
[3]*Service de Médecine Vasculaire, Bordeaux University Hospital, Bordeaux*
[4]*Department of Physiology and EA 3842, Faculty of Pharmacy, University of Limoges, Limoges*
[1,3,4]*France*
[2]*Spain*

1. Introduction

Systemic sclerosis (SSc) is characterized by a progressive fibrosis of the perivascular and interstitial connective tissues which can involve the skin, heart, lungs, kidneys, and the gastrointestinal tract. SSc is an uncommon, debilitating condition, associated to a vital risk linked to visceral extensions and has a high case-fatality rate among connectivitis. SSc begins in the vast majority of cases with a Raynaud's phenomenon, may have a limited or diffuse skin extension, and is often associated to arterial occlusions, digital ulcerations or necrosis. SSc clinical manifestations are heterogeneous and classifications distinguish limited to diffuse disease, depending on the distribution of the skin lesions and organ involvement [1-3]. There is today no curative treatment. Disease susceptibility differs according to sex, age and race, there is a notable familial clustering, and SSc incidence may be rising [4, 5]. The clinical management of the patients still remains a difficult challenge and the pharmacopeia offers limited choices to the clinician to bring relief to patients. Pulmonary, renal and myocardial complications have benefited from the introduction of angiotensin converting enzyme inhibitors, calcium pump inhibitors, prostacyclin analogs and endothelin antagonists. Based on recent pathophysiological insights, a number of novel agents are being developed [6-8].

2. SSc pathogenesis in 2011: An elusive mechanism

SSc pathogenesis remains obscure. Central features are an inflammatory vasculopathy, perivascular and interstitial sclerosis, altered angiogenesis and autoimmunity. Pathologic changes depend on whether they are observed at an early or late disease stage. The progression of the disease is typified by the accumulation of extra-cellular matrix (ECM) components in connective tissues. There are clinical and pathologic arguments to support the hypothesis that the vasculature is involved at an early step during disease progression.

Indeed, endothelium damage, perivascular edema and mononuclear cell infiltration are among earliest pathological changes that may precede the development of fibrosis [9-11]. Deregulated vascular tone, as evidenced by the Raynaud's phenomenon and morphological abnormalities of nail-fold capillary loops, as evidenced by capillaroscopy, also witness the underlying vasculopathy. In such a hypothetical vascular perspective, endothelial cell (EC) injury fuels other manifestations of the disease by the way of a deregulated inflammatory reaction. Whatever the primary target, a putative sequence of events leading to progression of the disease may follows microvascular injury leading in turn to perivascular and interstitial inflammation, autoimmunity leading to further endothelium injury, chronic progression of the inflammatory reaction, activation of interstitial fibroblasts, pericytes and other fibrocompetent cells leading to myofibroblast generation and subsequent persistent fibrogenic response [6, 12-18]. There are arguments to incriminate the genetic background in the disease susceptibility and progression. Genetic studies have underlined the inherent complexity of the disease, highlighting the involvement of the vasculature, the immune system and the ECM. Several polymorphisms in potential candidate genes have been identified [19-24]. The number of genes involved further underlines the disease spectrum heterogeneity. Environmental factors are linked to the disease, this being the case for exposure to silica, organic solvents or vinyl chloride. Infectious agents have been proposed to be involved, through endothelium damage, molecular mimicry-mediated autoimmune responses or other mechanisms [25, 26]. But how exposure to environmental risk factors combined to a permissive genetic background translates into initiation and progression of the disease is unclear. Therefore, fundamental questions remain currently unanswered with regard to key SSc features such as vascular, autoimmune and fibrotic events. The nature of the EC injury remains unknown. Several potential mechanisms have been explored, such as EC-specific T cells or auto-antibodies, vasculotropic viruses or environmental factors, oxidative stress, profibrotic and/or inflammatory cytokines. Altered angiogenesis is also a characteristic feature of SSc. Prevalent alterations of the capillary network in SSc include chaotic malformations with giant and bushy capillaries and reduced capillary density. There is, however, an insufficient angiogenic response, a defective vasculogenesis and a capillary loss in SSc [27]. Recent progresses have allowed progressive uncovering of the molecular mechanisms of tissue fibrosis. However, the widespread accumulation of ECM in SSc remain largely misunderstood, and therapeutic attempts to control fibrosis unfortunately remained unsuccessful [17, 18, 28-30].

3. SSc: A role for platelets?

A recent expansion of knowledge from basic research has illuminated the role of platelets in the inflammatory signalization network and underlined a hitherto unsuspected role for platelets in inflammatory diseases. Moreover, platelets are linked to endothelium homeostasis. They have been implicated in several vascular and fibrotic disorders. Hence, platelets stand as foreseeable contributors to SSc natural history. Indeed, there are signs of ongoing platelet activation in SSc but the underlying mechanisms remain ill-defined. First, it is not known how platelets could be activated during the course of the disease, through endothelium injury, immunological mechanisms or other reasons; second, it is not clear which platelet-derived mediators may specifically influence the progression of the disease. In the following sections are summarized some of the mechanisms linking platelets with inflammation, angiogenesis, vascular tone and fibrosis.

4. Platelets: Central actors of inflammation

4.1 Platelets transport bioactive mediators in the bloodstream

Platelets are cytoplasmic fragments that derive from the fragmentation of megakaryocytes (MKs) in the bone marrow sinuses. They harbor a unique store of secretory organelles having a distinct content in bioactive peptides. Alpha granules contain both soluble proteins destined to be secreted and membrane-bound proteins [31, 32]. Dense granules mostly contain an adenine nucleotide pool of ATP and ADP, bivalent cations calcium and magnesium and amines, including serotonin and histamine [33]. Platelet lysosomes contain a complex set of enzymes including acid proteases, such as cathepsin, carboxypeptidases, collagenases and various glycohydrolases [34]. Following platelet activation, the organelle content is released in a process termed secretion. The bulk of proteins secreted by platelets are remarkably large and diverse, as shown by proteomic studies on either platelet releasates or isolated granules. Classifications of the platelet secretome content with reference to biological effects pinpoint relations that platelets may encompass in various biological functions, including inflammation, tissue repair and angiogenesis [34-37]. Such a complexity has opened many new challenges with reference to the platelet role in human diseases.

In addition to MK biosynthesis, platelets also carry mediators that are endocytosed from plasma and possibly concentrated and/or modified within platelets. Such a plasma uptake has, for example, been demonstrated for fibrinogen, albumin, immunoglobulins, amino acids, and several inflammatory mediators including vascular endothelial growth factor (VEGF), histamine or serotonin [38, 39]. Passive and/or active mechanisms are responsible for the platelet uptake of plasma material. Platelets may be considered as mobile nodes, gathering (through endocytosis) and imparting information to target cells [40]. Apart from the rapid mobilization and release of granule content, platelets also express biomediators, including IL-1β, tissue factor, fibrinogen, thrombospondin, von Willebrand factor (vWF), GPIIb and GPIIIa, through a time-, translational-dependent pathway that is triggered upon platelet activation [41-45]. Finally, the traditional concept of platelet loss of function following activation is debated, as activated platelets circulate or persist in clots while keeping functional properties.

4.2 Platelet-derived microparticles recapitulate essential platelet functions

Activated platelets shed microparticles (MPs). Platelets are the major source of circulating MPs. MP biological roles recapitulate essential platelet functions as MPs represent a transport and delivery system of mediators participating to hemostasis, thrombosis, vascular repair and inflammation, acting both locally and systemically. MPs may transfer information to EC through adhesion and/or fusion, an event thought to contribute to the control of EC phenotype in inflammation [46-48].

4.3 Platelet-endothelium: A friend and foe relationship

4.3.1 Platelets maintain vascular integrity

One of the primary roles of platelets is to maintain vascular integrity [49]. At sites of vascular damage, platelets promptly adhere to exposed ECM [50], but also to activated EC (below), a first step in a sequence of events that result in platelet activation, initiation and propagation of hemostasis and thrombosis and in the release of key material contributing to wound repair and tissue regeneration, including ECM components and ECM remodeling proteins, matrix metalloproteinases (MMPs) and their inhibitors, the tissue inhibitors of metalloproteinases (TIMPs). Platelets also provide essential material for the angiogenic process, as summarized below. The role of platelets in tissue repair goes beyond vascular integrity. Indeed, platelets are essential for organ repair and regeneration as remarkably exemplified in the liver [37, 51-53].

4.3.2 The platelet/endothelium dialogue in inflammation

The dialogue between platelets and EC is a representative paradigm that has been extensively studied and reviewed because of its relevance in atherosclerosis [54]. Platelet-ECs interactions are critical in the initiation and progression of vascular inflammation. Platelet-derived inflammatory mediators turn EC phenotype to proinflammatory and procoagulant, and platelets facilitate leukocyte recruitment through the endothelium by providing chemotactic signals and platelet-bound ligands [49, 54]. Platelets are brought to inflammatory sites through vascular leakage, attachment to leukocytes but they also respond to chemotactic signals [55]. Coagulation and inflammation are intricately linked, and platelets represent an integrating platform for coagulation and inflammation cascades. For example, they anchor the procoagulant complex leading to the generation of thrombin a potent proinflammatory mediator. Platelets also contribute to other inflammatory cascades; for example, they propagate complement system activation [56]. Further readings may be found in [49, 54, 57-59].

The inflammatory reaction leads to platelet activation. ECM components, chemokines, triggering of platelet receptors with ligands on inflammatory cells activate platelets. Importantly, activated ECs bind and activate platelets, and the underlying mechanisms have been recently précised [50]. In resting conditions, the endothelium is not adhesive for platelets and prevents platelet activation through multiple mechanisms [60]. Activated ECs support platelet adhesion and activation. Endothelium denudation, resulting in ECM exposure, is not a prerequisite for platelet activation. Indeed, platelets roll and adhere on activated ECs, as shown, for example, after stimulation with Tumor Necrosis Factor-α, or following ischemia/reperfusion injury [61, 62]. EC activation (which can occurs through multiple mechanisms, inflammatory mediators, hypoxia, complement activation products, infectious agents...) results in the upregulation of adhesion molecules, including E- and P-selectin, $\alpha_v\beta_3$, intercellular adhesion molecule (ICAM)-1 or vWF, all ligands that mediate platelet rolling and firm adhesion in a process presenting profound analogies with the multistep-adhesion mechanisms of leukocytes on ECs [50, 54, 63-68]. Throughout the adhesion process platelets become activated. Activated platelets are a rich source of inflammatory mediators. They secrete a host of cytokines, chemokines, and lipid inflammatory mediators, deliver free acid arachidonic to bystander polymorphonuclear cells, allowing them to generate leukotriens. Activated platelets therefore contribute to generate a complex inflammatory milieu in their vicinity [37, 69, 70]. Platelet-derived inflammatory mediators deliver in turn activating signals to target cells including EC and leukocytes, resulting in the amplification of inflammation.

4.4 Platelets are a source of angiogenesis mediators

An important mechanism through which platelets control wound healing is linked to angiogenesis, as exemplified in tumor angiogenesis [71]. Platelets and platelet-derived MPs provide critical material for the generation and stabilization of the neo-angiogenic vessels; they secrete positive regulators and inhibitors of angiogenesis, including chemokines [72-

78]. Platelets also link coagulation to angiogenesis, through the proteolytic release of several cryptic angiogenic regulators [79]. VEGF is a critical angiogenic mediator in SSc (below) and its connections with platelets have been extensively studied. VEGF is transported by platelets [80]. Following binding to its receptor, VEGF induces EC survival, growth, permeability and migration. Other key angiogenic regulators secreted by platelets are platelet-derived growth factor (PDGF), transforming growth factor, (TGF)-β and angiopoietins. The angiogenic response is dependent on a complex regulated balance between the generation of pro- and anti-angiogenic molecules, with reference to magnitude and temporal production sequence [81]. The angiogenic activity of VEGF can only be appreciated by integrating the action of other mediators present in the EC environment [82, 83]. PDGF, TGF-β and angiopoietins are such mediators, acting in concert with VEGF for the stabilization of the vascular wall; their imbalanced expression has indeed been implicated in aberrant angiogenesis [82, 84]. Interestingly, there is a regulated differential secretion of pro- and anti-angiogenic mediators by platelets with reference to the nature of the agonist [85].

4.5 Platelet-derived mediators participate to vascular tone regulation

The blood flow is dependent on the constriction/dilation of resistance arteries. Endothelium and periarterial autonomic nervous plexus provide essential controls of the vascular tone [86, 87]. ECs are a source of vasoactive mediators that regulate blood flow, including the relaxing factors nitric oxid (NO), prostacyclin (PGI2) or endothelium-derived hyperpolarizing factor and vasoconstrictive factors including thromboxane A2 or endothelin-1 [88, 89]. Recent progress has highlighted the involvement of platelets and platelet-derived MPs in the control of the vascular tone. The integrity of the endothelium appears central to the vasomotor response to platelets; on intact endothelium, platelet derived mediators, including serotonin and ADP, cause the release of relaxing factors by the endothelium. If endothelium dysfunction has occurred, the absence of its protective role allows platelet-derived mediators, including serotonin and thromboxan A2 to induce vasoconstriction by directly acting on smooth muscle cells [90, 91]. Interestingly, VEGF may prove to have an increasing importance in vascular flow regulation, apart from its role in angiogenesis. Recent evidences indicate that it preserves the structure and function of neuro-effectors junctions [87].

4.6 Platelets are a source of fibrogenic mediators

Platelets are a rich source of pro-fibrotic molecules. Tissue fibrosis results from a deregulated wound-healing response to chronic injury. It is typically associated to a perpetuating inflammatory response, resulting for example from the persistence or repeated release of a tissue irritant, in contrast to the regulated acute inflammatory response that ends in a resolution step, repair of tissue damage and tissue homeostasis [92]. A central feature of tissue fibrosis is a quantitatively and qualitatively altered production of ECM. The increased biosynthesis of ECM components, particularly fibrillar collagens, by fibrocompetent cells contributes to generate a permanent and destructive tissue scarring that impairs organ function. Fibrocompetent cell activation is therefore at the root of the natural history of tissue fibrosis, and one of its decisive manifestations is transdifferentiation towards myofibroblasts, expressing α-smooth muscle actin (SMA), and harboring characteristic stress fibers and contractile phenotype [93]. It is generally accepted that the major source of myofibroblasts are local connective tissue fibroblasts. However, they can also be recruited from circulating fibrocytes and bone marrow-derived mesenchymal precursors, or they can derive from local epithelial and endothelial cells through the epithelial-mesenchymal transition [94-99]. Multiple soluble signals activate fibrocompetent cells. Among the most studied in SSc are the growth factors TGF-β1, PDGF, endothelin-1 and connective tissue growth factor. These mediators are potent fibroblast activators. TGF-β1 holds a peculiar position in SSc, as its deregulated expression represents a critical step. TGF-β1 promotes myofibroblastic transdifferentiation of quiescent fibroblasts, clearly demonstrated by the induction of α-SMA [100], stimulates their proliferation and the synthesis of ECM components, including fibrillar collagens. Epithelial-mesenchymal transition is linked to inflammation and fibrosis and several pro-fibrotic mediators induce the epithelial-mesenchymal transition [101]. A hierarchical induction of pro-fibrotic mediators in tissue fibrosis has been emphasized [102]. Chemokines, as monocyte chemotactic protein MCP-1, RANTES (regulated upon activation, normal T-cell expressed and secreted), interleukin (IL)-8, activate fibrogenic cells, including skin fibroblasts, stimulating their proliferation, chemotaxis, and ECM biosynthesis. The interaction between keratinocytes and fibroblasts is a critical step during the early phase of wound healing in the skin. Fibroblasts produce keratinocyte growth factor and, conversely, keratinocytes signal to fibroblasts leading to their activation, production of a variety of cytokines/chemokines/angiogenic mediators, induction of ECM component synthesis and α-SMA expression [102, 103]. There are important connections between vascular remodeling, angiogenesis and tissue fibrosis. Deregulated vascular remodeling is an important parameter in promoting the development of fibrosis and an imbalance between the production of angiogenic and antiangiogenic factors, such as CXC chemokines, at sites of tissue injury, is relevant to tissue fibrosis [17, 104-106]. Finally, a regulated balance between ECM production and degradation is a *sine qua non* condition for harmonious wound repair and tissue regeneration. Indeed, as shown in humans and in experimental tissue fibrosis models, the increased expression of some of TIMPs, a family of enzymes that control MMP activity through the inhibition of their proteolytic activity and the control of proform cleavage, leads to an altered MMP/TIMP balance, ECM homeostatic degradation/production disequilibrium, and ECM accumulation [107].

Platelets are essential actors in these mechanisms. They transport and secrete most of above -mentioned pro-fibrotic mediators, angiogenic and anti-angiogenic mediators, including CXC chemokines, ECM components and ECM remodeling proteins MMPs and TIMPs [108, 109]. Platelets influence cell growth and differentiation in a variety of situations [110]. They provide key control signals to angiogenesis. Persistent platelet activation in the microvascular bed may therefore contribute to tissue fibrosis [111-113]. However, few studies have considered their potential contribution. In fact, platelet-derived mediators have only recently being acknowledged as being of key importance in fibrosis as observed in liver and pulmonary diseases and, very recently, in SSc (below).

5. Evidence for platelet activation in SSc

There are signs of platelet activation in SSc, as indicated by measurements of various soluble and membrane-bound markers, circulating MPs and platelet- and platelet-leukocyte aggregates (Table 1). Soluble markers have been largely studied. As there are signs of ongoing EC injury in SSc, the specificity of these markers is an important point. P-selectin (CD62p) is a component of α-granules and of intracellular EC storage organelles. There has been debate whether the increase in plasma CD62p truly reflects platelet activation, as it is also expressed on activated ECs. It is however currently clear that most, if not all, measured plasma CD62p has a platelet origin [114, 115]. Activated ECs have also been discussed as potential contributors to soluble CD154 (sCD154). In fact, correlation studies demonstrated that it can be considered as mostly derived from platelets [116], but, recently, other cell sources have been described, that may potentially contribute to elevated circulating sCD154 levels [117]. Soluble P-selectin glycoprotein ligand-1 is elevated in SSc [118], which may also reflect some degree of platelet activation as it is expressed by platelets [119]. Chemokine (C-X-C motif) ligand-4 (CXCL4, Platelet Factor 4) is elevated in SSc; albeit until recently described as exclusively derived from platelets, other sources exist such as T-cells or macrophages that may be contributors to elevated circulating levels [120]. Tissue-plasminogen activator (tPA) has also been described as a marker of EC damage [121]. Studies of the expression of platelet membrane-bound activation markers also show that platelets are not globally activated, but that this activation concerns a fraction of their population [122]. Correlation studies in general do not evidence relations with clinical features of the disease, but this is a matter of debate as correlations were found for some markers such as sCD154, thromboxane B2 or MPs (Table 1). Finally, morphological electron microscopy-based studies also suggest platelet enhanced activability in SSc, and there are signs of platelet granule release [111, 123, 124]. A major point is that platelet activation may be prominently linked to the Raynaud's phenomenon. Indeed, features of platelet activation are also found in the primary Raynaud's phenomenon (below).

Platelet activation markers	Correlations with disease features	References
Circulating platelet aggregates	Not found	[125-127]
Platelet-leucocyte aggregates	Not found [128]	[128]
β-TG	Not found [122]; [130]	[122]; [125-127]; [129-134];
Serotonin	Not found	[135] (in the CREST variant); [136] (also in platelets)
CXCL4	Not found	[126]; [131]; [133]; Radstake Arthritis Rheum 2010;62 Suppl 10 :1210 (Abstract); [134]
Thromboxane B2 in plasma or urines (Thromboxane A2 metabolite)	Positive correlation with dSSc (Herrick 1996) [139]	[134]; [137-139];
TSP-1	Not found	[133]
tPA		[132]
Membrane CD62P	Not found	[122]; [128]
Soluble CD62P	Not found	[140]

Platelet activation markers	Correlations with disease features	References
sCD154	Positive correlation with lSSc, with digital ulcers and pulmonary arterial hypertension [141]	[141]; [142]
Platelet-derived MPs	Inverse correlation to the modified Rodnan thickness score [143]	[128]; [143]

Table 1. Markers of platelet activation in SSc
Platelet activation in SSc is documented by several studies. Markers have been measured in plasma or serum or on platelets (CD62P). The elevation of circulating tPA is not always found [139, 144]. Abbreviations: β-TG, β-thromboglobulin ; TSP-1, thrombospondin-1 ; dSSc, diffuse cutaneous SSc; lSSc, limited cutaneous SSc ([2]). Other abbreviations are spelled in the text.

6. Lack of platelet morphological abnormalities and count in SSc

There are no specific recognized abnormalities of the platelet count in SSc. Moderate thrombocytosis or thrombocytopenia are occasionally observed, and have been related to inflammation or microangiopathy, respectively [145, 146]. Platelet morphology is not altered.

7. Potential mechanisms mediating platelet activation in SSc

Mechanisms underlying platelet activation in SSc remain ill-defined. Questions that have been pursued are: (i) is there a platelet dysfunction in patients that would reduce the threshold level of platelet response to activating signals? (ii) are platelets activated in SSc as the result of EC injury, autoantibodies directed at platelets or other reasons? (iii) what is the role played by the Raynaud's phenomenon?

7.1 Is there a platelet disorder in SSc leading to platelet hyperactivability?

Several studies have examined the eventuality of platelet dysfunction in SSc (Table 2). Reports suggest augmented responsiveness of platelets to their physiological agonists, either strong agonists, such as thrombin or collagen, or weak agonists, such as serotonin, ADP, epinephrine or arachidonic acid, resulting in a reduced threshold of platelet aggregation to the agonist stimulus. Conversely, there is a reduced response to inhibitors of platelet activation such as prostacyclin. However, there are contradictory reports (Table 2). Platelet response to agonists as measured by the hyperactive phenotype is often difficult to interpret. There is a significant variability between individuals, as several genetic modifiers may influence platelet function and as platelet hyperactivity, as measured by aggregometry, can be detected in healthy individuals [147, 148]. Also, *in vivo*, platelet activation results from the combinational input of agonists that act in a complex synergistic way and vary from donor to donor [149-152]. The application of neural networks approaches for predicting platelet response to a complex milieu may represent a useful tool for studying platelet activation response to agonists in SSc. There are no straightforward interpretations of changes in platelet function in SSc. Interestingly, binding assays of radiolabelled collagen indicate a specific increase in the expression of the platelet collagen type 1 receptor in SSc patients [153], which would explain the enhanced response to collagen and indicate a primary or acquired defect. Proteomic studies on platelet compartments in SSc patients could help finding a potential primary or acquired platelet defects in this disease.

Platelet function changes	References
Hyperaggregability Spontaneous (in whole blood) In response to agonists	[126]; [131]; [154-158]
Enhanced adhesion to collagen	[159];
Reduced sensitivity to PGI2	[160]
Increased platelet sensitivity to collagen-induced aggregation	[138]; [157]
Increased expression of collagen type 1 receptor	[153]
Hyperaggregability not found	[161]

Table 2. Changes in platelet functions in SSc

7.2 Potential mechanisms mediating platelet activation in SSc

Platelet activation in SSc may first be the consequence of endothelium injury. Indeed, the canonical role of platelets is to react to endothelium damage, a circumstance that activates a bidirectional dialogue between ECs and platelets, initiating and sustaining inflammation. Through soluble and platelet-bound signals, activated platelets confer ECs a proinflammatory and procoagulant phenotype and, reciprocally, EC activation, as met in inflammation, leads to platelet activation resulting in a pro-inflammatory amplification loop. The balance of signals that keep platelet from being activated may be overcome in a variety of conditions. As summarized above, not only platelets react to the endothelial barrier loss of integrity with consequent exposure of the underneath collagen-rich matrix, but they also react to slighter features of EC activation, which do not lead *per se* to severe endothelium damage, as met for example in conditions in which ECs are activated by cytokines including TNFα, IL-1, VEGF, by oxidative stress or hypoxia [80, 162-165]. These signals induce the expression of a range of molecules promoting platelet adhesion on ECs. Platelets bind to these docking structures, an event that initiates their activation. These conditions also induce ECs to produce platelet agonists, such as multimeric vWF and ADP. Inflammation and coagulation are inextricably linked. Activated ECs express tissue factor, leading to the activation of coagulation, platelet activation, thrombin generation and further amplification of the inflammatory reaction. This is dramatically exemplified in renal involvement in SSc, characterized by thrombotic microangiopathy lesions. On electron microscopy studies, aggregates of platelets admixed with fibrin and fragmented red blood cells are observed within small interstitial vessels or glomerular capillaries. Hypoxia is a noxious stimulus that activates a range of inflammatory pathways, leading to EC activation through multiple mechanisms, including the production of angiogenic factors [166-168]. Hypoxia is thought to play a critical role in SSc. SSc-associated microangiopathy results in a disturbed blood flow in the capillaries with consequent hypoxia, which is likely to be aggravated by tissue fibrosis [169-172]. Hypoxia alters vascular endothelium but also directly activates platelets [173, 174] (our unpublished results). Altogether, conditions that turn EC phenotype to proinfammatory/prothrombotic are translated into platelet adhesion and activation, with the consequent release of inflammatory, mitogenic, angiogenic and fibrogenic platelet-derived mediators described above. These mediators further activate ECs, promoting the production of cytokine/chemokines, induction of adhesion and procoagulant molecules, and production and activation of MMPs. Moreover, ECs undergoing apoptosis become proadhesive for platelets [175], and activated platelets can in turn induce EC apoptosis [176].

In fact, endothelial injury in the microcirculation and arterioles is a predominant feature of SSc which has extensively been reviewed [13, 30, 177-180]. There are circulating stigmata of endothelial injury, including von Willebrand factor and supranormal (larger) vWF multimers [126, 131, 139, 181-184], soluble adhesion molecules, such as E-selectin or vascular cell adhesion molecule (VCAM)-1 and ICAM-1, thrombomodulin, tPA, or endothelin [185-188]. Increased nitrate in the plasma or serum of patients has been described, and been related to EC injury, as there are correlations with soluble E-selectin and soluble VCAM-1 [189, 190]. Elevated circulating ECs were also attributed to vascular damage in SSc [191]. EC apoptosis is a common and early feature in SSc [192]; however pathologic evidence for EC apoptosis remains controversial [177]. However there are inherent limitations to the interpretations of such biomarkers [193], these results show that there is an early insult to the vasculature during the course of the disease.

Importantly, the Raynaud's phenomenon itself, one, if not the first manifestation of SSc, preceding the onset of other symptoms of the disease [194-198], is associated with platelet activation [132]. The absence of endothelium abnormalities in the primary Raynaud's phenomenon is generally accepted, although limited morphological abnormalities have been described [199]. However, features of platelet activation are found in primary Raynaud's phenomenon [158, 200, 201] and platelet activation was proposed to play a role in its pathogenesis [135, 202]. Therefore, events responsible for the Raynaud's phenomenon lead to platelet activation in the absence of EC damage, a possible argument to place platelet activation as a very early pathogenic event in the reciprocal activation dialogue between platelets and ECs. Intriguingly, several factors that have been put forward as being potentially causative or susceptible to modify the progression of SSc, as exposure of extremities to cold, mechanical vibrations, exposure to organic solvents or silica, CMV infection are associated to some extent to platelet activation, and for some of them to trigger the Raynaud's phenomenon.

Finally, autoantibodies against platelet gpIIb/IIIa have been described in SSc [203]. However their role in platelet activation remains uncertain.

8. Platelet activation and the progression of SSc

SSc is a complex disease for which no specific causative mechanism has been identified. The disease may be initiated in the vasculature, as morphological changes are apparent before the onset of the disease; however, it is not clear how endothelium injury begins. Platelets play a large and complex physiological role in health and disease, as they contribute to hemostasis, inflammation, tissue repair, and to the innate and adaptative immunity, standing as essential links [69, 204]. Platelets establish intimate bidirectional relationship with the endothelium, making them potential contributors to SSc vasculopathy. The microcirculation is a characteristic target in SSc pathogenesis. Microcirculation hemorheologic conditions result in an intimate platelet/endothelium interface, characterized by a near capillary wall platelet concentration. Clearly, cross-interactions between ECs and platelets are inextricably linked under the form of feed-back activation loops and whether or not being a primary event, any condition leading to an endothelium insult drives platelet activation. Conversely, platelet activation drives to EC activation; the fact that platelet activation is observed in the primary Raynaud's phenomenon, in the absence of EC detectable damage, may signify that subtle early events activating platelets, such as disturbed blood flow or hypoxia, precede the onset of the disease. Following platelet activation in the microcirculation, as described above, a wide array of soluble and platelet-bound mediators with a pleiotropic range of actions are released that can contribute to several pathophysiological features of the disease including (i) vascular tone dysregulation, (ii) endothelium activation, (iii) inflammation, (iv) activation of the coagulation system, (v) fibrogenic response, (vi) altered angiogenesis. Apart from the possible deleterious cross-talk between endothelium and platelets, described above, two chief features of SSc progression that may be connected to platelets have been the subject of very recent reports. Altered angiogenesis and progressive perivascular and interstitial fibrosis are hallmarks of SSc [27]. First as summarized above, platelets are essential contributors to angiogenesis during wound healing, and ongoing platelet activation in capillary beds may be involved in the altered angiogenesis associated with SSc. In fact, in line with the major VEGF transporter role of platelets, platelet VEGF is increased in SSc patients. However, this is not the case for other angiogenic regulators, such as TGF-β1, PDGF-BB or angiopoietins [122]. VEGF, jointly with other mediators, determines the angiogenic or non-angiogenic status of the EC and an imbalance between the relative concentrations of angiogenic mediators is likely to alter angiogenesis homeostasis [170, 177]. Indeed, the deregulated expression of VEGF is thought to lead to abnormal angiogenesis, as exemplified by the resulting disorganization of the capillary network with large, leaky, fragile capillaries; dynamic parameters, such as the magnitude or the kinetics of VEGF release being critically important [170, 205-207]. Therefore platelet activation in the patient's microvascular beds may result in the release of inappropriate combinations of angiogenic and angiostatic mediators, and such disequilibrium may be relevant to the vascular disease in SSc [122, 208, 209]. Further, as summarized above, there are connections between angiogenesis, vascular remodeling and fibrosis and an unbalance between factors promoting and factors inhibiting angiogenesis may also be relevant to the progression of fibrosis. Second, as summarized above, platelets provide a cornucopia of mediators that may be relevant to the natural history of tissue fibrosis, i.e. through fibrocompetent cell activation. Sustained activation of fibrocompetent cells contribute to excessive ECM production in tissues. Indeed, fibroblasts expanded from the fibrotic skin or lungs from SSc patients have a myofibroblastic phenotype and there is a strong correlation between myofibroblast labeling in the lesional skin and the Rodnan skin score [210]. Crucial platelet links with tissue fibrosis have recently been emphasized in humans. In liver fibrosis the secretion of platelet-derived CXCL4 is instrumental [211]. In SSc, the role of platelet-derived serotonin in skin fibrosis is strongly suggested by the stimulation of the production of ECM by serotonin through binding to dermal fibroblasts serotonin receptor 5-HT_{2B}, increased expression of 5-HT_{2B} in the fibrotic skin of SSc patients and reduction of experimental fibrosis through pharmacological targeting of the 5-HT/5-HT_{2B} signaling and anti-platelet drugs [212].

9. Conclusion; Platelet activation in SSc: A deleterious loop?

The primary triggering event in SSc remains unclear. However, inflammation of the vasculature is a common denominator, whether resulting from an autoimmune response to a yet undefined antigen or other mechanisms. Whatever the primary target, inflammation leads to EC activation and, due to the reciprocal activating interplay between platelets and endothelium, EC activation in turn activates platelets and vice-versa. Platelet activation, through the release of cytokines, chemokines, angiogenic and chemotactic mediators...., amplifies the inflammatory reaction by triggering its many facets, including leukocyte recruitment, leading to further endothelium activation and perivascular inflammation, deregulated angiogenesis and, eventually, fibrosis (Figure 1). A chronic inflammatory scenario may contribute to fibrosis by the way of fibrocompetent cell activation, if the initial pathogenic trigger persists, either continuously or repetitively. Self-sustained myofibroblast-dependent fibrotic process takes place on the grounds of a chronic inflammation. Platelets may therefore stand at an important place in the ill-understood hierarchy of cell and soluble mediators interplay responsible for the disease. This scenario is evidently highly simplified due to the extreme complexity and heterogeneity of the disease pathophysiology. The lack of suitable animal models [213, 214] that would accurately recapitulate each steps of SSc progression remains a real handicap to understand the natural history of this disease.

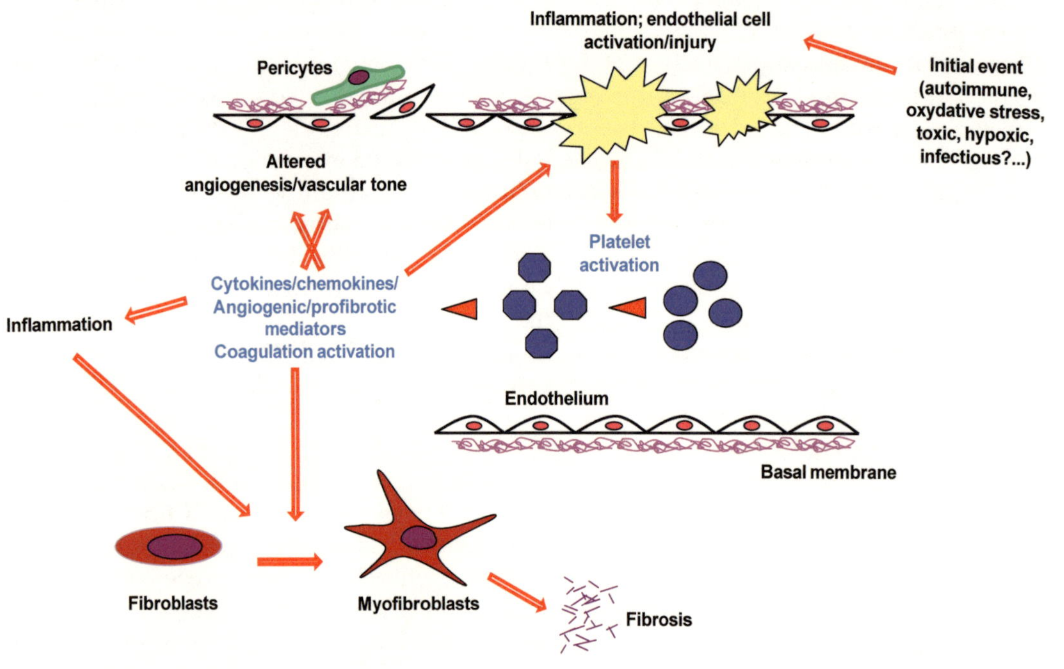

Fig. 1. Platelet activation in SSc: a deleterious loop?
This schematic model underlines the potential role that platelets may play in the initiation and progression of SSc; see text for details. The role of platelet-derived MPs may also be an important point to consider, as they recapitulate several platelet functions and may transfer platelet deleterious effects at sites distant from their generation.

10. Acknowledgments

Work supported by the Groupe Français de Recherche sur la Sclérodermie and the Association des Sclérodermiques de France. Julien Villeneuve is supported by an EMBO long term fellowship.

11. References

[1] Preliminary criteria for the classification of systemic sclerosis (scleroderma). Subcommittee for scleroderma criteria of the American Rheumatism Association Diagnostic and Therapeutic Criteria Committee. Arthritis Rheum. 1980;23:581-90.

[2] LeRoy EC, Black C, Fleischmajer R, Jablonska S, Krieg T, Medsger TA, Jr., et al. Scleroderma (systemic sclerosis): classification, subsets and pathogenesis. J Rheumatol. 1988;15:202-5.

[3] Matucci-Cerinic M, Steen V, Nash P, Hachulla E. The complexity of managing systemic sclerosis: screening and diagnosis. Rheumatology (Oxford). 2009;48 Suppl 3:iii8-13.

[4] Mayes MD, Lacey JV, Jr., Beebe-Dimmer J, Gillespie BW, Cooper B, Laing TJ, et al. Prevalence, incidence, survival, and disease characteristics of systemic sclerosis in a large US population. Arthritis Rheum. 2003;48:2246-55.

[5] Chifflot H, Fautrel B, Sordet C, Chatelus E, Sibilia J. Incidence and prevalence of systemic sclerosis: a systematic literature review. Semin Arthritis Rheum. 2008;37:223-35.

[6] Gabrielli A, Avvedimento EV, Krieg T. Scleroderma. N Engl J Med. 2009;360:1989-2003.

[7] Kowal-Bielecka O, Landewe R, Avouac J, Chwiesko S, Miniati I, Czirjak L, et al. EULAR recommendations for the treatment of systemic sclerosis: a report from the EULAR Scleroderma Trials and Research group (EUSTAR). Ann Rheum Dis. 2009;68:620-8.

[8] Quillinan NP, Denton CP. Disease-modifying treatment in systemic sclerosis: current status. Curr Opin Rheumatol. 2009;21:636-41.

[9] Freemont AJ, Hoyland J, Fielding P, Hodson N, Jayson MI. Studies of the microvascular endothelium in uninvolved skin of patients with systemic sclerosis: direct evidence for a generalized microangiopathy. Br J Dermatol. 1992;126:561-8.

[10] Prescott RJ, Freemont AJ, Jones CJ, Hoyland J, Fielding P. Sequential dermal microvascular and perivascular changes in the development of scleroderma. J Pathol. 1992;166:255-63.

[11] Trotta F, Biagini G, Cenacchi G, Ballardini G, Varotti C, Passarini B, et al. Microvascular changes in progressive systemic sclerosis: immunohistochemical and ultrastructural study. Clin Exp Rheumatol. 1984;2:209-15.

[12] Chizzolini C. Update on pathophysiology of scleroderma with special reference to immunoinflammatory events. Ann Med. 2007;39:42-53.

[13] Kahaleh B. Vascular disease in scleroderma: mechanisms of vascular injury. Rheum Dis Clin North Am. 2008;34:57-71; vi.

[14] Kahaleh MB, Sherer GK, LeRoy EC. Endothelial injury in scleroderma. J Exp Med. 1979;149:1326-35.

[15] Katsumoto TR, Whitfield ML, Connolly MK. The pathogenesis of systemic sclerosis. Annu Rev Pathol.2011;6:509-37.

[16] Varga J. Systemic sclerosis: an update. Bull NYU Hosp Jt Dis. 2008;66:198-202.

[17] Varga J, Abraham D. Systemic sclerosis: a prototypic multisystem fibrotic disorder. J Clin Invest. 2007;117:557-67.
[18] Varga JA, Trojanowska M. Fibrosis in systemic sclerosis. Rheum Dis Clin North Am. 2008;34:115-43; vii.
[19] Agarwal SK, Reveille JD. The genetics of scleroderma (systemic sclerosis). Curr Opin Rheumatol.2010;22:133-8.
[20] Radstake TR, Gorlova O, Rueda B, Martin JE, Alizadeh BZ, Palomino-Morales R, et al. Genome-wide association study of systemic sclerosis identifies CD247 as a new susceptibility locus. Nat Genet.2010;42:426-9.
[21] Whitfield ML, Finlay DR, Murray JI, Troyanskaya OG, Chi JT, Pergamenschikov A, et al. Systemic and cell type-specific gene expression patterns in scleroderma skin. Proc Natl Acad Sci U S A. 2003;100:12319-24.
[22] Gardner H, Shearstone JR, Bandaru R, Crowell T, Lynes M, Trojanowska M, et al. Gene profiling of scleroderma skin reveals robust signatures of disease that are imperfectly reflected in the transcript profiles of explanted fibroblasts. Arthritis Rheum. 2006;54:1961-73.
[23] Agarwal SK, Tan FK, Arnett FC. Genetics and genomic studies in scleroderma (systemic sclerosis). Rheum Dis Clin North Am. 2008;34:17-40; v.
[24] Milano A, Pendergrass SA, Sargent JL, George LK, McCalmont TH, Connolly MK, et al. Molecular subsets in the gene expression signatures of scleroderma skin. PLoS One. 2008;3:e2696.
[25] Hamamdzic D, Kasman LM, LeRoy EC. The role of infectious agents in the pathogenesis of systemic sclerosis. Curr Opin Rheumatol. 2002;14:694-8.
[26] Randone SB, Guiducci S, Cerinic MM. Systemic sclerosis and infections. Autoimmun Rev. 2008;8:36-40.
[27] Manetti M, Guiducci S, Ibba-Manneschi L, Matucci-Cerinic M. Mechanisms in the loss of capillaries in systemic sclerosis: angiogenesis versus vasculogenesis. J Cell Mol Med.2010;14:1241-54.
[28] Abraham DJ, Varga J. Scleroderma: from cell and molecular mechanisms to disease models. Trends Immunol. 2005;26:587-95.
[29] Gilliam AC. Scleroderma. Curr Dir Autoimmun. 2008;10:258-79.
[30] Abraham DJ, Krieg T, Distler J, Distler O. Overview of pathogenesis of systemic sclerosis. Rheumatology (Oxford). 2009;48 Suppl 3:iii3-7.
[31] Blair P, Flaumenhaft R. Platelet alpha-granules: basic biology and clinical correlates. Blood Rev. 2009;23:177-89.
[32] Harrison P, Cramer EM. Platelet alpha-granules. Blood Rev. 1993;7:52-62.
[33] McNicol A, Israels SJ. Platelet dense granules: structure, function and implications for haemostasis. Thromb Res. 1999;95:1-18.
[34] Rendu F, Brohard-Bohn B. The platelet release reaction: granules' constituents, secretion and functions. Platelets. 2001;12:261-73.
[35] Gnatenko DV, Perrotta PL, Bahou WF. Proteomic approaches to dissect platelet function: Half the story. Blood. 2006;108:3983-91.
[36] Maguire PB. Platelet proteomics: identification of potential therapeutic targets. Pathophysiol Haemost Thromb. 2003;33:481-6.
[37] Nurden AT, Nurden P, Sanchez M, Andia I, Anitua E. Platelets and wound healing. Front Biosci. 2008;13:3532-48.

[38] Handagama P, Rappolee DA, Werb Z, Levin J, Bainton DF. Platelet alpha-granule fibrinogen, albumin, and immunoglobulin G are not synthesized by rat and mouse megakaryocytes. J Clin Invest. 1990;86:1364-8.

[39] Mercado CP, Kilic F. Molecular mechanisms of SERT in platelets: regulation of plasma serotonin levels. Mol Interv. 2010;10:231-41.

[40] Warkentin TE, Aird WC, Rand JH. Platelet-endothelial interactions: sepsis, HIT, and antiphospholipid syndrome. Hematology Am Soc Hematol Educ Program. 2003:497-519.

[41] Booyse F, Rafelson ME, Jr. In vitro incorporation of amino-acids into the contractile protein of human blood platelets. Nature. 1967;215:283-4.

[42] Kieffer N, Guichard J, Farcet JP, Vainchenker W, Breton-Gorius J. Biosynthesis of major platelet proteins in human blood platelets. Eur J Biochem. 1987;164:189-95.

[43] Warshaw AL, Laster L, Shulman NR. Protein synthesis by human platelets. J Biol Chem. 1967;242:2094-7.

[44] Weyrich AS, Dixon DA, Pabla R, Elstad MR, McIntyre TM, Prescott SM, et al. Signal-dependent translation of a regulatory protein, Bcl-3, in activated human platelets. Proc Natl Acad Sci U S A. 1998;95:5556-61.

[45] Weyrich AS, Lindemann S, Tolley ND, Kraiss LW, Dixon DA, Mahoney TM, et al. Change in protein phenotype without a nucleus: translational control in platelets. Semin Thromb Hemost. 2004;30:491-8.

[46] Flaumenhaft R. Formation and fate of platelet microparticles. Blood Cells Mol Dis. 2006;36:182-7.

[47] Italiano JE, Jr., Mairuhu AT, Flaumenhaft R. Clinical relevance of microparticles from platelets and megakaryocytes. Curr Opin Hematol. 2010;17:578-84.

[48] Mause SF, Weber C. Microparticles: protagonists of a novel communication network for intercellular information exchange. Circ Res. 2010;107:1047-57.

[49] Smyth SS, McEver RP, Weyrich AS, Morrell CN, Hoffman MR, Arepally GM, et al. Platelet functions beyond hemostasis. J Thromb Haemost. 2009;7:1759-66.

[50] Gawaz M. Role of platelets in coronary thrombosis and reperfusion of ischemic myocardium. Cardiovasc Res. 2004;61:498-511.

[51] Lesurtel M, Graf R, Aleil B, Walther DJ, Tian Y, Jochum W, et al. Platelet-derived serotonin mediates liver regeneration. Science. 2006;312:104-7.

[52] Nocito A, Georgiev P, Dahm F, Jochum W, Bader M, Graf R, et al. Platelets and platelet-derived serotonin promote tissue repair after normothermic hepatic ischemia in mice. Hepatology. 2007;45:369-76.

[53] Stellos K, Kopf S, Paul A, Marquardt JU, Gawaz M, Huard J, et al. Platelets in regeneration. Semin Thromb Hemost. 2010;36:175-84.

[54] Gawaz M, Langer H, May AE. Platelets in inflammation and atherogenesis. J Clin Invest. 2005;115:3378-84.

[55] Czapiga M, Gao JL, Kirk A, Lekstrom-Himes J. Human platelets exhibit chemotaxis using functional N-formyl peptide receptors. Exp Hematol. 2005;33:73-84.

[56] Del Conde I, Cruz MA, Zhang H, Lopez JA, Afshar-Kharghan V. Platelet activation leads to activation and propagation of the complement system. J Exp Med. 2005;201:871-9.

[57] May AE, Seizer P, Gawaz M. Platelets: inflammatory firebugs of vascular walls. Arterioscler Thromb Vasc Biol. 2008;28:s5-10.

[58] Weber C. Platelets and chemokines in atherosclerosis: partners in crime. Circ Res. 2005;96:612-6.

[59] Weyrich AS, Zimmerman GA. Platelets: signaling cells in the immune continuum. Trends Immunol. 2004;25:489-95.

[60] Pober JS, Sessa WC. Evolving functions of endothelial cells in inflammation. Nat Rev Immunol. 2007;7:803-15.

[61] Frenette PS, Johnson RC, Hynes RO, Wagner DD. Platelets roll on stimulated endothelium in vivo: an interaction mediated by endothelial P-selectin. Proc Natl Acad Sci U S A. 1995;92:7450-4.

[62] Massberg S, Enders G, Leiderer R, Eisenmenger S, Vestweber D, Krombach F, et al. Platelet-endothelial cell interactions during ischemia/reperfusion: the role of P-selectin. Blood. 1998;92:507-15.

[63] Andre P, Denis CV, Ware J, Saffaripour S, Hynes RO, Ruggeri ZM, et al. Platelets adhere to and translocate on von Willebrand factor presented by endothelium in stimulated veins. Blood. 2000;96:3322-8.

[64] Bombeli T, Schwartz BR, Harlan JM. Adhesion of activated platelets to endothelial cells: evidence for a GPIIbIIIa-dependent bridging mechanism and novel roles for endothelial intercellular adhesion molecule 1 (ICAM-1), alphavbeta3 integrin, and GPIbalpha. J Exp Med. 1998;187:329-39.

[65] Defilippi P, Silengo L, Tarone G. Regulation of adhesion receptors expression in endothelial cells. Curr Top Microbiol Immunol. 1993;184:87-98.

[66] Gawaz M, Neumann FJ, Dickfeld T, Reininger A, Adelsberger H, Gebhardt A, et al. Vitronectin receptor (alpha(v)beta3) mediates platelet adhesion to the luminal aspect of endothelial cells: implications for reperfusion in acute myocardial infarction. Circulation. 1997;96:1809-18.

[67] Springer TA. Traffic signals for lymphocyte recirculation and leukocyte emigration: the multistep paradigm. Cell. 1994;76:301-14.

[68] Wagner DD, Burger PC. Platelets in inflammation and thrombosis. Arterioscler Thromb Vasc Biol. 2003;23:2131-7.

[69] [69] Gear AR, Camerini D. Platelet chemokines and chemokine receptors: linking hemostasis, inflammation, and host defense. Microcirculation. 2003;10:335-50.

[70] Klinger MH. Platelets and inflammation. Anat Embryol (Berl). 1997;196:1-11.

[71] Pinedo HM, Verheul HM, D'Amato RJ, Folkman J. Involvement of platelets in tumour angiogenesis? Lancet. 1998;352:1775-7.

[72] Brill A, Dashevsky O, Rivo J, Gozal Y, Varon D. Platelet-derived microparticles induce angiogenesis and stimulate post-ischemic revascularization. Cardiovasc Res. 2005;67:30-8.

[73] Carmeliet P. Angiogenesis in health and disease. Nat Med. 2003;9:653-60.

[74] Folkman J. Angiogenesis: an organizing principle for drug discovery? Nat Rev Drug Discov. 2007;6:273-86.

[75] Folkman J, Browder T, Palmblad J. Angiogenesis research: guidelines for translation to clinical application. Thromb Haemost. 2001;86:23-33.

[76] Jain RK. Molecular regulation of vessel maturation. Nat Med. 2003;9:685-93.

[77] Kisucka J, Butterfield CE, Duda DG, Eichenberger SC, Saffaripour S, Ware J, et al. Platelets and platelet adhesion support angiogenesis while preventing excessive hemorrhage. Proc Natl Acad Sci U S A. 2006;103:855-60.

[78] Mehrad B, Keane MP, Strieter RM. Chemokines as mediators of angiogenesis. Thromb Haemost. 2007;97:755-62.

[79] Browder T, Folkman J, Pirie-Shepherd S. The hemostatic system as a regulator of angiogenesis. J Biol Chem. 2000;275:1521-4.

[80] Verheul HM, Jorna AS, Hoekman K, Broxterman HJ, Gebbink MF, Pinedo HM. Vascular endothelial growth factor-stimulated endothelial cells promote adhesion and activation of platelets. Blood. 2000;96:4216-21.

[81] Carmeliet P, Jain RK. Angiogenesis in cancer and other diseases. Nature. 2000;407:249-57.

[82] Armulik A, Abramsson A, Betsholtz C. Endothelial/pericyte interactions. Circ Res. 2005;97:512-23.

[83] Hanahan D, Folkman J. Patterns and emerging mechanisms of the angiogenic switch during tumorigenesis. Cell. 1996;86:353-64.

[84] Carmeliet P. VEGF gene therapy: stimulating angiogenesis or angioma-genesis? Nat Med. 2000;6:1102-3.

[85] Italiano JE, Jr., Richardson JL, Patel-Hett S, Battinelli E, Zaslavsky A, Short S, et al. Angiogenesis is regulated by a novel mechanism: pro- and antiangiogenic proteins are organized into separate platelet alpha granules and differentially released. Blood. 2008;111:1227-33.

[86] Burnstock G. Autonomic neurotransmission: 60 years since sir Henry Dale. Annu Rev Pharmacol Toxicol. 2009;49:1-30.

[87] Storkebaum E, Carmeliet P. Paracrine control of vascular innervation in health and disease. Acta Physiol (Oxf). 2011, Jun 20

[88] Feletou M, Kohler R, Vanhoutte PM. Endothelium-derived vasoactive factors and hypertension: possible roles in pathogenesis and as treatment targets. Curr Hypertens Rep. 2010;12:267-75.

[89] Luscher TF, Boulanger CM, Dohi Y, Yang ZH. Endothelium-derived contracting factors. Hypertension. 1992;19:117-30.

[90] Vanhoutte PM. Endothelial control of vasomotor function: from health to coronary disease. Circ J. 2003;67:572-5.

[91] Vanhoutte PM, Houston DS. Platelets, endothelium, and vasospasm. Circulation. 1985;72:728-34.

[92] Serhan CN, Savill J. Resolution of inflammation: the beginning programs the end. Nat Immunol. 2005;6:1191-7.

[93] Tomasek JJ, Gabbiani G, Hinz B, Chaponnier C, Brown RA. Myofibroblasts and mechano-regulation of connective tissue remodelling. Nat Rev Mol Cell Biol. 2002;3:349-63.

[94] Karasek MA. Does transformation of microvascular endothelial cells into myofibroblasts play a key role in the etiology and pathology of fibrotic disease? Med Hypotheses. 2007;68:650-5.

[95] Keeley EC, Mehrad B, Strieter RM. Fibrocytes: bringing new insights into mechanisms of inflammation and fibrosis. Int J Biochem Cell Biol. 2010;42:535-42.

[96] Keeley EC, Mehrad B, Strieter RM. The role of circulating mesenchymal progenitor cells (fibrocytes) in the pathogenesis of fibrotic disorders. Thromb Haemost. 2009;101:613-8.

[97] Nakamura M, Tokura Y. Epithelial-mesenchymal transition in the skin. J Dermatol Sci. 2011;61:7-13.

[98] Opalenik SR, Davidson JM. Fibroblast differentiation of bone marrow-derived cells during wound repair. FASEB J. 2005;19:1561-3.

[99] Quan TE, Cowper SE, Bucala R. The role of circulating fibrocytes in fibrosis. Curr Rheumatol Rep. 2006;8:145-50.

[100] Desmouliere A, Geinoz A, Gabbiani F, Gabbiani G. Transforming growth factor-beta 1 induces alpha-smooth muscle actin expression in granulation tissue myofibroblasts and in quiescent and growing cultured fibroblasts. J Cell Biol. 1993;122:103-11.

[101] Kalluri R, Weinberg RA. The basics of epithelial-mesenchymal transition. J Clin Invest. 2009;119:1420-8.

[102] Krieg T, Abraham D, Lafyatis R. Fibrosis in connective tissue disease: the role of the myofibroblast and fibroblast-epithelial cell interactions. Arthritis Res Ther. 2007;9 Suppl 2:S4.

[103] Aden N, Nuttall A, Shiwen X, de Winter P, Leask A, Black CM, et al. Epithelial cells promote fibroblast activation via IL-1alpha in systemic sclerosis. J Invest Dermatol. 2010;130:2191-200.

[104] Friedlander M. Fibrosis and diseases of the eye. J Clin Invest. 2007;117:576-86.

[105] Strieter RM, Gomperts BN, Keane MP. The role of CXC chemokines in pulmonary fibrosis. J Clin Invest. 2007;117:549-56.

[106] Wynn TA. Common and unique mechanisms regulate fibrosis in various fibroproliferative diseases. J Clin Invest. 2007;117:524-9.

[107] Iredale JP. Models of liver fibrosis: exploring the dynamic nature of inflammation and repair in a solid organ. J Clin Invest. 2007;117:539-48.

[108] Anitua E, Andia I, Ardanza B, Nurden P, Nurden AT. Autologous platelets as a source of proteins for healing and tissue regeneration. Thromb Haemost. 2004;91:4-15.

[109] Villeneuve J, Block A, Le Bousse-Kerdiles MC, Lepreux S, Nurden P, Ripoche J, et al. Tissue inhibitors of matrix metalloproteinases in platelets and megakaryocytes: a novel organization for these secreted proteins. Exp Hematol. 2009;37:849-56.

[110] Nurden AT. Platelets and tissue remodeling: extending the role of the blood clotting system. Endocrinology. 2007;148:3053-5.

[111] Postlethwaite AE, Chiang TM. Platelet contributions to the pathogenesis of systemic sclerosis. Curr Opin Rheumatol. 2007;19:574-9.

[112] Katoh N. Platelets as versatile regulators of cutaneous inflammation. J Dermatol Sci. 2009;53:89-95.

[113] Andrae J, Gallini R, Betsholtz C. Role of platelet-derived growth factors in physiology and medicine. Genes Dev. 2008;22:1276-312.

[114] Blann AD, Lip GY, Beevers DG, McCollum CN. Soluble P-selectin in atherosclerosis: a comparison with endothelial cell and platelet markers. Thromb Haemost. 1997;77:1077-80.

[115] Fijnheer R, Frijns CJ, Korteweg J, Rommes H, Peters JH, Sixma JJ, et al. The origin of P-selectin as a circulating plasma protein. Thromb Haemost. 1997;77:1081-5.

[116] Viallard JF, Solanilla A, Gauthier B, Contin C, Dechanet J, Grosset C, et al. Increased soluble and platelet-associated CD40 ligand in essential thrombocythemia and reactive thrombocytosis. Blood. 2002;99:2612-4.

[117] Schonbeck U, Libby P. The CD40/CD154 receptor/ligand dyad. Cell Mol Life Sci. 2001;58:4-43.

[118] Yanaba K, Takehara K, Sato S. Serum concentrations of soluble P-selectin glycoprotein ligand-1 are increased in patients with systemic sclerosis: association with lower frequency of pulmonary fibrosis. Ann Rheum Dis. 2004;63:583-7.

[119] Frenette PS, Denis CV, Weiss L, Jurk K, Subbarao S, Kehrel B, et al. P-Selectin glycoprotein ligand 1 (PSGL-1) is expressed on platelets and can mediate platelet-endothelial interactions in vivo. J Exp Med. 2000;191:1413-22.

[120] Kasper B, Petersen F. Molecular pathways of platelet factor 4/CXCL4 signaling. Eur J Cell Biol. 2011;90:521-6.

[121] Marasini B, Cugno M, Bassani C, Stanzani M, Bottasso B, Agostoni A. Tissue-type plasminogen activator and von Willebrand factor plasma levels as markers of endothelial involvement in patients with Raynaud's phenomenon. Int J Microcirc Clin Exp. 1992;11:375-82.

[122] Solanilla A, Villeneuve J, Auguste P, Hugues M, Alioum A, Lepreux S, et al. The transport of high amounts of vascular endothelial growth factor by blood platelets underlines their potential contribution in systemic sclerosis angiogenesis. Rheumatology (Oxford). 2009;48:1036-44.

[123] Riddle JM, Bluhm GB, Pitchford WC, McElroy H, Jimenea C, Leisen J, et al. A comparative study of platelet reactivity in arthritis. Ann N Y Acad Sci. 1981;370:22-9.

[124] Maeda M, Kachi H, Mori S. Ultrastructural observation of platelets from patients with progressive systemic sclerosis (PSS). J Dermatol. 1998;25:222-30.

[125] Kahaleh MB, Osborn I, Leroy EC. Elevated levels of circulating platelet aggregates and beta-thromboglobulin in scleroderma. Ann Intern Med. 1982;96:610-3.

[126] Cuenca R, Fernandez-Cortijo J, Lima J, Fonollosa V, Simeon CP, Pico M, et al. [Platelet function study in primary Raynaud's phenomenon and Raynaud's phenomenon associated with scleroderma]. Med Clin (Barc). 1990;95:761-3.

[127] Kallenberg CG, Vellenga E, Wouda AA, The TH. Platelet activation, fibrinolytic activity and circulating immune complexes in Raynaud's phenomenon. J Rheumatol. 1982;9:878-84.

[128] Pamuk GE, Turgut B, Pamuk ON, Vural O, Demir M, Cakir N. Increased circulating platelet-leucocyte complexes in patients with primary Raynaud's phenomenon and Raynaud's phenomenon secondary to systemic sclerosis: a comparative study. Blood Coagul Fibrinolysis. 2007;18:297-302.

[129] Lee P, Norman CS, Sukenik S, Alderdice CA. The clinical significance of coagulation abnormalities in systemic sclerosis (scleroderma). J Rheumatol. 1985;12:514-7.

[130] Seibold JR, Harris JN. Plasma beta-thromboglobulin in the differential diagnosis of Raynaud's phenomenon. J Rheumatol. 1985;12:99-103.

[131] Lima J, Fonollosa V, Fernandez-Cortijo J, Ordi J, Cuenca R, Khamashta MA, et al. Platelet activation, endothelial cell dysfunction in the absence of anticardiolipin antibodies in systemic sclerosis. J Rheumatol. 1991;18:1833-6.

[132] Silveri F, De Angelis R, Poggi A, Muti S, Bonapace G, Argentati F, et al. Relative roles of endothelial cell damage and platelet activation in primary Raynaud's phenomenon (RP) and RP secondary to systemic sclerosis. Scand J Rheumatol. 2001;30:290-6.

[133] Macko RF, Gelber AC, Young BA, Lowitt MH, White B, Wigley FM, et al. Increased circulating concentrations of the counteradhesive proteins SPARC and

thrombospondin-1 in systemic sclerosis (scleroderma). Relationship to platelet and endothelial cell activation. J Rheumatol. 2002;29:2565-70.
[134] Maeda M, Kachi H, Mori S. Plasma levels of molecular markers of blood coagulation and fibrinolysis in progressive systemic sclerosis (PSS). J Dermatol Sci. 1996;11:223-7.
[135] Klimiuk PS, Grennan A, Weinkove C, Jayson MI. Platelet serotonin in systemic sclerosis. Ann Rheum Dis. 1989;48:586-9.
[136] Biondi ML, Marasini B, Bianchi E, Agostoni A. Plasma free and intraplatelet serotonin in patients with Raynaud's phenomenon. Int J Cardiol. 1988;19:335-9.
[137] Reilly IA, Roy L, Fitzgerald GA. Biosynthesis of thromboxane in patients with systemic sclerosis and Raynaud's phenomenon. Br Med J (Clin Res Ed). 1986;292:1037-9.
[138] Wilkinson D, Vowden P, Gilks L, Latif AB, Rajah SM, Kester RC. Plasma eicosanoids, platelet function and cold sensitivity. Br J Surg. 1989;76:401-5.
[139] Herrick AL, Illingworth K, Blann A, Hay CR, Hollis S, Jayson MI. Von Willebrand factor, thrombomodulin, thromboxane, beta-thromboglobulin and markers of fibrinolysis in primary Raynaud's phenomenon and systemic sclerosis. Ann Rheum Dis. 1996;55:122-7.
[140] Blann AD, Constans J, Carpentier P, Renard M, Satger B, Guerin V, et al. Soluble P selectin in systemic sclerosis: relationship with von Willebrand factor, autoantibodies and diffuse or localised/limited disease. Thromb Res. 2003;109:203-6.
[141] Allanore Y, Borderie D, Meune C, Lemarechal H, Weber S, Ekindjian OG, et al. Increased plasma soluble CD40 ligand concentrations in systemic sclerosis and association with pulmonary arterial hypertension and digital ulcers. Ann Rheum Dis. 2005;64:481-3.
[142] Komura K, Sato S, Hasegawa M, Fujimoto M, Takehara K. Elevated circulating CD40L concentrations in patients with systemic sclerosis. J Rheumatol. 2004;31:514-9.
[143] Guiducci S, Distler JH, Jungel A, Huscher D, Huber LC, Michel BA, et al. The relationship between plasma microparticles and disease manifestations in patients with systemic sclerosis. Arthritis Rheum. 2008;58:2845-53.
[144] Lau CS, McLaren M, Mackay I, Belch JJ. Baseline plasma fibrinolysis and its correlation with clinical manifestations in patients with Raynaud's phenomenon. Ann Rheum Dis. 1993;52:443-8.
[145] Frayha RA, Shulman LE, Stevens MB. Hematological abnormalities in scleroderma. A study of 180 cases. Acta Haematol. 1980;64:25-30.
[146] Valentini G, Chianese U, Tirri G, Giordano M. [Thrombocytosis in progressive generalized sclerosis (scleroderma) and in other rheumatic diseases]. Z Rheumatol. 1978;37:233-41.
[147] Smyth SS, Monroe DM, 3rd, Wysokinski WE, McBane RD, 2nd, Whiteheart SW, Becker RC, et al. Platelet activation and its patient-specific consequences. Thromb Res. 2008;122:435-41.
[148] Yee DL, Sun CW, Bergeron AL, Dong JF, Bray PF. Aggregometry detects platelet hyperreactivity in healthy individuals. Blood. 2005;106:2723-9.
[149] Chatterjee MS, Purvis JE, Brass LF, Diamond SL. Pairwise agonist scanning predicts cellular signaling responses to combinatorial stimuli. Nat Biotechnol. 2010;28:727-32.
[150] Huang EM, Detwiler TC. Characteristics of the synergistic actions of platelet agonists. Blood. 1981;57:685-91.

[151] Packham MA, Guccione MA, Chang PL, Mustard JF. Platelet aggregation and release: effects of low concentrations of thrombin or collagen. Am J Physiol. 1973;225:38-47.
[152] Ware JA, Smith M, Salzman EW. Synergism of platelet-aggregating agents. Role of elevation of cytoplasmic calcium. J Clin Invest. 1987;80:267-71.
[153] Chiang TM, Takayama H, Postlethwaite AE. Increase in platelet non-integrin type I collagen receptor in patients with systemic sclerosis. Thromb Res. 2006;117:299-306.
[154] Friedhoff LT, Seibold JR, Kim HC, Simester KS. Serotonin induced platelet aggregation in systemic sclerosis. Clin Exp Rheumatol. 1984;2:119-23.
[155] Goodfield MJ, Orchard MA, Rowell NR. Increased platelet sensitivity to collagen-induced aggregation in whole blood patients with systemic sclerosis. Clin Exp Rheumatol. 1988;6:285-8.
[156] Biondi ML, Marasini B. Abnormal platelet aggregation in patients with Raynaud's phenomenon. J Clin Pathol. 1989;42:716-8.
[157] Goodfield MJ, Orchard MA, Rowell NR. Whole blood platelet aggregation and coagulation factors in patients with systemic sclerosis. Br J Haematol. 1993;84:675-80.
[158] Lau CS, McLaren M, Saniabadi A, Belch JJ. Increased whole blood platelet aggregation in patients with Raynaud's phenomenon with or without systemic sclerosis. Scand J Rheumatol. 1993;22:97-101.
[159] Kahaleh MB, Scharstein KK, LeRoy EC. Enhanced platelet adhesion to collagen in scleroderma. Effect of scleroderma plasma and scleroderma platelets. J Rheumatol. 1985;12:468-71.
[160] Belch JJ, O'Dowd A, Forbes CD, Sturrock RD. Platelet sensitivity to a prostacyclin analogue in systemic sclerosis. Br J Rheumatol. 1985;24:346-50.
[161] Price JE, Klimiuk PS, Jayson MI. In vitro platelet aggregability studies: lack of evidence for platelet hyperactivity in systemic sclerosis. Ann Rheum Dis. 1991;50:567-71.
[162] Cook-Mills JM, Marchese ME, Abdala-Valencia H. Vascular Cell Adhesion Molecule-1 Expression and Signaling During Disease: Regulation by Reactive Oxygen Species and Antioxidants. Antioxid Redox Signal. 2011 May 11
[163] Pober JS. Endothelial activation: intracellular signaling pathways. Arthritis Res. 2002;4 Suppl 3:S109-16.
[164] Sellak H, Franzini E, Hakim J, Pasquier C. Reactive oxygen species rapidly increase endothelial ICAM-1 ability to bind neutrophils without detectable upregulation. Blood. 1994;83:2669-77.
[165] Takano M, Meneshian A, Sheikh E, Yamakawa Y, Wilkins KB, Hopkins EA, et al. Rapid upregulation of endothelial P-selectin expression via reactive oxygen species generation. Am J Physiol Heart Circ Physiol. 2002;283:H2054-61.
[166] Faller DV. Endothelial cell responses to hypoxic stress. Clin Exp Pharmacol Physiol. 1999;26:74-84.
[167] Michiels C, Arnould T, Remacle J. Endothelial cell responses to hypoxia: initiation of a cascade of cellular interactions. Biochim Biophys Acta. 2000;1497:1-10.
[168] Yamakawa M, Liu LX, Date T, Belanger AJ, Vincent KA, Akita GY, et al. Hypoxia-inducible factor-1 mediates activation of cultured vascular endothelial cells by inducing multiple angiogenic factors. Circ Res. 2003;93:664-73.
[169] Beyer C, Schett G, Gay S, Distler O, Distler JH. Hypoxia. Hypoxia in the pathogenesis of systemic sclerosis. Arthritis Res Ther. 2009;11:220.

[170] Distler O, Distler JH, Scheid A, Acker T, Hirth A, Rethage J, et al. Uncontrolled expression of vascular endothelial growth factor and its receptors leads to insufficient skin angiogenesis in patients with systemic sclerosis. Circ Res. 2004;95:109-16.

[171] Hunzelmann N, Krieg T. Scleroderma: from pathophysiology to novel therapeutic approaches. Exp Dermatol. 2010;19:393-400.

[172] Silverstein JL, Steen VD, Medsger TA, Jr., Falanga V. Cutaneous hypoxia in patients with systemic sclerosis (scleroderma). Arch Dermatol. 1988;124:1379-82.

[173] Bradford A. The role of hypoxia and platelets in air travel-related venous thromboembolism. Curr Pharm Des. 2007;13:2668-72.

[174] Bradley TD, Floras JS. Obstructive sleep apnoea and its cardiovascular consequences. Lancet. 2009;373:82-93.

[175] Bombeli T, Schwartz BR, Harlan JM. Endothelial cells undergoing apoptosis become proadhesive for nonactivated platelets. Blood. 1999;93:3831-8.

[176] Sindram D, Porte RJ, Hoffman MR, Bentley RC, Clavien PA. Platelets induce sinusoidal endothelial cell apoptosis upon reperfusion of the cold ischemic rat liver. Gastroenterology. 2000;118:183-91.

[177] Fleming JN, Schwartz SM. The pathology of scleroderma vascular disease. Rheum Dis Clin North Am. 2008;34:41-55; vi.

[178] Guiducci S, Distler O, Distler JH, Matucci-Cerinic M. Mechanisms of vascular damage in SSc--implications for vascular treatment strategies. Rheumatology (Oxford). 2008;47 Suppl 5:v18-20.

[179] Kahaleh B. The microvascular endothelium in scleroderma. Rheumatology (Oxford). 2008;47 Suppl 5:v14-5.

[180] Muller-Ladner U, Distler O, Ibba-Manneschi L, Neumann E, Gay S. Mechanisms of vascular damage in systemic sclerosis. Autoimmunity. 2009;42:587-95.

[181] Greaves M, Malia RG, Milford Ward A, Moult J, Holt CM, Lindsey N, et al. Elevated von Willebrand factor antigen in systemic sclerosis: relationship to visceral disease. Br J Rheumatol. 1988;27:281-5.

[182] Kahaleh MB, Osborn I, LeRoy EC. Increased factor VIII/von Willebrand factor antigen and von Willebrand factor activity in scleroderma and in Raynaud's phenomenon. Ann Intern Med. 1981;94:482-4.

[183] Mannucci PM, Lombardi R, Lattuada A, Perticucci E, Valsecchi R, Remuzzi G. Supranormal von Willebrand factor multimers in scleroderma. Blood. 1989;73:1586-91.

[184] Cuenca R, Fernadez-Cortijo J, Fonollosa V, Lima J, Simeon CP, Vilardell M, et al. von Willebrand factor activity in primary and in scleroderma-associated Raynaud's phenomenon. Lancet. 1990;335:1095.

[185] Kahaleh MB. Endothelin, an endothelial-dependent vasoconstrictor in scleroderma. Enhanced production and profibrotic action. Arthritis Rheum. 1991;34:978-83.

[186] Gruschwitz MS, Hornstein OP, von Den Driesch P. Correlation of soluble adhesion molecules in the peripheral blood of scleroderma patients with their in situ expression and with disease activity. Arthritis Rheum. 1995;38:184-9.

[187] Mercie P, Seigneur M, Conri C. Plasma thrombomodulin as a marker of vascular damage in systemic sclerosis. J Rheumatol. 1995;22:1440-1.

[188] Andersen GN, Caidahl K, Kazzam E, Petersson AS, Waldenstrom A, Mincheva-Nilsson L, et al. Correlation between increased nitric oxide production and markers of endothelial activation in systemic sclerosis: findings with the soluble adhesion molecules E-selectin, intercellular adhesion molecule 1, and vascular cell adhesion molecule 1. Arthritis Rheum. 2000;43:1085-93.

[189] van Gils JM, Zwaginga JJ, Hordijk PL. Molecular and functional interactions among monocytes, platelets, and endothelial cells and their relevance for cardiovascular diseases. J Leukoc Biol. 2009;85:195-204.

[190] Yamamoto T, Katayama I, Nishioka K. Nitric oxide production and inducible nitric oxide synthase expression in systemic sclerosis. J Rheumatol. 1998;25:314-7.

[191] Del Papa N, Colombo G, Fracchiolla N, Moronetti LM, Ingegnoli F, Maglione W, et al. Circulating endothelial cells as a marker of ongoing vascular disease in systemic sclerosis. Arthritis Rheum. 2004;50:1296-304.

[192] Jun JB, Kuechle M, Harlan JM, Elkon KB. Fibroblast and endothelial apoptosis in systemic sclerosis. Curr Opin Rheumatol. 2003;15:756-60.

[193] Hummers LK. Biomarkers of vascular disease in scleroderma. Rheumatology (Oxford). 2008;47 Suppl 5:v21-2.

[194] Flavahan NA, Flavahan S, Mitra S, Chotani MA. The vasculopathy of Raynaud's phenomenon and scleroderma. Rheum Dis Clin North Am. 2003;29:275-91, vi.

[195] Fonseca C, Abraham D, Ponticos M. Neuronal regulators and vascular dysfunction in Raynaud's phenomenon and systemic sclerosis. Curr Vasc Pharmacol. 2009;7:34-9.

[196] Generini S, Matucci Cerinic M. Raynaud's phenomenon and vascular disease in systemic sclerosis. Adv Exp Med Biol. 1999;455:93-100.

[197] Kahaleh MB. Raynaud's phenomenon and the vascular disease in scleroderma. Curr Opin Rheumatol. 1995;7:529-34.

[198] Sunderkotter C, Riemekasten G. Pathophysiology and clinical consequences of Raynaud's phenomenon related to systemic sclerosis. Rheumatology (Oxford). 2006;45 Suppl 3:iii33-5.

[199] Bukhari M, Herrick AL, Moore T, Manning J, Jayson MI. Increased nailfold capillary dimensions in primary Raynaud's phenomenon and systemic sclerosis. Br J Rheumatol. 1996;35:1127-31.

[200] Herrick AL. Pathogenesis of Raynaud's phenomenon. Rheumatology (Oxford). 2005;44:587-96.

[201] Polidoro L, Barnabei R, Giorgini P, Petrazzi L, Ferri C, Properzi G. Platelet activation in patients with the Raynaud's Phenomenon. Intern Med J. 2010 Dec 1

[202] Turton EP, Kent PJ, Kester RC. The aetiology of Raynaud's phenomenon. Cardiovasc Surg. 1998;6:431-40.

[203] Czirjak L, Molnar I, Csipo I, Szabolcs M, Mihaly A, Szegedi G. Anti-platelet antibodies against gpIIb/IIIa in systemic sclerosis. Clin Exp Rheumatol. 1994;12:527-9.

[204] Weyrich AS, Lindemann S, Zimmerman GA. The evolving role of platelets in inflammation. J Thromb Haemost. 2003;1:1897-905.

[205] Dor Y, Djonov V, Abramovitch R, Itin A, Fishman GI, Carmeliet P, et al. Conditional switching of VEGF provides new insights into adult neovascularization and pro-angiogenic therapy. EMBO J. 2002;21:1939-47.

[206] Lee RJ, Springer ML, Blanco-Bose WE, Shaw R, Ursell PC, Blau HM. VEGF gene delivery to myocardium: deleterious effects of unregulated expression. Circulation. 2000;102:898-901.

[207] Springer ML, Chen AS, Kraft PE, Bednarski M, Blau HM. VEGF gene delivery to muscle: potential role for vasculogenesis in adults. Mol Cell. 1998;2:549-58.

[208] Distler JH, Strapatsas T, Huscher D, Dees C, Akhmetshina A, Kiener HP, et al. Dysbalance of angiogenic and angiostatic mediators in patients with mixed connective tissue disease. Ann Rheum Dis. 2011;70:1197-202.

[209] Trojanowska M. Cellular and molecular aspects of vascular dysfunction in systemic sclerosis. Nat Rev Rheumatol. 2010;6:453-60.

[210] Kissin EY, Merkel PA, Lafyatis R. Myofibroblasts and hyalinized collagen as markers of skin disease in systemic sclerosis. Arthritis Rheum. 2006;54:3655-60.

[211] Zaldivar MM, Pauels K, von Hundelshausen P, Berres ML, Schmitz P, Bornemann J, et al. CXC chemokine ligand 4 (Cxcl4) is a platelet-derived mediator of experimental liver fibrosis. Hepatology. 2010;51:1345-53.

[212] Dees C, Akhmetshina A, Zerr P, Reich N, Palumbo K, Horn A, et al. Platelet-derived serotonin links vascular disease and tissue fibrosis. J Exp Med. 2011;208:961-72.

[213] Artlett CM. Animal models of scleroderma: fresh insights. Curr Opin Rheumatol. 2010;22:677-82.

[214] Beyer C, Schett G, Distler O, Distler JH. Animal models of systemic sclerosis: prospects and limitations. Arthritis Rheum. 2010;62:2831-44.

3

Using Proteomic Analysis for Studying the Skin Fibroblast Protein Profile in Systemic Sclerosis

P. Coral-Alvarado[1], G. Quintana[1,2] et al.*
[1]*Rheumatology Section Fundacion Santa Fe de Bogota, Medicine School, Universidad de los Andes*
[2]*Rheumatology Unit, Medicine School Universidad Nacional de Colombia*
Colombia

1. Introduction

Increased efforts have been made during the last few decades to develop new technologies capable of identifying and quantifying the expression proteome in different cellular systems in physiological and physiopathological conditions for determining illness biomarkers, pharmaceutical targets and/or posttranslational modifications (PTM) by means of proteomic techniques. 2D gel electrophoresis, with immobilized pH gradients, associated with mass spectrometry, is one of the fundamentals steps in studying proteomics. The 2D technique can be used in studying the quantitative expression of protein profiles according to iso-electric point (Ip), molecular weight (Mr), protein solubility and the relative abundance of the above. This methodology provides a protein profile reflecting changes in protein expression levels, isoforms and PTM.

Proteins can be classified into those known by their structure and function, those recognized by determined domains and about which there is some knowledge, and those whose function is still not known. Proteomics is defined as the large-scale study of proteins expressed for a specific tissue from a genome, (global proteomics) or differentially expressed proteins (differential proteomics). Determining differentially expressed proteins, or proteins suffering a change in physiological circumstances, is the clue to understanding such pathology's cellular mechanisms. Although an expressed gene in specific tissues (as an answer to biologic alterations) could be analyzed by a mRNA expression study (transcriptomics), these results do not always coincide with the expected expression profiles since the number and activity of proteins associated with the same regulation in different stages could be modified. Genomic data integration is required, as well as transcritomics,

*C. Cardozo[3], J. Iriarte[2], Y. Sanchez[4], S. Bravo[5], J. Castano[6], M.F. Garces[7], L. Cepeda[7], A. Iglesias-Gamarra[2] and J.E. Caminos[7].
[1]*Rheumatology Section Fundacion Santa Fe de Bogota, Medicine School, Universidad de los Andes, Colombia*
[2]*Rheumatology Unit, Medicine School Universidad Nacional de Colombia, Colombia*
[3]*Biothechnology Department, Universidad Nacional de Colombia, Colombia*
[4] *Pathology Department, Universidad Nacional de Colombia, Colombia*
[5]*Phisiology Department, Universidad de Santiago de Compostela-Espana, Espana*
[6]*Cellular biology, physiology and immunology Department, Universidad de Cordoba-Espana, Espana*
[7]*Biochemistry Unit, Universidad Nacional de Colombia, Colombia*

proteomics, variome, peptidomics, and metabolome to understand physiological phenomenon in a comprehensive manner.

Systemic sclerosis (SSc) is a chronic illness of the connective tissue having unknown etiology; it has a variable course and severity and is characterized by intercellular matrix alterations and secondary fibrosis of enormous amounts of connective tissue. This results in hardening and thickening of the skin, alterations in the microvasculature and the large vessels, secondary to changes in the endothelial cells together with Raynaud's phenomenon, self-immunity alterations, and musculoskeletal and visceral degenerative fibrotic changes (1).

Despite recent advances having been made in understanding some molecular pathways involved in SSc, its etiopathogenesis remains unknown. Treatment for these patients has had very limited effectiveness, and the natural course of the illness inevitably leads to a fatal outcome. A better understanding of the illness' physiopathology is required to be able to orientate suitable therapeutic measures, carry out effective monitoring of its response, and determine severity criteria indicating a bad prognosis for the illness. This is where genomics, micro-array analysis and proteomics appear as valuable therapeutic and diagnosis tools.

Several groups have reported gene expression profiles for SSc-patient's tissues and cells (2-6).

Zhou found that fibroblasts in SSc patients showed different RNAm expression profiles for fibrilarine autoantigens, B centromere protein, P27 centromeric autoantigen , RNA polymerase I , DNA topoisomerase I, and PMScl (2). Luzina found high chemokine and cytokine levels in bronchoalveolar lavage (LAB) in SSc patients (3). Whitfield examined skin biopsies in four SSc patients, identifying 2,776 genes which expressed themselves in different ways to that of healthy controls (4).Tan (using a fibroblast culture) identified 62 genes which expressed themselves in different ways in SSc (5). Zhou reported fibroblast micro-array analysis results for fibroblasts from 18 sets of discordant twins in SSc (6,7).

Protein analysis using two-dimensional electrophoresis electrophoresis on polyacrylamide gel (2D PAG) will contribute to and extend the knowledge produced by analyzing gene expression, especially for proteins undergoing crucial PTM in their function.

Proteomic analysis involves many methodologies orientated towards identifying and characterizing altered proteins as a result of illness. Thousands of proteins are evaluated in just one trial in such studies, leading to detecting expression profiles as a consequence of abnormality in cell function or interaction. Traditional methods used in proteome analysis have included 2D PAG where proteins are first separated according to their electric charge and then by their mass in the second direction before being stained, thus allowing mixtures of 1,000 to 3,000 proteins to be visualized. The development of special software and the use of Internet have allowed multiple genes and databases to be compared. When being combined with mass spectrometry, a separation appears which allows efficient identification of proteins of interest, including many of their PTM. This analysis can be applied in comparative studies of expression profiles during different stages of the illness or healthy tissue compared to affected tissue, thus being able to identify the different modifications in the protein characteristics of clinical interest in different illnesses (8).

Clinical proteomics is aimed at identifying proteins involved in pathological processes, as well as evaluating changes in their expression during different stages of an illness.

Proteomics in clinical practice offers the technical skill for identifying biomarkers for diagnosis and therapeutic intervention. Potential biomarkers developed from proteomic analysis will have further specificity and sensitivity in clinical trials, since they measure protein alteration involved in an illness (9). A good understanding of data management, correlation, interpretation, and validation is crucial in obtaining precise results contributing towards understanding cellular alterations which could be involved in developing SSc.

Only two proteomic studies were found in the current literature. Rottoli has analyzed the type of immune response and protein composition in pulmonary fibrosis patients' LBA medium associated with SSc, sarcoidosis and idiopathic pulmonary fibrosis. Proteomic analysis revealed quantitative differences between the three illnesses, finding increased SSc in plasmatic proteins such as alpha1-beta glycoprotein, C3 complement, alpha 1-antitrypsin, beta- haptoglobin, and prothrombin (10,11). Czubaty has used a commercial cell line (HeLa S3) for proteomic analysis of Topoisomerase I protein patterns by comparing co-immunoprecipitation with mass spectrometry and identified 36 new proteins which were associated with Topoisomerase I and their possible interaction site in the RRM domain (12). However, these studies have been carried out in a not very specific medium, such as LBA.

A two-phase fibroblast proteomic study was thus proposed (pre-treatment and post-treatment) in fibroblasts, these being the cells initially involved in SSc physiopathology in one of its most important expressions: fibrosis. Fibrosis is one of the pathognomonic pathological findings for SSc, representing one of the most exemplary phenotypes.

Characteristically, there is uncontrollable collagen production and that of other extracellular matrix proteins due to resident fibroblasts in the skin, lungs and other vital organs leading to an excessive accumulation of connective tissue. As the illness progresses, this increased deposit of connective tissue alters the tissues' normal architecture, ending in a functional alteration of the latter and determining a very significant involvement in morbidity-mortality of patients suffering fibrosis-related SSc (13).

Protein expression pattern was observed when carrying out a proteomic analysis on SSc patients' fibroblasts during different stages of the illness and comparing them to healthy individuals' fibroblasts. Their appearance was analyzed and thus an increase, decrease, or absence of their profiles was determined, looking for an association of the proteins found with phases and serological and clinical characteristics. Proteins involved in the illness' etiopathology during its different stages were isolated as this could have therapeutic implications in an illness in which current treatment is very limited and not very efficient.

2. Materials and methods

2.1 Patients

This was a cases and controls study in which 11 patients who fulfilled with American College of Rheumatology SSc criteria were included during different phases of the illness (14,15) and subdivided into two groups: limited SSc and diffuse SSc, according to the parameters proposed by Le Roy (1). Table 1.

The cutaneous involvement of the skin was evaluated according to the modified Rodnan index (16) which ranges from 0 (normal) to 3 (severe), measured in 17 different body areas (maximum possible score is 51).

Clinical features	SSc Patients (n=11)
Age at onset/yrs	44.75 ±10
Female/male ratio	3:01
Disease duration yrs	9,65 ± 4
SSc subtype	
lSSc	7
dSSc	3
Morphea	1
Raynaud phenomenon %	90
Raynaud duration, yrs	9.1 ± 4
Rodnan Score	22.1 ± 9
Calcinosis %	45
Telangiectsias %	64
Renal Crisis %	0
Digital ulcers %	0
Gastrointestinal involvement %	20
Pulmonary involvement %	0
Antibodies Anticentromere %	60
Antibodies Anti SL-70 %	30
Antibodies Antinuclear %	90

Table 1. General characteristics of SSc patients

Patients had no treatment or had suspended 4 weeks before taking the biopsy (a treatment scheme was defined as involving any of the following medications, alone or combined: prednisone, D-penicillamine, colchicine, micophenolate mofetil, methotrexate, cyclophosphamide).
Healthy controls were individuals without an autoimmune illness or who had not undergone previous immunodepressor treatment.
Registration forms were completed; they then contained SSc patients' demographic data, clinical characteristics and antibody levels.
All individuals involved in the study signed the participation consent form according to established ethical norms.

2.2 Skin biopsy

Following the cutaneous biopsy technique's guidelines by means of punch (17), two skin biopsies were taken from each SSc patient: a skin sample with SSc involvement obtained from the body area having the maximum Rodan score and another clinically healthy skin sample having a zero Rodan score. The same technique was used for a skin biopsy of healthy individuals taken from a non-esthetic non-visible area. The material was prepared for cell culture.

2.3 Obtaining fibroblasts from skin biopsies from healthy controls and SSc patients

This stage of the study, as well as the rest of the procedures, had been previously agreed on by the interdisciplinary team for which the critical route in each process was determined. Clear coordination of activities was needed to guarantee that:

- The patients were appropriately and conveniently informed about the investigation and the lab procedures that would be carried out for analyzing samples;
- The biopsies would arrive at the lab immediately after samples had been taken to ensure rapid processing; and
- Serum taken from patients was convenient and suitable for lab procedures.
- According to previously-defined protocols, the sample should have arrived at the lab on the day the sample was taken as follows (18):
- Tubes marked with the names of the patients, indicating whether the fragment of skin had been taken from a clinically healthy area or from a clinically sick one; and
- Dry tubes to take the blood sample from the same patient.

The following procedures had been previously carried out in the lab:

- Preparation of the means of transport for the biopsy: A DMEM medium was used with a F-12 medium supplemented with an antibiotic solution (100ug/ml streptomycin, 0.25ug/ml B anphotericin) at 3% in sealed sterile glasses; and
- Preparation of the material and supplies for the culture: a culture medium was prepared to be supplemented with autologous human serum.

The skin biopsies immersed in the transport medium and the serums were transported at 4°C and taken to a lab specializing in human fibroblast cultures. Once in the lab, the samples were processed in the white zone, cell culture room, in the safety cabin following management protocols for these areas, according to the Lab Quality Manual.

- Each sample was washed three times with HANK´s saline solution supplemented at 3% with antibiotic and antimycotic solution (100mg/ml penicillin, 100ug/ml streptomycin, 0.25ug/ml B anphotericine);
- The samples were cut by a scalpel into small explants (half millimeter maximum size). The fragments so obtained were planted as explants in six-well culture plates;
- A total blood sample was taken from each patient in a dry tube to obtain serum by centrifuging at 2,500 rpm for 20 minutes at room temperature, with which the fibroblast culture medium would be autologously supplemented;
- 2ml DNEM culture medium with F-12 supplemented at 20% with autologous serum and 1% antimycotic antibiotic solution was added to each well; and
- Each sample was identified with a number for each patient, followed by whether the sample was healthy or unhealthy.

The cultures were monitored daily under an inverted microscope at 10X by 40X enlargement:

- Observations and photographs were registered;
- The culture medium was changed every third day; and
- The first cells began to be observed during the second week after culture.

Confluence was obtained around the fourth week.

Cell preparation for obtaining the proteins was carried out, following the following steps:

- Cells were previously washed with 1X PBS solution;
- Once the washing solution had been removed, 600 ul extraction protein buffer was added to each well as described in the protocol for 2D electrophoresis or Trizol study for obtaining NRA; and
- The fibroblasts were incubated for 10 minutes and then homogenized with the help of a rake. Cell separation was confirmed with an inverted microscope and each well's content was placed in a 1.5 ml Eppendorf tube and stored at -80°C until proteins were analyzed.

3. 2D electrophoresis for analyzing human fibroblast proteins in SSc patients and controls

14 fibroblast culture samples were studied by 2D-SD PAGE obtained from skin biopsies from three healthy controls and skin from a healthy and unhealthy region in 11 SSc patients. A recognition code was assigned. All individuals involved in the study signed the participation consent form, according to the ethical standards for such protocol.

The fibroblasts were lysed in a 600 ul protein extraction buffer made up of 7M thiourea, 2M ABS-14 detergent (1%), 40 mM Tris base and 0.001% bromophenol, all of which form part of BIO RAD protein extraction kit (cat. 163-2086). Anpholites (pH 3-10) were added at 200 mM final concentration before starting the lysis for reducing cysteine disulphide links.

The samples suspended in lysis buffer were initially sonified on ice to break up the genomic DNA cells and fragments (10%). The product was spun at 16,000 g for 20 minutes, separating proteins from the remains of cells and other macromolecules. These samples were stored at -80°C until subsequent analysis.

The Lowry method (RC DC, assay protein, Bio-Rad) was used for protein quantification; uni-dimensional electrophoresis was carried out by means of Laemmli's method to obtain an electrophoretic map and thus guarantee the integrity of proteins from fibroblast lysates. Once protein concentration and integrity had been verified, 2D PAG SDS electrophoresis trials were carried out. Electrophoresis was carried out on 10% and 12% acrylamide gels (30%/0.8v/v acrylamide/bisacrylamide), best results being obtained at 12%.

Isoelectrofocusing (IEF) followed BIO RAD's recommended method (cat.163-2105); 7 cm IPG strips, pH 3-10 and pH 4-7 ranks were selected. The latter were placed on trays to hold samples of interest suspended in rehydration buffer (125ul total volume); this buffer contained (m urea, 2% CHAPS, 50 Mm dithiethreitol (DTT), 3-10 anpholites (0.2%) and blue bromophenol traces. The fibroblast lysates were left (for one or two hours) and it was verified that the gel was totally covered by the previous solution, after which mineral oil was placed on the strip to avoid evaporation. The samples were covered and incubated for sixteen hours. Two functions were fulfilled in this step: the strips were hydrated and the samples were absorbed by the pH strip gel (which is why time taken and conditions for this procedure were so important).

Human fibroblast culture protein IEF was carried out on Protean IEF Cell equipment (BIO RAD), initially on a linear gradient until reaching 250V for 30 minutes, then at 4,000V for 2 hours on a linear gradient and finally on a fast ramp until the equipment reached 12,000V when the IEF finished. Small wicks of filter paper were placed before passing the strip from the hydration tray to the IEF equipment; they were moistened with ultrapure water and the strip was then placed. However, everything had to be covered with mineral oil so as to avoid evaporation before starting the process.

The 2D in which the proteins were separated according to weight was developed on 12% gels according to the preliminary analysis. Once the IEF was finished, the strips were separated from the electrode and placed in the equilibrium solution trays again, with 2% of equilibrium buffer I (6M urea, 2% SDS, 0.375M Tris-HCl (pH 8.8), 20% glycerol and 2% DTT). They were incubated for 10 minutes, the disulphur groups thus being reduced. The strips were then incubated for 10 minutes in equilibrium II buffer (6M urea, 2% SDS, 0.375M Tris-HCl (pH 8.8), 20% glycerol and 0.5g iodoacetamide). The sulphidryl groups were

removed to avoid reduction reversibility. This step was repeated, but this time the strips were placed in the 2D running buffer (tri/glycine/SDS at pH 8.8).
Meanwhile the 2D gel was placed in low fusion point agarose solution which was dissolved in SDS_PAGE running buffer. The proteins were separated in BIO RAD chambers, whether with Mini-Protean 3 cell (cat165-3301/02) or Mini-Protean Tetra cell (CAT 165-8000/01); the procedure began with a 40V voltage and was slowly increased to 60V voltage.
Once the proteins had been separated in 2D, they were silver stained according to manufacturer's recommendations (Invitrogen, Silver Express staining kit, cat.LC 61000).
The gels were documented with Quantity One 1-D Analysis Software and differential expression points were found with PDQuest 2-D Analysis Software.
The spots or differential expression points between controls and patients were analyzed with MALDI-TOF/TOF (4700 Proteomics Analyzer, Applied Biosystems). Four points were split and sent to the Córdoba University's central research support service (SCAI) proteomics unit in Spain.
It should be pointed out that the best results obtained in separating proteins from fibroblasts in patients and controls by means of 2D electrophoresis were on 4-7 pH strips and 12% gels. All 2D electrophoresis trials were carried out from the same human fibroblast culture lysate for both patients' samples and triplicate controls.

4. Statistical study

The results were presented descriptively with measurements, medians and interquartile ranges expressed according to expected variables. Association measurements having binominal categorical variables were presented in the analysis, depending on population distribution. A Wilcoxon or Mann-Whitney chi square test was used and association was measured by odds ratio (OR). Controls having similar conditions to the chosen patient cases regarding age and gender were sought to avoid differential expression which could have been explained by a physiological condition associated with these two variables and which could have increased or decreased potential associations.

5. Results

Proteins in cells from silver stained fibroblast cultures were observed in representative 2D SD-Page electrophoresis. The trials were carried out on 12% gel and IPG strips having pH4-7. Standardization studies were carried out on strips having pH 3-10 but most proteins were located in the pH 4-7 range where better resolution appeared. Each fibroblast sample was analyzed by 2D electrophoresis in triplicate.
2D electrophoresis images of human fibroblast proteins from controls and SSc patients were analyzed by PDQest software allowing the gels to be normalized. Proteins (spots) which were differentially expressed in controls and scleroderma patients (marked with arrows and numbers on each gel in Figure 1) were isolated, digested with trypsin and the peptides so produced were analyzed by mass spectrometry (peptide mass fingerprints) (MALDI-TOF). The analyzed spots from silver stained gels as well as isolated ones stained with Coomasie blue were mainly from different haptoglobin protein isoforms (Table 2), having greater than

SPOT	PROTEIN	SPECIE	WEIGHT MOLECULAR (KDA)	PROTEIN SCORE	**PROTEIN SCORE CI** %	NUMBER OF MATCHED PEPTIDES	ION SCORE TOTAL	ION SCORE CI %	ACCESSION NO.
1	haptoglobin precursor [Homo sapiens]	Homo sapiens	45859.8	91	99.997	8	44	99.611	gi|306882
1	haptoglobin, isoform CRA_a [Homo sapiens]	Homo sapiens	47377.6	90	99.997	8	44	99.611	gi|119579598
1	haptoglobin [Homo sapiens]	Homo sapiens	38722.4	88	99.995	8	44	99.611	gi|3337390
1	haptoglobin isoform 2 preproprotein [Homo sapiens]	Homo sapiens	38940.5	88	99.995	8	44	99.611	gi|186910296
1	haptoglobin, isoform CRA_d [Homo sapiens]	Homo sapiens	40457.3	87	99.993	8	44	99.611	gi|119579601
1	haptoglobin, isoform CRA_c [Homo sapiens]	Homo sapiens	40528.3	87	99.993	8	44	99.611	gi|119579600

<table>
<tr><th>SPOT</th><th>PROTEIN</th><th>SPECIE</th><th>WEIGHT MOLECULAR (KDA)</th><th>PROTEIN SCORE</th><th>PROTEIN SCORE CI %</th><th>NUMBER OF MATCHED PEPTIDES</th><th>ION SCORE TOTAL</th><th>ION SCORE CI %</th><th>ACCESSION NO.</th></tr>
<tr><td>2</td><td>haptoglobin precursor [Homo sapiens]</td><td>Homo sapiens</td><td>45859.8</td><td>159</td><td>100</td><td>8</td><td>109</td><td>100</td><td>gi|306882</td></tr>
<tr><td>2</td><td>haptoglobin, isoform CRA_a [Homo sapiens]</td><td>Homo sapiens</td><td>47377.6</td><td>158</td><td>100</td><td>8</td><td>109</td><td>100</td><td>gi|119579598</td></tr>
<tr><td>2</td><td>haptoglobin isoform 2 preproprotein [Homo sapiens]</td><td>Homo sapiens</td><td>38940.5</td><td>156</td><td>100</td><td>8</td><td>109</td><td>100</td><td>gi|186910296</td></tr>
<tr><td>2</td><td>haptoglobin, isoform CRA_c [Homo sapiens]</td><td>Homo sapiens</td><td>40528.3</td><td>155</td><td>100</td><td>8</td><td>109</td><td>100</td><td>gi|119579600</td></tr>
<tr><td>2</td><td>haptoglobin Hp2</td><td>Homo sapiens</td><td>42344.1</td><td>153</td><td>100</td><td>7</td><td>109</td><td>100</td><td>gi|223976</td></tr>
<tr><td>2</td><td>haptoglobin, isoform CRA_b [Homo sapiens]</td><td>Homo sapiens</td><td>51387.5</td><td>152</td><td>100</td><td>8</td><td>108</td><td>100</td><td>gi|119579599</td></tr>
<tr><td>3</td><td>haptoglobin precursor [Homo sapiens]</td><td>Homo sapiens</td><td>45859.8</td><td>116</td><td>100</td><td>9</td><td>61</td><td>99.988</td><td>gi|306882</td></tr>
</table>

SPOT	PROTEIN	SPECIE	WEIGHT MOLECULAR (KDA)	PROTEIN SCORE	**PROTEIN SCORE CI** %	NUMBER OF MATCHED PEPTIDES	ION SCORE TOTAL	ION SCORE CI %	ACCESSION NO.
3	haptoglobin, isoform CRA_a [Homo sapiens]	Homo sapiens	47377.6	115	100	9	61	99.988	gi|119579598
3	haptoglobin [Homo sapiens]	Homo sapiens	38722.4	114	100	9	61	99.988	gi|3337390
3	100 haptoglobin isoform 2 preproprotein [Homo sapiens]	Homo sapiens	38940.5	113	100	9	61	99.988	gi|186910296
3	haptoglobin, isoform CRA_c [Homo sapiens]	Homo sapiens	40528.3	112	100	9	61	99.988	gi|119579600
3	haptoglobin Hp2	Homo sapiens	42344.1	110	100	8	61	99.988	gi|223976
3	haptoglobin, isoform CRA_b [Homo sapiens]	Homo sapiens	51387.5	109	100	9	60	99.985	gi|119579599
3	HP protein [Homo sapiens]	Homo sapiens	38868.5	104	100	8	61	99.988	gi|78174390

SPOT	PROTEIN	SPECIE	WEIGHT MOLECULAR (KDA)	PROTEIN SCORE	PROTEIN SCORE CI %	NUMBER OF MATCHED PEPTIDES	ION SCORE TOTAL	ION SCORE CI %	ACCESSION NO.
4	haptoglobin [Homo sapiens]	Homo sapiens	38722.4	79	99.957	7	42	99.676	gi|3337390
4	haptoglobin [Homo sapiens]	Homo sapiens	38940.5	79	99.956	7	42	99.676	gi|1212947
4	haptoglobin, isoform CRA_c [Homo sapiens] 42	Homo sapiens	40528.3	78	99.943	7	42	99.676	gi|119579600
4	haptoglobin isoform 1 preproprotein [Homo sapiens]	Homo sapiens	45860.8	75	99.892	7	42	99.676	gi|4826762
4	haptoglobin, isoform CRA_a [Homo sapiens]	Homo sapiens	47377.6	74	99.867	7	42	99.676	gi|119579598

Table 2. Proteins identified by mass spectrometry (MALDI/TOF- TOF) which were separated by 2 D electrophoresis and obtained from cultures of human fibroblasts from SSc patients and healthy subjects. The proteins corresponding to isolated spots in Figure 1, which differ in expression profile between controls subjects and patients.

99% protein score confidence interval (the search will be more credible the nearer this is to 100 but confirmation must be above 99%). The protein score is a score given by a search engine (MASCOT) to each identified peptide, according to the probabilistic system based on peptide mass distribution, depending on the mass of the protein to which they belong (Mowse System). These were identified by comparing the MALDI-TOF peptide map to the theoretic value calculated for peptides from all SWISS-PROT database proteins and the TrEMBLE database for human sequences and by applying Mascot software. Proteins corresponding to spots identified by MALDI-TOF (Table 2) were correlated with their molecular weights and isoelectric points when located on the 2D gels (Figure 1 and 2)

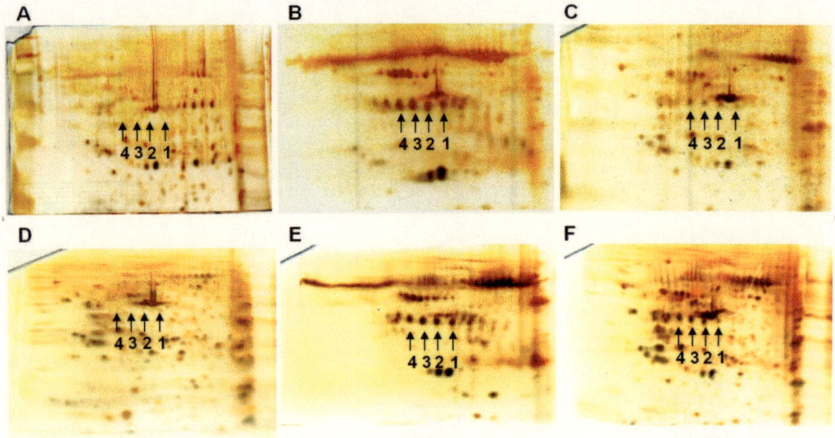

Fig. 1. Representative electrophoresis of proteins obtained from isolated lysates human fibroblasts cultures from skin biopsies of healthy and Scleroderma patients using 2D SDS - PAGE (12%). Healthy controls (A, D) SSc patient F11, healthy skin (B) and diseased skin (C) SSc patient F7, healthy skin (E) and sick skin (F). IPGs strips were used (pH 4-) and staining of the gels were developed with silver reagent.

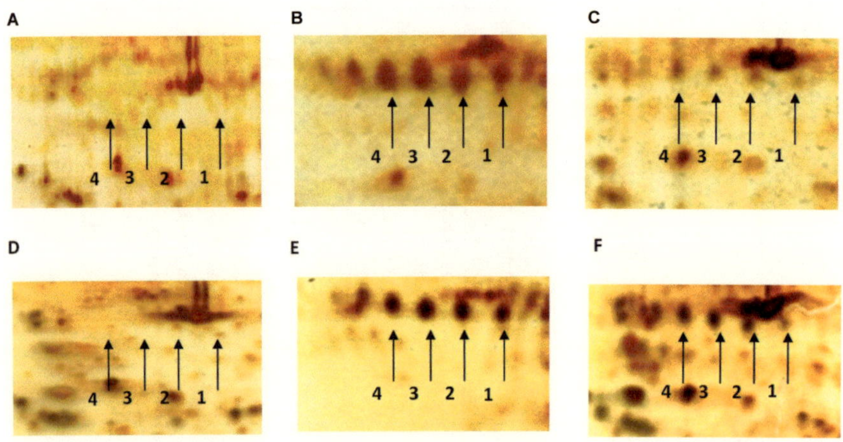

Fig. 2. Amplified region noted in Figure 1. 2D electrophoresis of human fibroblast proteins corresponding to differentially expressed spots were identified by MALDI-TOF/TOF (4700 Proteomics Analyzer, Applied Biosystems). Healthy controls (A, D) SSc patient F11, healthy region (B) and diseased region (C) SSc patient F7, healthy region (E) and sick region (F).

#	Age	Disease	Raynaud	Raynaud	Antibodies	Pattern	Levels	Rodnan	Microstomy	Calcinosis	clerodactili	erpigmenta	opopigmenta	elangiectasia	Finger edema	PSAP	Diagnosis	Spots	Spots
Patient	at onset, yrs	Duration, yrs		Duration, yrs	Antinuclears			Score										Health skin	sick skin
1	29	7	Absent	0	Negative	Negativo	0	0	Absent	Absent	Absent	Absent	Absent	Absent	Absent	25	Morphea	**	***
2	42	3	Present	6	Positive	Centromere	40	16	Present	Absent	Present	Present	Present	Present	Present	30	lSSc	****	***
3	27	1	Present	8	Positive	Centromere	1260	26	Present	Absent	Present	Present	Present	Present	Present	35	dSSc	0	*
4	48	7	Present	10	Positive	Centromere	1260	18	Present	Present	Present	Present	Present	Present	Absent	34	lSSc	*	**
5	39	9	Present	5	Positive	Centromero	1260	12	Present	Present	Present	Absent	Absent	Present	Present	28	lSSc	0	0
6	50	10	Present	12	Positive	Homogeneus	1260	9	Present	Absent	Absent	Absent	Absent	Absent	Present	30	lSSc	*	**
7	49	9	Present	8	Positive	Nucleolar	640	12	Absent	Absent	Absent	Absent	Absent	Absent	Present	26	lSSc	*	**
8	41	4	Present	18	Positive	Nucleolar	40	8	Absent	Absent	Absent	Present	Absent	Absent	Present	30	lSSc	0	0
9	45	3	Present	3	Positive	Nucleolar	1260	20	Present	Present	Present	Present	Present	Present	Present	38	lSSc	****	***
10	20	20	Present	20	Positive	Centromere	1240	23	Present	Present	Present	Present	Present	Present	Present	45	dSSc	0	0
11	48	14	Present	15	Positive	Centromere	160	23	Present	Present	Present	Absent	Absent	Present	Present	25	dSSc	**	*

Table 3. Main clinical and serological variables and intensity of expression of the spots in Colombian patients suffering SSc

presenting approximately identical molecular weight but having a different isoelectric point, thus reflecting different protein processing mechanisms as previously described in scleroderma patients. Table 2 shows the identity of haptoglobin isoforms in scleroderma-derived human fibroblasts in scleroderma patients.
It was determined whether there were any associations between the clinical and serologic variables and the intensity of the spots' expression. Gender, initiation age, Raynaud's disease duration, pulmonary hypertension, antinuclear antibodies' pattern and dilution, modified Rodnan index, microstomy, calcinoses, telangiectasia and classification of the illness were then categorically and quantitatively evaluated with dominant spots' expression intensity, without finding any type of association (Table 3 and 4).

Characteristic	Health Skin	Sick Skin
Microstomy	0,72	0,821
Antibodies antinuclear	0,465	0,602
Calcinosis	0,97	0,821
Sclerodactilia	0,43	0,502
Hyperpigmentation	0,152	0,821
Hypopigmentation	0,233	0,821
Telangiectasia	0,437	0,502
SSc Subtype	0,151	0,119
PAH	0,181	0,978

Table 4. Association between clinical characteristics and expression of the spots. Measured by the intensity of protein electrophoresis. Determined by Chi square - p value

6. Discussion

Despite recent advances in understanding some molecular paths involved in SSc, its etiopathogenesis still remains unknown. Treating these patients has very limited effectiveness and the disease's natural course inevitably leads to a fatal outcome. A better understanding of its physiopathology is required to orientate suitable therapeutic treatment for efficiently monitoring its response and determining severity criteria indicating a poor prognosis for the illness. Genomics, micro-array analysis and proteomics thus appear as valuable diagnostic and therapeutic tools.
Proteomic analysis uses many methodologies orientated towards identifying and characterizing altered proteins as a result of illness. Millions of proteins are evaluated in one trial in these studies, leading to the detection of expression profiles as a consequence of abnormal function or cell interaction. The traditionally-used methods in proteomic analysis include 2D electrophoresis on polyacrylamide gel where proteins are separated first depending on their electric charge and then by their mass in the second direction and finally stained, visualizing 1,000 to 3,000 proteins. Special software having been developed and the use of internet have led to many genes and databases being compared. Separation is achieved when combined with mass spectrometry leading to the efficient identification of proteins of interest, including many of their PTMs. Such analysis can be applied to comparative expression profile studies during different stages of the illness or comparing

healthy tissues to unhealthy tissues, thereby identifying modifications in the characteristics of t proteins of clinical interest in different illnesses.

Haptoglobin was identified in the current study after proteomic analysis in fibroblasts from SSc patients during different stages of the illness as being a protein which expressed itself in a different but constant way in all SSc patients by contrast with healthy individuals.

Haptoglobin is an acute phase protein, indicative of different pathological conditions such as forms of cancer, hepatic cirrhosis and hepatitis C. This protein appears with around 6 phenotypes, besides combinations in PTM, such as glycolization and deamination, thus increasing the number of presentation forms (19).

Recent studies have demonstrated that idiopathic pulmonary fibrosis is caused by alteration of protein expression involved in different processes such as matrix remodeling, inflammation and tissue damage and repair. Similar studies to the current study (carried out in LBA in pulmonary fibrosis by proteomics) have demonstrated that this protein's expression significantly increased (20). However, the advantage of this study was the identification of this protein in a fibroblast culture, cells directly involved in the illness's physiopathology and whose increase did not correlate to the illness' severity but to its presence, thereby assuming that high haptoglobin values can predict SSc development.

Once haptoglobin has been identified as a protein present in untreated SSc patients, proteomic studies must be carried out to analyze this protein's behavior when influenced by different therapeutic schemes. Such study is currently taking place.

7. Conclusion

Identifying haptoglobin in a fibroblast culture in untreated SSc patients did not correlate with the severity of the illness but with its presence. It could thus become a predictive tool for SSc development. However, it is worth studying its behavior in the same patients using different therapeutic schemes and prospective studies are needed including a bigger population to verify these observations.

8. References

[1] LeRoy EC, Black C, Fleischmajer R, Jablonska S, Krieg T, Medsger TA, Jr., et al. Scleroderma (systemic sclerosis): classification, subsets and pathogenesis. J Rheumatol. 1988;15:202-5.

[2] Zhou X, Tan FK, Xiong M. Systemic sclerosis (scleroderma): specific autoantigen genes are selectively overexpressed in scleroderma fibroblasts. J Immunol 2001, 167:7126–33.

[3] Luzina IG, Atamas SP, Wise R. Gene expression in bronchoalveolar lavage cells from scleroderma patients. Am J Respir Cell Mol Biol 2002, 26:549–57.

[4] Whitfield ML, Finlay DR, Murray JI. Systemic and cell type-specific gene expression patterns in scleroderma skin. Proc Natl Acad Sci U S A 2003; 100:12319–24.

[5] Tan F, Hildebrand B, Lester M. Classification analysis of the transcriptosome of dermal fibroblasts from systemic sclerosis (SSc) patients. Arthritis Rheum 2004;50:S621.

[6] Zhou X, Arnett FC, Xiong M, Feghali-Bostwick CA. Gene expression profiling of dermal fibroblasts from twins discordant for systemic sclerosis. Arthritis Rheum 2004;50:S629.

[7] Feghali-Bostwick C. Genetics and Proteomics in Scleroderma. Curr Rheumatol Rep 2005;7:129-34.

[8] Kalbas M, Lueking A, Kowald A, Muellner S. New analytical tools for Studying Autoimmune Diseases. Current Pharmaceutical Design, 2006; 12:3735-42.

[9] Dominguez D, Lopes R, Torres L. Proteomics: Clinical Applications. Clin Lab Sci 2007;20:245-48.

[10] Rottoli P, Magi B, Perari M, Liberatori S, Nikiforakis N, Bargagli E, Cianti R, Bini L, Pallini V. Cytokine profile and proteome analysis in bronchoalveolar lavage of patients with sarcoidosis, pulmonary fibrosis associated with systemic sclerosis and idiopathic pulmonary fibrosis. Proteomics 2005, 5, 1423–30.

[11] Rottoli P, Magi B, Cianti R, Bargagli E,Vagaggini C, Nikiforakis N, Pallini V and Bini L.Carbonylated proteins in bronchoalveolar lavage of patients with sarcoidosis, pulmonary fibrosis associated with systemic sclerosis and idiopathic pulmonary fibrosis. Proteomics 2005, 5, 2612–18.

[12] Czubaty A, Girstun A, Kowalska-Loth B, Trzcinska A, Purta E, Winczura A, Grajkowski W, Staron K. Proteomic analysis of complexes formed by human topoisomerase I. Biochimica et Biophysica Acta 2005; 1749: 133–41.

[13] Varga J, Trojanowska M. Fibrosis in Systemic Sclerosis. Rheum Dis Clin N Am 2008; 34:115–43.

[14] Preliminary criteria for the classification of systemic sclerosis (scleroderma). Subcommittee for scleroderma criteria of the American Rheumatism Association Diagnostic and Therapeutic Criteria Committee. Arthritis and rheumatism. 1980 May;23:581-90.

[15] Medsger T. Natural history of systemic sclerosis and the assessment of disease activity, severity, functional status, and psychologic well-being. Rheum Dis Clin N Am 2003; 29: 255–73.

[16] Furst DE, Clements PJ, Steen VD, Medsger TA Jr, Masi AT, D'Angelo WA. The modified Rodnan skin score is an accurate reflection of skin biopsy thickness in systemic sclerosis. J Rheumatol 1998;25:84–8.

[17] Keyes EL. The cutaneous punch. J Cutan Genito-Urin Dis 1989; 195: 98–101.

[18] Arvelo F, Perez P y Cotte C. Obtención De Laminas De Piel Humana Mediante Ingenieria De Tejidos. ACV. 2004: 55:74-82.

[19] Shah A, Singh H, Sachdev V, Lee J, Yotsukura S, Salgia R, Bharti A. Differential Serum Level Of Specific Haptoglobin Isoforms In Small Cell Lung Cancer. Curr Proteomics. 2010 Apr 1;7(1):49-65.

[20] Kim TH, Lee YH, Kim KH, Lee SH, Cha JY, Shin EK, Jung S, Jang AS, Park SW, Uh ST, Kim YH, Park JS, Sin HG, Youm W, Koh ES, Cho SY, Paik YK, Rhim TY, Park CS. Role of Lung Apolipoprotein A1 in Idiopathic Pulmonary Fibrosis: Anti-inflammatory and Anti-fibrotic Effect on Experimental Lung Injury/Fibrosis. Am J Respir Crit Care Med. 2010; 182(5): 633-642.

4

Apoptosis of T Lymphocytes in Systemic Sclerosis

M. Szymanek, G. Chodorowska, A. Pietrzak and D. Krasowska
Department of Dermatology, Venereology and Paediatric Dermatology, Medical University of Lublin, Lublin, Poland

1. Introduction

Systemic sclerosis (SSc) is a systemic, autoimmune, chronic inflammatory disease affecting the connective tissue. SSc is mainly characterised by progressive fibrosis of the skin, subcutaneous tissue and internal organs, leading to their failure (1). In the majority of cases, lesions involve the osteoarticular, gastrointestinal or cardiovascular system, lungs, kidneys, and nervous system (2-4). The disease occurs in all ethnic groups and mainly affects women; its peak incidence is observed in the 5th and 6th decade of life. Occasionally, lesions develop in childhood (about 3% of cases) (5).

The aetiology and pathogenesis of SSc have not been fully elucidated. The immune system activation appears to be essential for the development of disease (6-8). By releasing cytokines and growth factors, the immune response markedly affects the growth and differentiation of fibroblasts as well as synthesis of collagen (9). The study findings demonstrate that the extent of lymphocytic infiltrates in the affected skin of SSc patients correlates with the severity and degree of skin hardening (10). In the early stages of SSc, inflammatory infiltrates in the skin composed of T lymphocytes, macrophages, mast cells, eosinophils, basophils, and, although less frequently, of B lymphocytes, precede the histological features of fibrosis (7,11). With the progression of fibrosis, inflammatory infiltrates tend to regress (12).

2. The role of T lymphocytes in SSc

T lymphocytes are essential for the pathogenesis of immunological abnormalities in systemic sclerosis. CD4+ T lymphocytes and macrophages are most abundant in the skin whereas CD8+ T lymphocytes are abundant in the lungs (13). The total number of lymphocytes in the peripheral blood is normal or slightly decreased; however, the ratio of circulating CD4/CD8 lymphocytes and the percentage of CD4+25+ T cells are increased while the number of CD8+ T lymphocytes is reduced. Additionally, increased concentration of the soluble CD8 molecule (sCD8) in peripheral blood is suggestive of enhanced activation of lymphocytes in systemic sclerosis (14-16). In the inflammatory stage of SSc, the activated T lymphocytes induce fibrotic processes through the production of cytokines or through direct contact with fibroblasts. The mediators secreted by Th1 lymphocytes (IL-2, IL-12, IL-18, IFN-γ), Th2 lymphocytes (IL-4, IL-5, IL-6, IL-10, IL-13, IL-17) and macrophages are of particular importance (17-19). Serum levels of IL-4, IL-10, IL-13, IL-17 secreted by Th2 lymphocytes are elevated. IL-4 appears to be essential for fibrosis. It increases the synthesis of collagen in fibroblasts and induces the production of TGF-β, which stimulates the synthesis of various types of collagen, proteoglycans and fibronectin, and inhibits their synthesis by increasing the production of a tissue inhibitor of matrix metalloproteinases. Moreover, a negative correlation between the serum concentration of IL-10, severity of skin lesions and duration of vasomotor disorders has been demonstrated (20). Through the inhibition of IFN-γ and TNF activities, IL-10 is most likely to stimulate indirectly the processes of tissue fibrosis (16), because both IFN-γ and TNF are important SSc mediators. IFN-γ is secreted by Th1 lymphocytes and, to a lesser degree, by NK cells, CD8 lymphocytes, macrophages and dendritic cells. IFN-γ is one of the key inhibitors of collagen synthesis. It decreases the levels of procollagen I, II and III, inhibits proliferation of fibroblasts and stimulating effects of TGF-β. Its involvement in the pathogenesis of systemic sclerosis is supported by significantly lower levels of this cytokine in serum of patients compared to controls (19). TNF, on the other hand, affects directly and indirectly the growth of fibroblasts, synthesis of collagen and activation of the endothelial cells. Increased concentrations of the soluble CD30 molecule (sCD30), belonging to the TNF receptor family, are suggestive of activation of Th2 cells and are directly proportionally correlated with the severity of skin lesions (16).

The involvement of T lymphocytes in the pathogenesis of systemic sclerosis is also confirmed by changes in concentration of these mediators secreted by immune response cells. Increased levels of IL-2 were found in serum of SSc patients, which correlated with the extent of skin involvement and progression of the disease, as IL-2, a pro-inflammatory cytokine, stimulates monocytes and macrophages to increased synthesis of TGF-β, which in turn stimulates fibroblasts to secrete the extracellular matrix (3,20). Furthermore, elevated levels of a soluble IL-2 receptor (sIL2R) were observed; the relation between the duration of Raynaud`s phenomenon and sIL2R concentrations in patients with lSSc was found to be inversely proportional whereas in dSSc patients directly proportional (10). Elevated levels of IL-1, IL-6, IL-13 and the connective tissue growth factor (CTGF) were detected in serum and tissues of SSc patients. IL-17 was found to be overexpressed in the peripheral blood and skin of SSc patients. IL-17 is synthesized by Th1 and Th2 lymphocytes. It induces the endothelial cells to produce IL-1, IL-6 and stimulates the expression of adhesive molecules ICAM-1 and VCAM-1 (12,21). Moreover, it stimulates proliferation of fibroblasts and activates macrophages to produce TNF and IL-1, which in turn induces fibroblasts to produce collagen, IL-6 and the platelet-derived growth factor (PDGF) (7).

Since cytokines are essential for the activation of mediators and humoral immune response, their impaired production by Th1 and Th2 lymphocytes may be the key factor for the development of systemic sclerosis. Noteworthy, cytokines secreted by Th2 cells stimulate whereas those secreted by Th1 cells inhibit the synthesis of collagen. However, some studies demonstrate the inhibiting effects of Th2 cells on synthesis of type I collagen (14).

Furthermore, the most recent reports indicate significant involvement of B lymphocytes in the pathogenesis of systemic sclerosis (18). The activation of B lymphocytes in SSc is manifested by hypergammaglobulinaemia, presence of autoantibodies, stimulation of polyclonal B cells and overexpression of CD 19 molecules on naive and memory B lymphocytes (22,23). Noteworthy, homeostasis of the peripheral B lymphocyte subpopulation is impaired in systemic sclerosis. Increased activity of naive B lymphocytes and decreased numbers of memory cells as well as plasmoblasts are observed. Despite their reduced numbers, memory lymphocytes are activated continuously, which is most likely associated with CD 19 overexpression (13). Overexpression of CD 19 appears to be specific for systemic sclerosis (24). It has not been demonstrated in other autoimmune diseases, such as systemic lupus erythematosus or dermatomyositis (18). The detection of autoantibodies in over 90% of SSc patients is a relevant diagnostic and prognostic marker of internal organ involvement and severity of disease (25). In systemic sclerosis, antinuclear antibodies react mainly with the nucleolar antigens and are directed against one antigen (26). A close genetic relationship of autoantibodies with the HLA system suggests the involvement of immunogenetic mechanisms in the development of SSc (1). T lymphocytes have been shown to affect the synthesis of anti-DNA topoisomerase antibodies, other autoantibodies and accumulation of B lymphocytes in skin lesions. This confirms the hypothesis that interactions between T and B lymphocytes are likely to play a significant role in the pathogenesis of systemic sclerosis (7,27).

The cause of lymphocyte activation in systemic sclerosis is not known. Genetic predisposition (haplotypes DR3, DR5, DRw52) and environmental factors are considered (28). Moreover, microchimerism, exposure to organic solvents and toxins (toluene, benzene, xylene, aliphatic hydrocarbons, epoxy resins), infective factors, particularly human cytomegalovirus, some drugs, including bleomycin, vitamin K, penicillamine, beta-blockers, pentazocine, and genetically-determined individual susceptibility to oxidative stress, combined with secretion of free radicals, are also implicated (1,29-32). Recent studies stress the role of impaired or deregulated apoptosis in the pathogenesis of SSc immune changes regarding compromised ability to eliminate autoreactive T or B lymphocytes (2,13,33).

According to the recent findings, the abnormal ratio of CD4/CD8 lymphocytes, associated with excessive loss of CD8+ T lymphocytes, may result not only from the activity of lymphocytotoxic antibodies and anti-lymphocyte antibodies blocking determinants but also from enhanced apoptosis of CD8+ T cells (34). Noteworthy, inhibition of apoptosis in systemic sclerosis leads to excessive activation of T and B lymphocytes, contributing to overproduction of antibodies (35).

The objective of the present review is to discuss the selected parameters of T lymphocyte apoptosis in patients with systemic sclerosis.

3. Apoptosis – genetically programmed cell death

Apoptosis (from Greek - "dropping off" of leaves) is an active, programmed process of morphological and biochemical changes determined by the expression of appropriate genes leading to cell death. It enables the elimination of cells without inducing inflammation and damage to the surrounding tissues (36). Apoptosis always involves single cells although their overall number may be high. As a genetically programmed cell death, apoptosis plays a key role in maintaining proliferation and homeostasis of multicellular organisms. It counteracts excessive proliferation and ensures the choice of cells with an optimal set of receptors in the immune system. Moreover, it conditions the precise control of the number and type of cells during ontogenesis and organogenesis, and eliminates excessively produced embryonic and damaged cells, whose survival would not be beneficial for the organism (37-39). The process of apoptosis was discovered by Alastair Currie, John Kerr and Andrew Wyllie in 1972 (40). Morphologically, apoptosis is characterized by shrinkage of the cytoplasm, condensation of the cell nucleus followed by its fragmentation (41); due to such changes, the microvilli are lost and apoptotic bodies formed, composed of morphologically intact nuclear fragments or other cell organelles. Finally, the apoptotic bodies are phagocytised by the adjacent scavenger cells (Fig.1) (42). The biochemical changes observed during apoptosis involve a decrease in mitochondrial potential, release of cytochrome c from mitochondria, an increase in intracellular concentration of calcium ions, formation of free radicals, activation of caspases, loss of asymmetric distribution of phospholipids in the cell membrane and enzymatic degradation of DNA. Due to gradual suppression of metabolic activity and increased permeability of the cell membrane, the cell, whose nucleus shows apoptotic changes, dies within several hours (43). Normal apoptosis neither impairs the tissue structure and function nor generates the immune response (44).

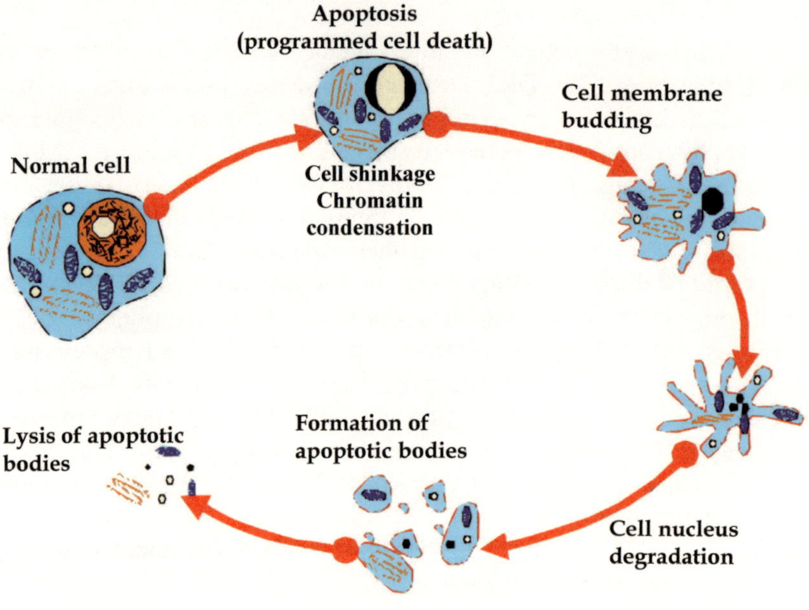

Fig. 1. Morphological cell changes during apoptosis (42)

There are several stages of programmed cell death: initiation, effector, and destruction (45). The initiation stage involves cell damage in response to a death signal, which leads to critical DNA damage, metabolic stress or activation of programmed cell death receptors. A relevant element of initiation is protein p53, which decides whether the signal received is strong enough to initiate apoptosis or if there is still a possibility to inhibit the cell cycle at phase G1 and activate the repair mechanisms. When the signal is strong enough, the cell enters the effector stage, which determines the irreversibility of changes. At this stage, however, internal regulation (e.g. mediated by Bcl proteins) is possible. The activation of caspase cascade initiates the destruction stage - irreversible structural and functional changes leading to cell death. The remaining parts of a damaged cell are phagocytised, most commonly by tissue macrophages (44,46).

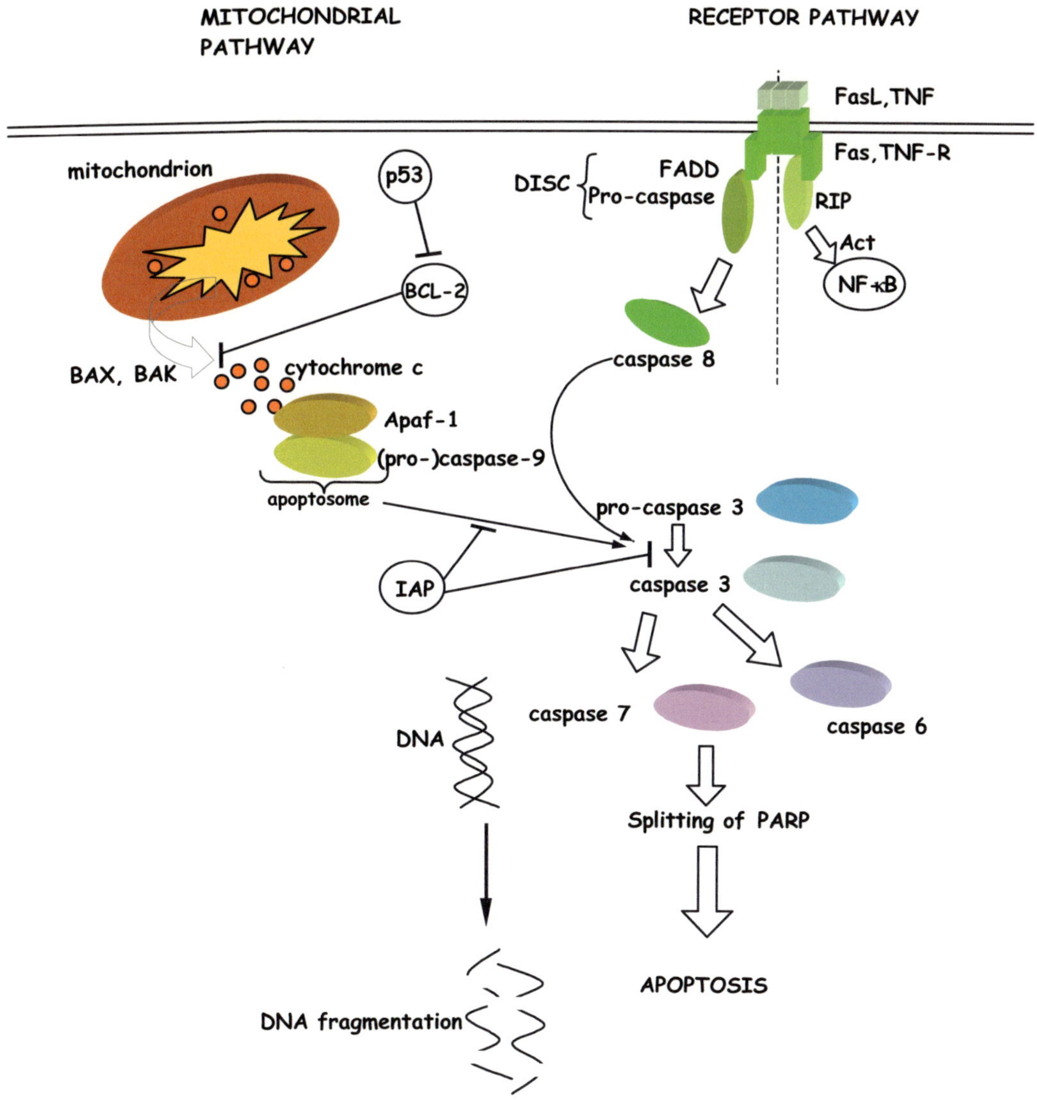

Fig. 2. Pathways of apoptosis induction (based on literature data)

Apoptosis may be induced by direct DNA damage caused by intrinsic (e.g. cytokines) or extrinsic factors (e.g. hyperthermia, ionizing radiation). The physiological activators of apoptosis are considered to be the tumour necrosis factor (TNF), transforming growth factor β (TGF-β), some neurotransmitters (e.g. dopamine), calcium, glucocorticosteroids, NK cells or cytotoxic T lymphocytes. Moreover, apoptosis is induced by loss of cell-extracellular matrix contact. The pathological factors inducing apoptosis include some bacterial toxins, free radicals, metabolites and some viruses. Apoptosis can also be triggered by physical factors, e.g. ultraviolet radiation, gamma radiation, thermal shock or hypoxia (43,47,48). The pharmacological inducers of apoptosis include chemotherapeutics such as cisplatin, doxorubicin, bleomycin, cytosine arabinoside, methotrexate, vincristine, inhibitors of DNA

topoisomerase I (from the camptothecin family) and inhibitors of DNA topoisomerase II (etoposide, teniposide) (49).
Apoptosis can be induced via the intrinsic (mitochondrial) or extrinsic (receptor) pathway. The dominating mitochondrial pathway is connected with caspase cascade activation. The permeability of the outer mitochondrial membrane is increased resulting in translocation of proteins from the perimitochondrial space to the cytoplasm. The mitochondria release the programmed cell death-inducing factors: cytochrome c, apoptosis-inducing factor (AIF), the second mitochondria-derived activator of caspase/direct inhibitor of apoptosis-binding protein with low pi (Smac/Diablo), Omi/HtrA2 serine protease (high temperature requirement) and endonuclease G. This results in decreased mitochondrial potential – the marker of early apoptosis, autocatalytic activation of pro-caspase 9 and effector caspases, which induces proteolysis of various nuclear and cytoplasmic proteins (44,50,51). The extrinsic (receptor) pathway induces apoptosis through binding of a specific ligand by the receptor on the cell surface. The receptors in question are the TNF receptors (TNF-R, Fas), binding TNF and FasL, respectively. The ligands are protein death signals sent by other cells. The activated ligand-bound receptor binds adaptor proteins, which results in autocatalytic activation of pro-caspase 8 and other effector caspases, ultimately leading to cell death (Fig.2) (44,52).

4. The role of Bcl in SSc apoptosis

The best-known products of cellular oncogenes regulating apoptosis are Bcl proteins. The family includes both proteins inhibiting (Bcl-2, Bcl-X_L, Bcl-w, Mcl-1, BAG-1) and initiating (Bax, Bcl-x_s, Bak, Bik, Bad, Bid, Bim, NOXA) apoptosis (40). The basic functional elements of Bcl proteins are p26, responsible for binding the protein with intracellular membranes, and at least one of the four Bcl-2 homology domains (BH 1-4). The BH1 subunit determines the regulation of apoptosis, BH2 is responsible for formation of homo- or heterodimers with other Bcl proteins, BH3 occurs also in other proteins regulating the process of programmed cell death whereas BH4 enables the anti-apoptotic action (53,54). According to the function and structure of Bcl-2 constituents, the proteins can be divided into three groups: 1- proteins with all four domains and anti-apoptotic effects (e.g. Bcl-2, Bcl-X_l); 2 – pro-apoptotic proteins (e.g. Bax, Bak), deprived of the BH4 domain (except for Bcl- x_s); and 3 - pro-apoptotic proteins containing only the BH3 domain (e.g. Bim, Bid, Bik, Bad) (46,55).
B cell lymphoma/leukaemia 2 (Bcl-2) is the product of bcl-2 gene localized on chromosome 18. It is detected in the inner mitochondrial membrane, endoplasmic reticulum and nuclear membrane, albeit in smaller amounts. Bcl-2 shows the anti-apoptotic action; therefore, under physiological conditions, its expression is observed in the cells of all three embryonic germ layers, non-renewable cells (e.g. neurons) and epithelial basilar cells (56,57). Bcl-2 acts anti-apoptotically thanks to formation of heterodimers with the molecules enhancing apoptosis (Bax) (46). In addition to blocking pro-apoptotic proteins, Bcl-2 stabilizes the cell membranes contributing to increased membranous potential, increased adenosine triphosphate (ATP) synthesis and inhibition of calcium ion escape. Moreover, it activates the regulatory proteins of G1 phase (including p53) (58).
In systemic sclerosis, the effects of Bcl-2 on T lymphocytes are regulated by various cytokines, such as IL-2, IL-4, IL-7, IL-13, and IL-15 (59). The study conducted by Stummvoll

et al. in 39 SSc patients, demonstrated significantly higher expression of Bcl-2 in CD4+ lymphocytes compared to the control group of 47 healthy individuals. There were, however, no significant differences in the expression of Bcl-2 in CD8+ lymphocytes, which suggests that increased expression of Bcl-2 exerts protective effects on CD4+ lymphocytes, hence promotes increased loss of CD8+ lymphocytes and increased ratio of CD4+/CD8+ (in favour of CD4+) (60). Kessel et al., who studied 27 SSc patients, did not find significant differences in Bcl-2 expression in CD8+ lymphocytes compared to the control group (28 healthy individuals), which strongly suggests that anti-apoptotic effects of Bcl-2 do not involve CD8+ lymphocytes (61). Furthermore, Czuwara et al. observed increased apoptosis and impaired expression of Bcl-2 in mononuclear cells of peripheral blood in SSc patients as well as reduced response to camptothecin. They demonstrated that camptothecin, an inhibitor of topoisomerase I, stimulated the process of programmed cell death resulting in decreased expression of Bcl-2. In mononuclear cells of peripheral blood of SSc patients, this effect was markedly lesser compared to the control group of healthy individuals (62).

Bcl-2 is an anti-apoptotic protein, which prevents programmed cell death both via the intrinsic pathway, inhibiting the release of pro-apoptotic particles from the mitochondria and via the receptor pathway, inducing the anti-apoptotic action of NF-κB (45,63).

Extremely enhanced spontaneous expression of Bcl-2 in peripheral mononuclear cells and its high increase mediated by camptothecin and IL-2 were demonstrated in a female patient with systemic sclerosis and breast cancer. Increased expression of Bcl-2 was likely to be caused by the coexistence of two diseases. The authors suggest that further studies involving a larger population of patients are required to interpret explicitly the pathogenetic and diagnostic role of Bcl-2 (62).

The findings reported by Stummvoll et al., who studied 17 patients with diffuse and 22 patients with limited SSc, did not reveal significant differences in Bcl-2 expression in CD4+ and CD8+ lymphocytes. The authors suggest that expression of Bcl-2, as a marker of apoptosis, may not be dependent on the clinical form of systemic sclerosis (60). Similar results were presented by Cipriani et al. in 17 patients with dSSc and 5 with lSSc, which is likely to indicate that Bcl-2-mediated apoptosis is not dependent on the clinical form of SSc (59). Moreover, there were no significant relations between the expression Bcl-2 in peripheral blood lymphocytes in SSc patients and the duration of disease, its activity, degree and extent of skin lesions, duration of sclerotic microangiopathy, organ changes, antinuclear antibodies or treatment applied (59,60).

The Bcl-2 – Bax ratio is thought to be essential for apoptosis - due to antagonistic effects of these proteins, the ratio decides about cell survival or otherwise (64).

The Bcl-2-associated X protein (Bax) is one of the best-known proteins of the Bcl family. It has an important function in pro-apoptotic regulation of programmed cell death via the mitochondrial pathway. In its inactive form, it is localized in the cytoplasm. Having stimulated the cell to apoptotic death, Bcl-2 translocates to the outer mitochondrial membrane, where it is oligomerised (63). The functional molecule is the 21 kDa protein of the structure similar to Bcl-2. The action of p53 results in increased amounts of Bax and decreased amounts of Bcl-2, which leads to their imbalance and formation of Bax-Bax homodimers. This results in formation of the mitochondrial membranous channel, release of cytochrome c to the cytoplasm, activation of caspases and disintegration of cell structures (40,46). Moreover, Bax accelerates the transition of the cell into the phase of genetic material replication, which suggests its relevant role in proliferative processes, i.e. promoting neoplasia. This could explain worse prognosis in neoplasms with high Bax expression and better prognosis in cancers with low Bcl-2/Bax ratio (46).

According to the study carried out by Stummvoll et al. in 39 SSc patients and 47 healthy controls, there were no significant differences in Bax expression in CD4+ and CD8+ lymphocytes, which is likely to suggest that Bax does not play any significant role in apoptosis regulation in SSc patients. Moreover, there were no significant differences in Bax expression in relation to the clinical subtype, duration of disease, or immunosuppressive therapy administered (60). Our findings in 40 patients with systemic sclerosis revealed higher expression of Bax in CD8+ lymphocytes in patients with active disease (65). This enhanced Bax expression in CD8+ lymphocytes may suggest the increased loss of these cells through the process of apoptosis. The pathogenesis of SSc is associated with increased proliferation of CD4+ and loss of CD8+ lymphocytes. Apoptosis appears to be one of the possible mechanism for CD8+ loss (14).

5. The role of NF-κB in SSc apoptosis

Another relevant transcription factor responsible for activation and regulation of expression of genes involved in apoptosis is the nuclear factor κB (NF-κB) (66). It plays a crucial role in regulation of the immune response, inflammatory processes, oncogenesis, and virus replication. Moreover, it is necessary for activation of lymphocytes, proliferation and expression of cytokines (61). The NF-κB–activated genes include genes encoding cytokines IL-1, IL-2, IL-6, IL-12, TNF, LTα/β), granulocyte macrophage-colony stimulating factors (GM-CSF), immunoreceptors (with the MHC ligand), cell adhesion molecules (ICAM, VCAM, ELAM), acute phase proteins (SAA - serum amyloid), enzymes (inducible nitric oxide synthase - iNOS, cyclooxygenase-2 - COX-2) and genes encoding oncogenesis-involved factors (cIAP1, cIAP2, fasl, c-myc, p53, cyclin D1) (67). To date, ten various transcription factors belonging to the NF-κB family (Rel) have been identified in mammals. Five of them are transcription regulators: Rel/NF-κB (p50/p105 – NF-κB1, p52/p100 – NF-κB2, c-Rel-Rel, RelA – p65 and RelB); the remaining ones have inhibitory properties (IκB-IκBa, IκBb, IκBg-p105, IκBd-p100, Bcl-3) (68). All regulatory factors contain the rel homology domain (RHD), composed of 300 amino acids, which is responsible for formation of dimmers, their permeation to the nucleus and binding to an appropriate DNA fragment (69). The terminal fragment of RHD contains a nuclear location sequence (NLS), which permits binding to the nucleus (67).

The NF-κB proteins may be homo- and heterodimers (except for RelB). The majority of homodimers are not capable of inducing transcription whereas heterodimeric structures contain transactivating domains indispensible for induction of genes involved in the immune response (68,70). The best-known heterodimer is p50/Ril, composed of two subunits, p50, a product of NF-κB1 gene, and p65, a product of RelA gene (67).

NF-κB, found bound to IκB in all cells, except for lymphocytes B, is activated in the cytoplasm, following the cell exposure to pro-inflammatory factors, e.g. lipopolysaccharides, (LPS), the tumour necrosis factor (TNF-α, TNF-β), epidermal growth factor (EGF), free radicals, cytokines, viruses, ionizing or ultraviolet radiation. NF-κB, released during IκB degradation, is translocated to the nucleus, where it binds to DNA and activates suitable genes, e.g. mediators of inflammation, carcinogenesis or IκB mediators (68, 70).

Numerous data highlight a significant regulatory role of NF-κB in the process of apoptosis. Being involved in various pathways of programmed cell death, NF-κB exerts anti- and pro-apoptotic effects, which is most likely dependent on the predominance of factors activating or inhibiting the expression of the cascade of apoptotic events. Apoptosis is inhibited due to NF-κB-induced transcription of Bcl anti-apoptotic genes (Bcl-xl, BFl/A1) and inhibitors of apoptosis (cIAP1, cIAP2) (which indirectly reduces the activity of cytochrome c). Moreover, the mechanism of activation of tumour receptor-associated factors (TRAF1, TRAF2) and IAPs (cIAP1, cIAP2, XIAP), resulting in inhibition of the caspase cascade, is involved; caspase 8 is deactivated by TRAF1, TRAF2, cIAP1, cIAP2, whereas caspase 3 mainly by activated proteins cIAP1 and cIAP2 (Fig.3) (61,66,71,72).

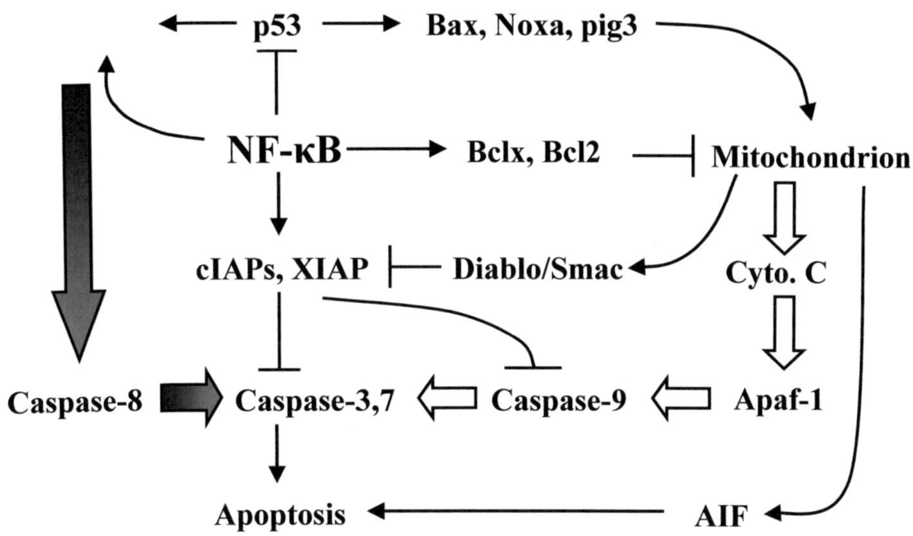

Fig. 3. Possible pathways of NF-κB anti-apoptotic action (66)

An example of NF-κB anti-apoptotic action is its involvement in transcriptional regulation of genes associated with liver regeneration after partial hepatectomy or protection of cortical neurons against apoptotic effects of β-amyloid (exposure of cortical neurons to β-amyloid is connected with an increase in IκB-α mRNA level, which reduces the NF-κB activity) (73,74).

On the other hand, the role of NF-κB in transcriptional regulation of several pro-apoptotic genes is noteworthy. It is highly likely that this process results from rapid activation of NF-κB in response to the apoptotic signal and from effects of NF-κB on expression of some genes associated with programmed cell death, e.g. TNF, c-myc or fasl genes (66). By increasing the expression of FasL, NF-κB enhances the Fas-FasL interactions. Moreover, as demonstrated earlier, the transcription factor RelA (p65) is essential for activation of the promoter fragment FasL (75,76). It should be emphasized, however, that some researches do not confirm possible NF-κB-activated apoptosis mediated by expression of Fasl gene (77,78).

Another indirect example of pro-apoptotic NF-κB action is activation of nitric oxide synthase required for production of nitric oxide. The process results in inhibition of caspase cascade, which leads to cell apoptosis (61). It is worth noting that apoptosis may be regulated by the antagonistic action of protein p53 towards NK-κB, which compete for binding to the co-activator p300 (33).

The involvement of NF-κB in cell cycle regulation involves facilitation of transition from phase G1 to S through inhibition of activation or function of p53 and increased expression of the cyclin D1. Additionally, NF-κB can activate the transition from phase G2 to M by inhibiting the expression of the growth arrest DNA-damage protein 45 (GADD45), which blocks the cyclin B/CDK2 complex (66).

The ability of transcription factor NF-κB proteins to suppress apoptosis and regulate the cell cycle indicates that NF-κB may play an essential role in oncogenesis. Enhanced expression of NF-κB has been demonstrated in numerous neoplastic diseases, e.g. breast, lung or thyroid cancer, T and B cell leukaemia, malignant melanoma, prostate, gallbladder, head and neck cancer (34,35,79-82).

In the study performed in 27 SSc patients and 28 healthy controls, Kassel et al. observed reduced expression of NF-κB in CD8+ lymphocytes of SSc patients compared to controls; additionally, an inverse correlation was found between the percentage of anti-apoptotic CD8+ T lymphocytes and NF-κB expression. The authors believe that decreased NF-κB expression in CD8+ lymphocytes in peripheral blood is likely to be one of the mechanisms of enhanced apoptosis of CD8+ lymphocytes in SSc patients. This weighs in favour of the anti-apoptotic action of NF-κB in systemic sclerosis and thus confirms an important role of NF-κB in regulation of homeostasis and tolerance of T lymphocytes (61, 83). The exact mechanism leading to decreased NF-κB expression in CD8+ lymphocytes in SSc patients has not been fully explained. The ability of NF-κB to regulate the expression of anti-apoptotic genes, such as cellular inhibitors of apoptosis (c-IAP1, c-IAP2, IXAP), TNF receptor-associated factors (TRAF1 and TRAF2) as well as Bcl-2 proteins, appears to be crucial (83,72). Importantly, NF-κB, as a nuclear transcription factor, and pathways of its anti-apoptotic action can be activated by various factors: cytokines, free radicals, lipopolysaccharides, or directly acting receptors, e.g. TNF receptor (61). The NF-κB involvement in regulation of apoptosis has been confirmed in experimental studies carried out for over ten years. Numerous reports indicate that NF-κB activation is necessary for protection of lymphocytes against apoptosis induced by various factors (83). In 1997, Ivanov et al. suggested a possible relevant role of NF-κB in the regulation of Fas receptor-induced apoptosis of T lymphocytes (84). Two years later, Dudley et al. confirmed protective effects of NF-κB on T lymphocytes against Fas receptor- and TNF-induced apoptosis (85). The recent reports demonstrate that NF-κB activation is indispensible for protection of T lymphocytes against apoptosis induced by mutagens and anti-Fas antibodies (78).

According to Auphan et al. and Lanza et al., steroid preparations are likely to contribute to NF-κB inactivation, hence increasing the percentage of apoptotic cells. Glucocorticosteroids, as one of the most powerful anti-inflammatory and immunosuppressive agents, inhibit the synthesis of cytokines and many cell surface molecules required for induction of immune responses. NF-κB is inactivated due to steroid-induced increased synthesis of IκB. IκB, a nuclear factor inhibitor, retains NF-κB in the cytoplasm in the form of inactive complexes (86,87).

6. The role of mitochondrial membrane potential in SSc apoptosis

Many researchers stress an important role of mitochondria in programmed cell death (88-90). The majority of human cells undergo apoptosis via the intrinsic pathway (91). It has been shown that the key point in induction of mitochondrial pathway of apoptosis is increased permeability of the outer mitochondrial membrane, usually accompanied by decreased potential of inner mitochondrial membrane ($\Delta\Psi m$). The differences result from metabolic features of membranes. High values of inner mitochondrial membrane ($\Delta\psi m$) have to be maintained for proper mitochondrial energetic processes, which lead to the formation of adenosine triphosphate (ATP). In normal cells, the inner mitochondrial membrane is virtually impermeable; however, it is equipped with transport systems for selected metabolites, whose weight does not exceed 1.5 kDa. Thanks to the presence of voltage-dependent anion channels (VDACs), the outer mitochondrial membrane acts as a molecular sieve, which is permeable to the majority of ions and low-molecular substances dissolved in water of a molecular weight below 5 kDa. VDACs are characterized by reversibility and selectivity, both for anions and cations; at low voltages, they are open for anion metabolites. Thus, under normal conditions they are impermeable to positively charged cytochrome c. The mechanism for opening and closing of VDACs is regulated by Bcl proteins (55,63,92-94).

The results of studies in patients with chronic B-cell leukaemia reveal that decreased mitochondrial potential is a marker of early apoptosis mediated by the mitochondrial permeability transition pores (MPTPs) formed in the inner mitochondrial membrane. The major constituents of MPTPs are adenine nucleotide translocase (ANT) and cyclophilin D, located in the inner mitochondrial membrane as well as VDACs and the peripheral benzodiazepine receptor located in the outer membrane. In normal mitochondria, VDACs and ANTs form a macromolecular complex responsible for transport of adenine nucleotides from the site of ATP production within the mitochondrial matrix to that of ATP consumption in the cytosol. Since apoptosis is relevant for the development of systemic sclerosis, impaired production of ATP should be expected in T lymphocytes of SSc patients. It is known that the mitochondria are essential for apoptosis, which results from the fact that permeability of the mitochondrial membrane and activation of caspases determine irreversibility of the process. Interestingly, permeability of the outer mitochondrial membrane is a constant feature of apoptosis. The opening of several MPTPs, or even one of them, leads to depolarization of mitochondria, impaired oxidative phosphorylation and marked swelling of mitochondria. With progression of programmed cell death, the mitochondrial potential decreases, which results in the release of proteins closed within the intermembrane space (e.g. cytochrome c, apoptosis-inducing factor (AIF), pro-caspase 2, 3, 9, adenylate kinase, the second mitochondrial activator of caspases). The outflow of these molecules is necessary for quick activation of the cascade of programmed cell death events (95,96).

In contrast to the outer membrane, apoptotic permeability of the inner membrane is not a constant feature of apoptosis and does not cause such an intense release of proteins from the matrix. An increase in inner membrane permeability to dissolved molecules of molecular weight of about 1.5 kDa is a characteristic feature, which is associated with dispersion of the proton gradient responsible for mitochondrial transmembrane potential ($\Delta\Psi_m$) (97,98).

The available literature lacks studies assessing the mitochondrial membrane potential in the population of CD4+ and CD8+ lymphocytes. In our study, the percentage of apoptotic cells was analysed using chloromethyl-X-rosamine (CMXRos) (65). The method assesses the

mitochondrial potential, an indicator of the induction of an intrinsic apoptotic pathway. The method was chosen as it enabled the assessment of the very early stages of apoptosis, before the cells undergoing apoptosis are eliminated from the circulation through phagocytosis (89).
Our findings show higher percentages of CD4+ and CD8+ lymphocytes with reduced mitochondrial membrane potential (ΔΨm) in patients compared to healthy controls, which is likely to suggest the activation of early CD8+ T lymphocyte apoptosis through the mitochondrial pathway in patients with systemic sclerosis (65). It is noteworthy to mention that a decrease in mitochondrial potential is characterized by specificity, as the process involves only the cells entering apoptosis, and universality, as it regards all cells entering the programmed cell death pathway. Moreover, decreased mitochondrial potential is characterized by irreversibility since the cells of decreased ΔΨm undergo apoptosis even when the triggering stimulus is removed (99,100). Thus, the measurement of mitochondrial potential seems to be an extremely sensitive and precise method for assessment of apoptotic cell percentages.

7. The role of Fas receptor and Fas ligand in SSc apoptosis

The role of the soluble Fas (sFas) in initiation of programmed cell death is illuminated by the results of studies in patients with systemic sclerosis and other autoimmune diseases (101). The Fas receptor (APO-1, CD95) and Fas ligand (FasL) belong to the family of TNF receptors (102). Soluble Fas (sFas) is a 4 kDa glycosylated type I membrane protein, whereas FasL is synthesized as a 40 kDa type II transmembrane protein. The Fas receptor is expressed on the surface of various types of normal and neoplastic human cell lines, e.g. T and B lymphocytes, macrophages, hepatocytes or thymocytes. FasL is produced by activated CD4+, CD8+ T lymphocytes and NK cells; it is expressed in the eyes and testes and is characterized by high cytotoxic activity towards the Fas receptor-bearing cells. The activity of FasL is stimulated by UV radiation, gamma radiation and some drugs, e.g. bleomycin, anisomycin and doxorubicin, and inhibited by cyclic adenosine monophosphate (cAMP), retinoic acid, nitric oxide and vitamin D_3 (39,75,76,103).
In response to an apoptotic signal, FasL binds to the Fas receptor, which results in Fas trimerisation. The interactions between Fas and FasL are relevant for induction of lymphoid line apoptosis and systemic immune response. The pro-apoptotic action is possible thanks to the complex of adaptor proteins, the mediators of the reaction, or to cell contact. This happens because Fas receptor fragments are deprived of catalytic domains. One of the adaptor proteins contains the death domain (DD) - the sequence of specific amino acids, which enables interactions of FADD protein with the cytoplasmic fragment of activated Fas receptor. Consequently, the death-inducing signalling complex (DISC) is formed. In addition to DD, the FADD protein has the death effector domain (DED), to which pro-caspase 8 binds with its DED. This complex is necessary for autocatalytic activation of pro-caspase 8. At this stage, two pathways of further signalling leading to apoptosis are possible. In the first one, active caspase 8 is sufficient to activate pro-caspase 3, which finally leads to condensation of nuclear chromatin and DNA degradation. The cells characterized by this signalling on the extrinsic pathway are called type I cells. In contrast, in type II cells, activation of caspase 8 is insufficient for induction of apoptosis as it is usually weak, and thus does not lead to formation of sufficient amounts of the product. The signal has to be enhanced on the mitochondria-dependent intrinsic pathway. A link between both apoptotic pathways is the Bid protein (Fig.4) (39,76,104,105).

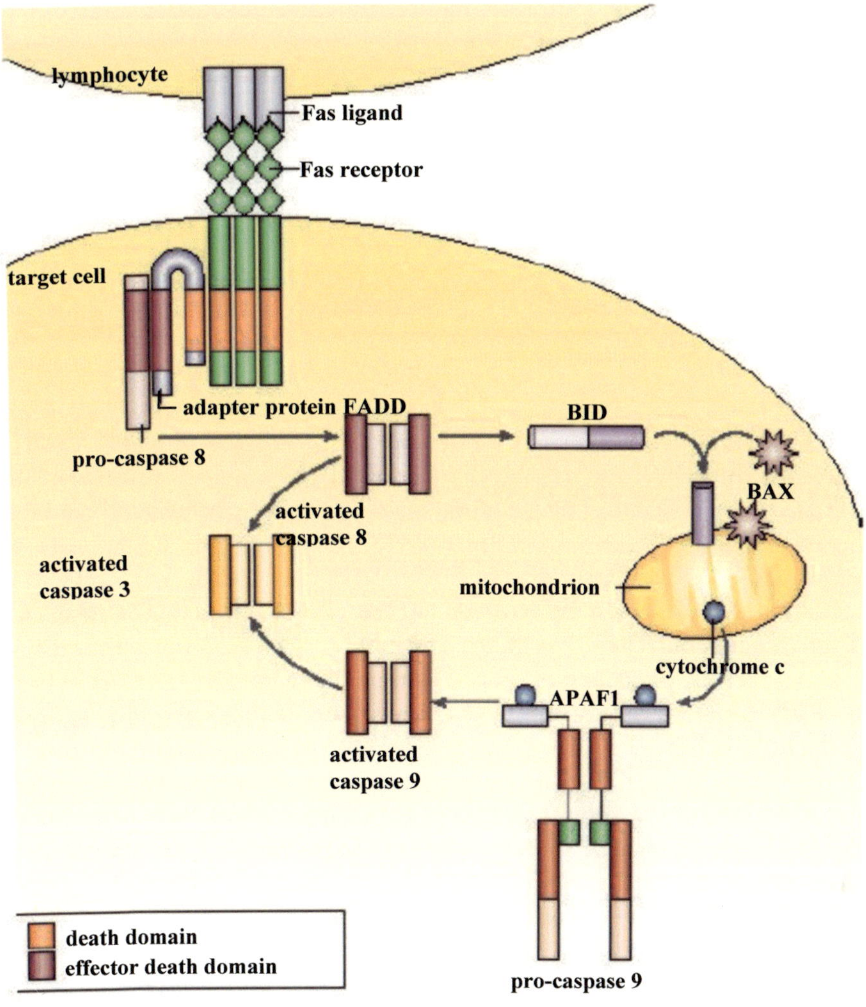

Fig. 4. The pathway of apoptotic events induced by FasL (39)

Wetzig et al. demonstrated significantly increased levels of sFas in the group of 30 patients with systemic sclerosis compared to 15 healthy controls. The authors suggested that increased sFas levels might be an important marker of prevention of T lymphocyte apoptosis in systemic sclerosis (103). Similar results were reported by Dziankowska-Bartkowiak et al., who studied the group of 29 SSc patients and 10 healthy controls and found significantly higher levels of sFas in SSc patients, which is likely to implicate an important role of sFas in apoptosis prevention in systemic sclerosis (106). By affecting FasL-Fas coupling sFas may prevent the induction of apoptosis, thus promote the activation of T lymphocytes in systemic sclerosis. The available results suggest that sFas may be essential for inhibition of apoptosis in the pathogenesis of systemic sclerosis. By preventing the initiation of programmed cell death, sFas is likely to increase the proliferative response of lymphocytes to autoantigenes, ultimately leading to excessive activation of T lymphocytes (14,101,107). Stummvoll et al. observed statistically significantly higher concentrations of sFas in serum of SSc patients compared to healthy controls. Additionally, they showed higher Fas expression in CD8+ lymphocytes in SSc patients compared to controls, which is likely to suggest increased apoptosis of these lymphocytes. However, they did not observe any significant differences in Fas expression in CD4+ lymphocytes. Abnormal serum sFas levels in SSc patients are likely to be a marker of T lymphocyte activation during systemic sclerosis (60). Cipriani et al. demonstrated significantly higher serum sFas concentrations in 22 SSc patients in comparison with healthy controls, which also seems to confirm the earlier implicated role of the receptor pathway of apoptosis in the pathogenesis of systemic sclerosis (59). Moreover, elevated sFas levels in SSc patients compared to healthy controls were observed by Nozawa et al., yet the differences were not statistically significant, which may be associated with the smaller population of patients included in their study (only 16 patients) (108).

The literary data indicates that SSc patients are characterized not only by increased numbers of activated T lymphocytes but also by the enhanced expression of Fas receptors in these cells, compared with healthy controls (60). This shows that increased serum levels of sFas in SSc patients may protect autoreactive T lymphocytes against apoptosis induced by the Fas-ligand system and lead to excessive activation of T lymphocytes (14,101,107). Increased concentrations of sFas may be indicative of inhibition of apoptosis induction by the receptor pathway, and thus contributes to the activation of T lymphocytes in this disease.

It is worth mentioning, however, that there are studies in which no significant differences in serum sFas levels in SSc patients were found compared to healthy controls, which may be associated with different study designs, differences in disease activity or therapy administered (101,109,110).

Apoptosis appears to be mediated by the Fas receptor pathway in both forms of disease; nevertheless, considering the clinical picture of both forms, higher levels of sFas should be expected in SSc patients, whose disease develops more rapidly and affects the internal organs, especially in early stages (103,111-113). In the study by Wetzig et al., involving 16 lSSc and 14 dSSc patients, there were no significant differences in sFas levels according to the clinical form of disease (103). Similar results were reported by Stummvoll et al. Additionally, they demonstrated a positive correlation between Fas receptor expression and the age of the patients. Their findings, showing statistically significant differences in Fas expression and sFas concentration, are likely to indicate enhanced activation of T cells resulting from impaired apoptosis of lymphocytes (60). Otherwise, the findings reported by Dziankowska-Bartkowiak et al. revealed statistically significant differences in sFas levels depending on the disease form. Their study involved two size-comparable groups of patients (15 dSSc and 14 lSSc patients). The sFas concentrations in dSSc patients were found higher in comparison with lSSc patients (52,106). According to Ingegnoli et al., expression of Fas receptor in CD4+ and CD8+ lymphocytes was significantly higher in dSSc patients. These findings are likely to confirm impaired lymphocyte homeostasis in systemic sclerosis. The authors suggested that enhanced Fas expression in dSSc patients might lead to the development of autoregulation mechanisms due to abnormal immune response. sFas-induced excessive activation of T lymphocytes is likely to lead finally to the elimination of autoreactive lymphocytes through Fas receptor-activated apoptotic pathways (16).

In the studies carried out by Wetzig et al. in SSc patients, only a slight correlation between sFas concentration and disease activity was found. The activity of disease was assessed based on elevated CRP, SR and/or presence of immune complexes, leucocytosis and clinical markers of skin involvement (swelling, redness, or tenderness). The diagnostic criteria of inactive disease included normal SR and CRP, as well as skin sclerosis without swelling or atrophies. Elevated sFas levels were more common in patients with active disease, although in single cases high sFas levels were also observed in patients with inactive SSc (103).

Ates et al. found no significant correlations between sFas concentration and degree or extent of skin involvement in SSc patients. They assessed the severity and extent of sclerosis using the 4-degree (0-3) scoring method of Kahaleh et al. in 15 body areas (101). Different results were reported by Dziankowska-Bartkowiak et al, who also used the Kahaleh scale and observed a positive correlation between sFas concentration and severity of skin lesions and a directly proportional relation between the serum sFas level and osteoarticular involvement. The authors suggest that elevated sFas levels in systemic sclerosis may be a marker of skin and osteoarticular involvement (106).

Ates et al. did not show significant differences in serum sFas concentrations of patients with lung fibrosis and those without HRCT-detected chest lesions. Moreover, they did not observe significant correlations between serum sFas levels and lung diffusion capacity (101). Similar results were presented by Luzin et al. and Wetzig et al. (103,114). However, there are also reports stressing the role of sFas in the development of interstitial lung disease in SSc patients. The evidence can be found in studies devoted to the role of apoptosis in the pathogenesis of systemic sclerosis induced by bleomycin. According to Kuwano et al., anti-FasL antibodies administered in injections may prevent lung fibrosis induced by bleomycin in SSc patients. Anti-FasL antibodies are most likely to lead to inhibition of apoptosis induced via the Fas-FasL pathway (115). This mechanism, however, does not seem sufficiently protective as lung fibrotic processes are induced not only through the ligand-receptor pathway (49).

Taking into account the treatment used, Ates et al. demonstrated significantly higher serum sFas levels in untreated SSc patients in comparison to healthy controls and patients undergoing therapy (101).

The available literature does not provide evidence for significant correlations between Fas protein concentrations and disease duration or presence of oesophageal or cardiac lesions (59,103).

8. The role of cytochrome c in SSc apoptosis

Furthermore, the role of cytochrome c in apoptosis should be highlighted. Cytochrome c is a water-soluble 15 kDa haem protein, consisting of a 104 amino acid-long peptide chain combined with the haem molecule. It plays an essential role in oxygen phosphorylation and apoptosis, being involved in caspase 3 activation and DNA fragmentation (94,116,117). Like the majority of mitochondrial proteins, cytochrome c is encoded by the nuclear gene and synthesized in the cytoplasm as a precursor 12 kDa molecule, called apocytochrome c. It translocates from the cytoplasm, independently of the receptors, along the outer mitochondrial membrane to the perimitochondrial space where functionally active molecules of cytochrome c are formed mediated by the inner mitochondrial membrane enzyme - cytochrome c haem lyase. During programmed cell death, cytochrome c translocates from the mitochondria to the cytosol in response to the apoptotic signal. The molecular mechanism of this translocation is not fully explained. As demonstrated earlier, it results from decreased membranous mitochondrial potential characteristic of early stages of apoptosis. The release of cytochrome c during apoptosis is regulated by Bcl proteins. Under normal conditions, VDAC, formed in the outer mitochondrial membrane by the mitochondrial channel protein porin, is impermeable to cytochrome c. Mediated by pro-apoptotic proteins (Bax, Bak, tBid), VDAC opens and releases cytochrome c from the intermembrane space, whereas anti-apoptotic proteins, e.g. Bcl-xl, close the channel retaining cytochrome c within the mitochondria. Cytochrome c in the cytoplasm initiates programmed cell death events through the caspase cascade-dependent pathway (44). By catalysing the heptameric complex of caspase 9 and apoptosis protease activating factor 1 (Apaf 1), a proenzyme of caspase 9, cytochrome c acts as a cofactor of the reaction. Cytochrome c binds Apaf 1 without the involvement of deoxyadenosine triphosphate (dATP); subsequently, in the presence of cytochrome c and with dATP involved, pro-caspase 9 can bind to Apaf 1, which results in caspase 9 activation. In cases of cytochrome c deficiency, even if dATP is available, this reaction is infeasible, which points to the relevant role of cytochrome c in initiation of the cascade of caspases - executors of the death signal. The consequence of caspase 9 activation is indirect involvement of cytochrome c in activation of caspase 3, which leads to DNA fragmentation and cell death (Fig.5) (45,117,118).

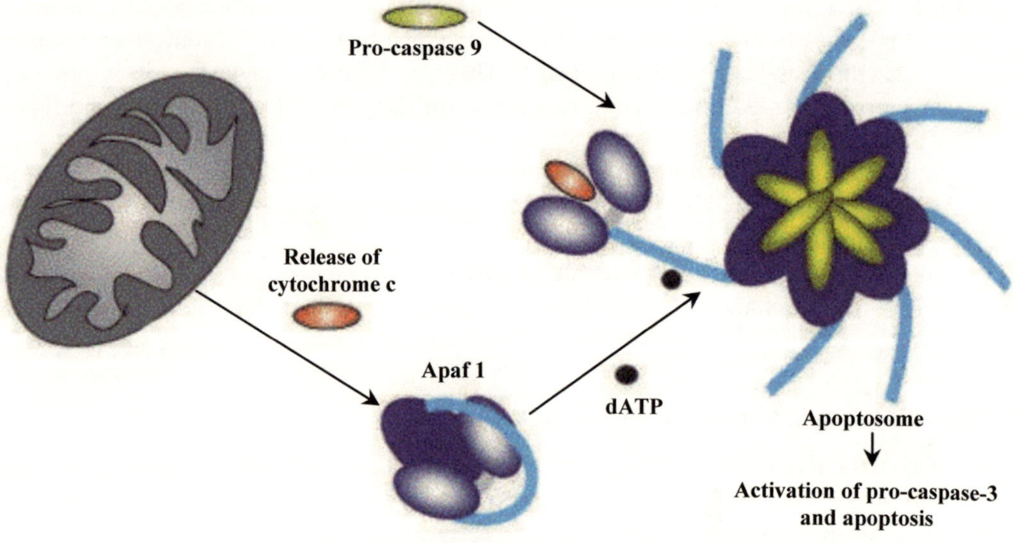

Fig. 5. The role of cytochrome c in apoptosis (117)

9. The role of caspase 9 in SSc apoptosis

Caspase 9 (ICE-LAP6, Mch6) belongs to the intracellular proteases of cysteine, whose common feature is hydrolysis of protein substrates at the place of asparagine acid carboxyl residue. These enzymes play a key role in apoptosis; capable of destroying the enzymatic and effector proteins, they ultimately lead to complete cell disintegration. Caspase 9 is synthesized in its pro-enzymatic form as a zymogene. Unlike other caspases, the caspase 9 zymogene shows high chemical activity, which may suggest that pro-caspase 9 proteolysis is not necessary for enzyme activation (119,120). Like other cysteine proteases, pro-caspase 9 has a N-terminal pro-domain consisting of a larger subunit - p20 (20kDa) and a smaller subunit - p10 (about 10 kDa), joined with a short linker. This pro-domain is involved in dimerisation of pro-caspase molecules and their maintenance in inactive forms. According to its structure, caspase 9 is a caspase with a long pro-domain, with the caspase activation and recruitment domain (CARD). The enzyme is activated due to binding of the homological fragment of 85 amino acids of NH_2- terminal fragment of Apaf to CARD 1 in the presence of cytochrome c and dATP and due to the effects of caspase 3 and granzyme B on the pro-caspase 9 molecule, which was demonstrated under in vitro conditions (118,121-124). Caspase 9 can also be activated with involvement of active caspase 8 during Bid disintegration, which results in the release of cytochrome c to the cytosol. Moreover, pro-caspase 9 may be proteolysed through the apoptosome-independent pathway using caspase 12 (125,126). The enzymatically active caspase 9 acts as a tetramer formed of two heterodimers consisting of a small and large subunit ($p20_2$ – $p10_2$) (40,127-129). Ultimately, it is located in the cytosol, where to pro-caspase 9 translocates from the perimitochondrial space of various organs in response to the apoptosis-inducing stimulus. High expression of caspase 9 was shown in the heart, ovaries and testes. Its presence was also detected in the liver, kidneys, brain, spleen and lymphoid cell lines and neuroblastoma lines (45,130).

In the process of apoptosis, caspase 9 plays an important role in induction of caspase cascade - the pathway of biochemical events directly responsible for programmed cell death. By activating the effector caspase 3 and 7, it substantially contributes to degradation and fragmentation of cytoplasmic and nuclear proteins. Additionally, since it can be activated by caspase 3, caspase 9, as an active enzyme, is crucially involved in irreversible changes occurring in the cells during apoptosis (128,130,131). The caspase 9 involvement in apoptosis is regulated by specific inhibitors, such as the tumour-up-regulated CARD-containing antagonist of caspase nine (TUCAN) protein, Akt kinase (protein kinase B), anti-apoptotic Bcl proteins and IAPs (132).

The role of cytochrome c and caspase 9 in apoptosis has not been fully elucidated; therefore, further research is required.

10. Key points

1. The Bcl family appears to play a significant role in the regulation of T lymphocyte apoptosis in SSc patients. Enhanced expression of Bax in CD8+ lymphocytes in patients with active disease suggests increased loss of these lymphocytes through intensified apoptosis.
2. Decreased expression of NF-κB in activated CD8+ lymphocytes in peripheral blood is likely to be one of the mechanisms potentiating apoptosis of CD8+ lymphocytes in patients with systemic sclerosis.
3. Measurements of mitochondrial potential appear relevant for assessment of early stages of apoptosis in patients with systemic sclerosis.
4. Fas is likely to play an important role in prevention of T lymphocyte apoptosis during systemic sclerosis.

11. References

[1] Abraham D.J., Varga J. Scleroderma: from cell and molecular mechanisms to disease models. Trends Immunol. 2005, 26, 587-595.

[2] Denton C.P., Black C.M. Scleroderma - clinical and pathological advances. Best Pract Res Clin Rheumatol. 2004, 18, 271-290.

[3] Haustein U.F. Systemic sclerosis-scleroderma. Dermatol Online J. 2002, 8, 3.

[4] Latsi P.I., Wells A.U. Evaluation and management of alveolitis and interstitial lung disease in scleroderma. Curr Opin Rheumatol. 2003, 15, 748-755.

[5] Ozcelik O., Haytac M.C., Ergin M., Antmen B., Seydaoglu G. The immunohistochemical analysis of vascular endothelial growth factors A and C and microvessel density in gingival tissues of systemic sclerosis patients: their possible effects on gingival inflammation. Oral Surg Oral Med Oral Pathol Oral Radiol Endod. 2008, 105, 481-485.

[6] Trojanowska M., Varga J. Molecular pathways as novel therapeutic targets in systemic sclerosis. Curr Opin Rheumatol. 2007, 19, 568-573.

[7] Zhivotovsky B., Samali A., Gahm A., Orrenius S. Caspases: their intracellular localization and translocation during apoptosis. Cell Death Differ. 1999, 6, 644-651.

[8] Zuber J.P., Spertini F. Immunological basis of systemic sclerosis. Rheumatology (Oxford). 2006, 45, iii23-iii25.

[9] Morgiel E., Krywejko J., Wiland P. Immunological aspects of systemic sclerosis and new strategies in therapy. Adv Clin Exp Med. 2008, 17, 441-446.

[10] Jimenez S.A., Derk C.T. Following the molecular pathways toward an understanding of the pathogenesis of systemic sclerosis. Ann Intern Med. 2004, 140, 37-50.

[11] Tamby M.C., Chanseaud Y., Guillevin L., Mouthon L. New insights into the pathogenesis of systemic sclerosis. Autoimmun Rev. 2003, 2, 152-157.

[12] Sakkas L.I. New developments in the pathogenesis of systemic sclerosis. Autoimmunity. 2005, 38, 113-116.

[13] Gu Y.S., Kong J., Cheema G.S., Keen C.L., Wick G., Gershwin M.E. The immunobiology of systemic sclerosis. Semin Arthritis Rheum. 2008, 38, 132-160.

[14] Gindzieńska-Sieśkiewicz E., Klimiuk P.A., Kowal-Bielecka O., Sierakowski S. Aspekty immuno-patologiczne twardziny układowej. Pol Merk Lek. 2005, 19, 800-803.

[15] Gustafsson R., Tötterman T.H., Klareskog L., Hällgren R. Increase in activated T cells and reduction in suppressor inducer T cells in systemic sclerosis. Ann Rheum Dis. 1990, 49, 40-45.

[16] Ingegnoli F., Trabattoni D., Saresella M., Fantini F., Clerici M. Distinct immune profiles characterize patients with diffuse or limited systemic sclerosis. Clin Immunol. 2003, 108, 21-28.

[17] Degiannis D., Seibold J.R., Czarnecki M., Raskova J., Raska K. Jr. Soluble and cellular markers of immune activation in patients with systemic sclerosis. Clin Immunol Immunopathol. 1990, 56, 259-270.

[18] Hasegawa M., Fujimoto M., Takehara K., Sato S. Pathogenesis of systemic sclerosis: altered B cell function in the key linking systemic autoimmunity and tissue fibrosis. J Dermatol Sci. 2005, 39, 1-7.

[19] Wojas-Pelc A., Lipko-Godlewska S. INF-γ w surowicy chorych na twardzinę układową i skórną - badanie porównawcze. Przeg Derm. 2008, 95, 371-378.

[20] Dziankowska-Bartkowiak B., Zalewska A., Sysa-Jedrzejowska A. Duration of Raynaud's phenomenon is negatively correlated with serum levels of interleukin 10 (IL-10), soluble receptor of interleukin 2 (sIL2R), and sFas in systemic sclerosis patients. Med Sci Monit. 2004, 10, CR202-208.

[21] Kurasawa K., Hirose K., Sano H., Endo H., Shinkai H., Nawata Y., Takabayashi K., Iwamoto I. Increased interleukin-17 production in patients with systemic sclerosis. Arthritis Rheum. 2000, 43, 2455-2463.
[22] Gorla R., Airò P., Malagoli A., Carella G., Prati E., Brugnoni D., Franceschini F., Cattaneo R. CD4+ and CD8+ subsets: naive and memory cells in the peripheral blood of patients with systemic sclerosis. Clin Rheumatol. 1994, 13, 83-87.
[23] Yanaba K., Bouaziz J.D., Matsushita T., Magro C.M., St Clair E.W., Tedder T.F. B-lymphocyte contributions to human autoimmune disease. Immunol Rev. 2008, 223, 284-299.
[24] Sato S., Fujimoto M., Hasegawa M., Takehara K. Altered blood B lymphocyte homeostasis in systemic sclerosis: expanded naive B cells and diminished but activated memory B cells. Arthritis Rheum. 2004, 50, 1918-1927.
[25] Nikpour M., Stevens W.M., Herrick A.L, Proudman S.M. Epidemiology of systemic sclerosis. Best Pract Res Clin Rheumatol. 2010, 24, 857-869.
[26] Puszczewicz M. Przeciwciała przeciwjądrowe w twardzinie układowej - charakterystyka antygenowa i znaczenie kliniczne. Reumatologia. 2006, 44, 169-175.
[27] Harris M.L., Rosen A. Autoimmunity in scleroderma: the origin, pathogenetic role, and clinical significance of autoantibodies. Curr Opin Rheumatol. 2003, 15, 778-784.
[28] Haustein U.F., Anderegg U. Pathophysiology of scleroderma: an update. J Eur Acad Dermatol Venereol. 1998, 11, 1-8.
[29] Herrick A.L., Matucci Cerinic M. The emerging problem of oxidative stress and the role of antioxidants in systemic sclerosis. Clin Exp Rheumatol. 2001, 19, 4-8.
[30] Jimenez S.A., Artlett C.M. Microchimerism and systemic sclerosis. Curr Opin Rheumatol. 2005, 17, 86-90.
[31] Riccieri V., Spadaro A., Fuksa L., Firuzi O., Saso L., Valesini G. Specific oxidative stress parameters differently correlate with nailfold capillaroscopy changes and organ involvement in systemic sclerosis. Clin Rheumatol. 2008, 27, 225-230.
[32] Sfrent-Cornateanu R., Mihai C., Stoian I., Lixandru D., Bara C., Moldoveanu E. Antioxidant defense capacity in scleroderma patients. Clin Chem Lab Med. 2008, 46, 836-841.
[33] Wadgaonkar R., Phelps K.M., Haque Z., Williams A.J., Silverman E.S., Collins T. CREB-binding protein is a nuclear integrator of nuclear factor-kappa B and p53 signaling. J Biol Chem. 1999, 274, 1879-1882.
[34] Sovak M.A., Bellas R.E., Kim D.W., Zanieski G.J., Rogers A.E., Traish A.M., Sonenshein G.E. Aberrant nuclear factor-kappaB/Rel expression and the pathogenesis of breast cancer. J Clin Invest.1997, 100, 2952-2960.
[35] Mukhopadhyay T., Roth J.A., Maxwell S.A. Altered expression of the p50 subunit of the NF-kappa B transcription factor complex in non-small cell lung carcinoma. Oncogene. 1995, 11, 999-1003.
[36] Kern P., Keilholz L., Forster C., Seegenschmiedt M.H., Sauer R., Herrmann M. In vitro apoptosis in peripheral blood mononuclear cells induced by low-dose radiotherapy displays a discontinuous dose-dependence. Int J Radiat Biol. 1999, 75, 995-1003.
[37] Baś M., Cywińska A., Sokołowska J., Krzyżowska M. Apoptoza - programowana śmierć komórki. Część III. Rola apoptozy w procesach fizjologicznych i patologicznych. Życie Weterynaryjne. 2004, 79, 671-675.
[38] Honing L.S., Rosengerg R.N. Apoptosis and neurologic disease. Am J Med. 2000, 108, 317-330.
[39] Nagata S. Fas ligand-induced apoptosis. Annu Rev Genet. 1999, 33, 29-55.

[40] Horodyjewska A., Pasternak K. Apoptotyczna śmierć komórki. Adv Clin Exp Med. 2005, 14, 545-554.

[41] Wyllie A.H. Apoptosis: an overview. Br Med Bull. 1997, 53, 451-465.

[42] Kalmakoff J., Ward V. Baculovirus-Host Interactions. University of Otago, Dunedin, New Zealand, 2003. http://www.microbiologybytes.com.

[43] Raskin C.A. Apoptosis and cutaneous biology. J Am Acad Dermatol. 1997, 36, 885-896.

[44] Szpringer E., Lutnicki K. Znaczenie apoptozy w wybranych chorobach w dermatologii. Nowa Med. 2002, 3, 24-32.

[45] Dziankowska-Bartkowiak B., Waszczykowska E., Sysa-Jędrzejowska A. Ocena zjawiska apoptozy u chorych na twardzinę układową. Przeg Derm. 2003, 1, 17-23.

[46] Faran G., Dworakowska D., Jassem E. Kliniczne znaczenie immunohistochemicznej ekspresji białek p53, Bcl-2 i Bax u chorych na niedrobnokomórkowego raka płuca. Współcz Onkol. 2004, 8, 328-337.

[47] Krammer P.H., Behrmann I., Daniel P., Dhein J., Debatin K.M. Regulation of apoptosis in the immune system. Curr Opin Immunol. 1994, 6, 279-289.

[48] Williams GT. Apoptosis in the immune system. J Pathol. 1994, 173, 1-4.

[49] Yamamoto T., Nishioka K.: Possible role of apoptosis in the pathogenesis of bleomycin-induced scleroderma. J Invest Dermatol. 2004, 122, 44-50.

[50] Hengartner MO. The biochemistry of apoptosis. Nature. 2000, 407, 770-776.

[51] Rich T., Allen R.L., Wyllie A.H. defying death after DNA damage. Nature. 2000, 407, 777-783.

[52] Susin S.A., Lorenzo H.K., Zamzami N., Marzo I., Brenner C., Larochette N., Prévost M.C., Alzari P.M., Kroemer G. Mitochondrial release of caspase-2 and –9 during the apoptotic process. J Exp Med. 1999, 189, 381-394.

[53] Usuda J., Chiu S.M., Murphy E.S., Lam M., Nieminen A.L., Oleinick N.L. Domain-dependent photodamage to Bcl-2. A membrane anchorage region is needed to form the target of phthalocyanine photosensitization. J Biol Chem. 2003, 278, 2021-2029.

[54] Yao P.L., Lin Y.C., Sawhney P., Richburg J.H. Transcriptional regulation of FasL expression and participation of sTNF-alpha in response to sertoli cell injury. J Biol Chem. 2007, 282, 5420-5431.

[55] Rupniewska Z., Bojarska-Junak A. Apoptoza: przepuszczalność błony mitochondrialnej i rola pełniona przez białka z rodziny Bcl-2. Postepy Hig Med Dosw. 2004, 58, 538-547.

[56] Borner M.M., Brousset P., Pfanner-Meyer B., Bacchi M., Vonlanthen S., Hotz M.A., Altermatt H.J., Schlaifer D., Reed J.C., Betticher D.C. Expression of apoptosis regulatory proteins of the Bcl-2 family and p53 in primary resected non-small-cell lung cancer. Br J Cancer. 1999, 79, 952-958.

[57] Hockenbery D.M., Zutter M., Hickey W., Nahm M., Korsmeyer S.J. BCL2 protein is topographically restricted in tissues characterized by apoptotic cell death. Proc Natl Acad Sci U S A. 1991, 88, 6961-6965.

[58] Reed J.C. Bcl-2 and the regulation of programmed cell death. J Cell Biol. 1994, 124, 1-6.

[59] Cipriani P., Fulminis A., Pingiotti E., Marrelli A., Liakouli V., Perricone R., Pignone A., Matucci-Cerinic M., Giacomelli R. Resistance to apoptosis in circulating alpha/beta and gamma/delta T lymphocytes from patients with systemic sclerosis. J Rheumatol. 2006, 33, 2003-2014.

[60] Stummvoll G.H., Aringer M., Smolen J.S., Köller M., Kiener H.P., Steiner C.W., Bohle B., Knobler R., Graninger W.B. Derangement of apoptosis-related lymphocyte homeostasis in systemic sclerosis. Rheumatology (Oxford). 2000, 39, 1341-1350.

[61] Kessel A., Rosner I., Rozenbaum M., Zisman D., Sagiv A., Shmuel Z., Sabo E., Toubi E. Increased CD8+ T cell apoptosis in scleroderma is associated with low levels of NF-kappa B. J Clin Immunol. 2004, 24, 30-36.

[62] Czuwara J., Makieła B., Nowicka U., Barusińska A., Górkiewicz-Petkow A., Majewski S., Jabłońska S., Rudnicka L. Apoptoza w komórkach jednojądrowych krwi obwodowej pacjentów z twardziną układową. Prz Derm. 1996, 83, 461-467.

[63] Skalska J., Dębska-Vielhaber G., Głąb M., Kulawiak B., Malińska D., Koszela-Piotrowska I., Bednarczyk P. Dołowy K., Szewczyk A. Mitochondrialne kanały jonowe. Post Bioch. 2006, 52, 137-144.

[64] Brown R. The bcl-2 family of proteins. Br Med Bull. 1997, 53, 466-477.

[65] Szymanek M. Research of the choosen apoptosis parameters in patients with systemic sclerosis. Doctoral thesis. Promoter –dr hab. D. Krasowska. Lublin 2009.

[66] Chen F., Castranova V., Shi X. New insights into the role of nuclear factor-kappaB in cell growth regulation. Am J Pathol. 2001, 159, 387-397.

[67] Starska K. Rola rodziny cząsteczek transkrypcyjnego czynnika jądrowego NF-κB w regulacji cyklu komórkowego i zjawiska apoptozy w przebiegu onkogenezy i progresji nowotworu. Otorynolaryngologia. 2006, 5, 51-56.

[68] Wydmuch Z., Więcławek A., Besser P., Mazurek U., Pytel A., Pacha J. Leki przeciwzapalne blokujące aktywność czynnika transkrypcyjnego NKκB. Poradnik farmaceutyczny. 2005, 5, 1-4.

[69] Siebenlist U., Franzoso G., Brown K. Structure, regulation and function of NF-kappa B. Annu Rev Cell Biol. 1994, 10, 405-455

[70] Wong H.K., Kammer G.M., Dennis G., Tsokos G.C. Abnormal NF-kappa B activity in T lymphocytes from patients with systemic lupus erythematosus is associated with decreased p65-RelA protein expression. J Immunol. 1999, 163, 1682-1689.

[71] Duval H., Harris M., Li J., Johnson N., Print C.: New insights into the function and regulation of endothelial cell apoptosis. Angiogenesis 2003, 6, 171-183.

[72] Wang C.Y., Guttridge D.C., Mayo M.W., Baldwin A.S. Jr. NF-kappaB induces expression of the Bcl-2 homologue A1/Bfl-1 to preferentially suppress chemotherapy-induced apoptosis. Mol Cell Biol. 1999, 19, 5923-5929.

[73] Fausto N., Laird A.D., Webber E.M. Liver regeneration. 2. Role of growth factors and cytokines in hepatic regeneration. FASEB J. 1995, 9, 1527-1536.

[74] Guo Q., Robinson N., Mattson M.P. Secreted beta-amyloid precursor protein counteracts the pro-apoptotic action of mutant presenilin-1 by activation of NF-kappaB and stabilization of calcium homeostasis. J Biol Chem. 1998, 273, 12341-12351.

[75] Hsu S.C., Gavrilin M.A., Lee H.H., Wu C.C., Han S.H., Lai M.Z. NF-kappa B-dependent Fas ligand expression. Eur J Immuno. 1999, 29, 2948-2956.

[76] Kavurma M.M., Khachigian L.M. Signaling and transcriptional control of Fas ligand gene expression. Cell Death Differ. 2003, 10, 36-44.

[77] Latinis K.M., Norian L.A., Eliason S.L., Koretzky G.A. Two NFAT transcription factor binding sites participate in the regulation of CD95 (Fas) ligand expression in activated human T cells. J Biol Chem. 1997, 272, 31427-31434.

[78] Rivera-Walsh I., Cvijic M.E., Xiao G., Sun S.C. The NF-kappa B signaling pathway is not required for Fas ligand gene induction but mediates protection from activation-induced cell death. J Biol Chem. 2000, 275, 25222-25230.

[79] Dejardin E., Deregowski V., Chapelier M., Jacobs N., Gielen J., Merville M.P., Bours V. Regulation of NF-kappaB activity by I kappaB-related proteins in adenocarcinoma cells. Oncogene. 1999, 18, 2567-2577.

[80] Devalaraja M.N., Wang D.Z., Ballard D.W., Richmond A. Elevated constitutive IkappaB kinase activity and IkappaB-alpha phosphorylation in Hs294T melanoma cells lead to increased basal MGSA/GRO-alpha transcription. Cancer Res. 1999, 59, 1372-1377.

[81] Gilmore T.D., Koedood M., Piffat K.A., White D.W. Rel/NF-kappaB/IkappaB proteins and cancer. Oncogene. 1996, 13, 1367-1378.

[82] Yang J., Liu X., Bhalla K., Kim C.N., Ibrado A.M., Cai J., Peng T.I., Jones D.P., Wang X. Prevention of apoptosis by Bcl-2: release of cytochrome c from mitochondria blocked. Science. 1997, 275, 1129-1132.

[83] Liang Y., Zhou Y., Shen P. NF-κB and its regulation on the immune system. Cell Mol Immunol. 2004, 1, 343-350.

[84] Ivanov V.N., Lee R.K., Podack E.R., Malek T.R. Regulation of Fas-dependent activation-induced T cell apoptosis by cAMP signaling: a potential role for transcription factor NF-kappa B. Oncogene. 1997, 14, 2455-2464.

[85] Dudley E., Hornung F., Zheng L., Scherer D., Ballard D., Lenardo M. NF-kappaB regulates Fas/APO-1/CD95- and TCR- mediated apoptosis of T lymphocytes. Eur J Immunol. 1999, 29, 878-886.

[86] Auphan N., DiDonato J.A., Rosette C., Helmberg A., Karin M. Immunosuppression by glucocorticoids: inhibition of NF-kappa B activity through induction of I kappa B synthesis. Science. 1995, 270, 286-290.

[87] Macho A., Decaudin D., Castedo M., Hirsch T., Susin S.A., Zamzami N., Kroemer G. Chloromethyl-X-rosamine – a fluorochrome for the determination of the mitochondrial transmembrane potential. Cytometry. 1998, 31, 75.

[88] Rasola A., Geuna M. A flow cytometry assay simultaneously detects independent apoptotic parameters. Cytometry. 2001, 45, 151-157.

[89] Stahnke K., Fulda S., Friesen C., Strauss G., Debatin K.M. Activation of apoptosis pathways in peripheral blood lymphocytes by in vivo chemotherapy. Blood. 2001, 98, 3066-3073.

[90] Vermes I., Haanen C., Reutelingsperger C. Flow cytometry of apoptotic cell death. J Immunol Methods. 2000, 243, 167-190.

[91] Green D.R., Kroemer G. Pharmacological manipulation of cell death: clinical applications in sight? J Clin Invest. 2005, 115, 2610-2617.

[92] Rostovtseva T., Colombini M. VDAC channels mediate and gate the flow of ATP: implications for the regulation of mitochondrial function. Biophys J. 1997, 72, 1954-1962.

[93] Rostovtseva T.K., Komarov A., Bezrukov S.M., Colombini M. VDAC channels differentiate between natural metabolites and synthetic molecules. J Membr Biol. 2002, 187, 147-156.

[94] Bossy-Wetzel E., Newmeyer D.D., Green D.R. Mitochondrial cytochrome c release in apoptosis occurs upstream of DEVD – specific caspase activation and independently of mitochondrial transmembrane depolarization. EMBO (Eur Mol Biol Organ) J. 1998, 17, 37-49.

[95] Helewski K.J., Kowalczyk-Ziomek G.I., Konecki J. Apoptoza i martwica – dwie drogi do jednego celu. Wiad Lek. 2006, 59, 679-684.

[96] Martinou J.C., Green D.R. Breaking the mitochondrial barrier. Nat Rev Mol Cell Biol. 2001, 2, 63-67.

[97] Bernardi P., Scorrano L., Colonna R., Petronilli V., Di Lisa F. Mitochondria and cell death. Mechanistic aspects and methodological issues. Eur J Biochem. 1999, 264, 687-701.
[98] Brenner C., Kroemer G. Apoptosis. Mitochondria--the death signal integrators. Science. 2000, 289, 1150-1151.
[99] Lanza L., Scudeletti M., Puppo F., Bosco O., Peirano L., Filaci G., Fecarotta E., Vidali G., Indiveri F. Prednisone increases apoptosis in in vitro activated human peripheral blood T lymphocytes. Clin Exp Immunol. 1996, 103, 482-490.
[100] Macho A., Decaudin D., Castedo M., Hirsch T., Susin S.A., Zamzami N., Kroemer G. Chloromethyl-X-rosamine is an aldehyde-fixable potential-sensitive fluorochrome for the detection of early apoptosis. Cytometry. 1996, 25, 333-340.
[101] Ateş A., Kinikli G., Turgay M., Duman M. The levels of serum-soluble Fas in patients with rheumatoid arthritis and systemic sclerosis. Clin Rheumatol. 2004, 23, 421-425.
[102] Takata-Tomokuni A., Ueki A., Shiwa M., Isozaki Y., Hatayama T., Katsuyama H., Hyodoh F., Fujimoto W., Ueki H., Kusaka M., Arikuni H., Otsuki T. Detection, epitope-mapping and function of anti-Fas autoantibody in patients with silicosis. Immunology. 2005, 116, 21-29.
[103] Wetzig T., Petri J.B., Mittag M., Haustein U.F. serum levels of soluble Fas/APO-1 receptor are increased in systemic sclerosis. Arch Dermatol Res. 1998, 290, 187-190.
[104] Arai H., Gordon D., Nabel E.G., Nabel G.J. Gene transfer of Fas ligand induces tumor regression in vivo. Proc Natl Acad Sci U S A. 1997, 94, 13862-13867.
[105] Watzlik A., Dufter C., Jung M., Opelz G., Terness P. Fas ligand gene-carrying adeno-5 AdE-asy viruses can be efficiently propagated in apoptosis-sensitive human embryonic retinoblast 911 cells. Gene Ther. 2000, 7, 70-74.
[106] Dziankowska-Bartkowiak B., Waszczykowska E., Zalewska A., Sysa-Jedrzejowska A. Evaluation of caspase 1 and sFas serum levels in patients with systemic sclerosis: correlation with lung dysfunction, joint and bone involvement. Mediators Inflamm. 2003, 12, 339-343.
[107] Cheng J., Zhou T., Liu C. Protection from Fas-mediated apoptosis by a soluble form of the Fas molecule. Science. 1994, 263, 1759-1762.
[108] Nozawa K., Kayagaki N., Tokano Y., Yagita H., Okumura K., Hasimoto H. Soluble Fas (APO-1, CD95) and soluble Fas ligand in rheumatic diseases. Arthritis Rheum. 1997, 40, 1126-1129.
[109] Goel N., Ulrich D.T., Clair W.S., Fleming J.A., Lynch D.H., Seldin M.F. Lack of correlation between serum soluble Fas/APO-1 levels and autoimmune disease. Arthritis Rheum. 1995, 38, 1738-1743.
[110] Tomokuni A., Aikoh T., Matsuki T., Isozaki Y., Otsuki T., Kita S., Ueki H., Kusaka M., Kishimoto T., Ueki A. Elevated soluble Fas/APO-1 (CD95) levels in silicosis patients without clinical symptoms of autoimmune diseases or malignant tumours. Clin Exp Immunol. 1997, 110, 303-309.
[111] Chung L., Lin J., Furst D.E., Fiorentino D. Systemic and localized scleroderma. Clin Dermatol. 2006, 24, 374-392.
[112] LeRoy E.C., Black C., Fleischmajer R., Jabłońska S., Krieg T., Medsger T.A. Jr, Rowell N., Wollheim F. Scleroderma (systemic sclerosis): classification, subsets and pathogenesis. J Rheumatol. 1988, 15, 202-205.
[113] LeRoy E.C., Medsger T.A. Jr. Criteria for the classification of early systemic sclerosis. J Rheumatol. 2001, 28, 1573-1576.
[114] Luzina I.G., Papadimitriou J.C., Anderson R., Pochetuhen K., Atamas S.P. Induction of prolonged infiltration of T lymphocytes and transient T lymphocyte-dependent

collagen deposition in mouse lungs following adenoviral gene transfer of CCL18. Arthritis Rheum. 2006, 54, 2643-2655.

[115] Kuwano K., Hagimoto N., Kawasaki M., Yatomi T., Nakamura N., Nagata S., Suda T., Kunitake R., Maeyama T., Miyazaki H., Hara N. Essential roles of the Fas-Fas ligand pathway in the development of pulmonary fibrosis. J Clin Invest. 1999, 104, 13-19.

[116] Reed J.C. Cytochrome c: can't live with it--can't live without it. Cell. 1997, 91, 559-562.

[117] Vempati U.D., Diaz F., Barrientos A., Narisawa S., Mian A.M., Millán J.L., Boise L.H., Moraes C.T. Role of cytochrome C in apoptosis: increased sensitivity to tumor necrosis factor alpha is associated with respiratory defects but not with lack of cytochrome C release. Mol Cell Biol. 2007, 27, 1771-1783.

[118] Li P., Nijhawan D., Budihardjo I., Srinivasula S.M., Ahmad M., Alnemri E.S., Wang X. Cytochrome c and dATP-dependent formation of Apaf-1/caspase-9 complex initiates an apoptotic protease cascade. Cell. 1997, 91, 479-489.

[119] Gupta S. Molecular steps of death receptor and mitochondrial pathways of apoptosis. Life Sci. 2001, 69, 2957-2964.

[120] Yao P.L., Lin Y.C., Sawhney P., Richburg J.H. Transcriptional regulation of FasL expression and participation of sTNF-alpha in response to sertoli cell injury. J Biol Chem. 2007, 282, 5420-5431.

[121] Hofmann K., Bucher P., Tschopp J. The CARD domain: a new apoptotic signalling motif. Trends Biochem Sci. 1997, 22, 155-156

[122] Johnson C.R., Jarvis W.D. Caspase-9 regulation: an update. Apoptosis. 2004, 9, 423-427.

[123] Kuida K. Caspase-9. Int J Biochem Cell Biol. 2000, 32, 121-124.

[124] Wang P., Shi T., Ma D. Cloning of a novel human caspase-9 splice variant containing only the CARD domain. Life Sci. 2006, 79, 934-940.

[125] Marsden V.S., O'Connor L., O'Reilly L.A., Silke J., Metcalf D., Ekert P.G., Huang D.C., Cecconi F., Kuida K., Tomaselli K.J., Roy S., Nicholson D.W., Vaux D.L., Bouillet P., Adams J.M., Strasser A. Apoptosis initiated by Bcl-2-regulated caspase activation independently of the cytochrome c/Apaf-1/caspase-9 apoptosome. Nature. 2002, 419, 634-637.

[126] Rao R.V., Castro-Obregon S., Frankowski H., Schuler M., Stoka V., del Rio G., Bredesen D.E., Ellerby H.M. Coupling endoplasmic reticulum stress to the cell death program. An Apaf-1-independent intrinsic pathway. J Biol Chem. 2002, 277, 21836-21842.

[127] Ho P.K., Hawkins C.J. Mammalian initiator apoptotic caspases. FEBS J. 2005, 272, 5436-5453.

[128] Korzeniewska-Dyl I. Kaspazy – struktura i funkcja. Pol Merk Lek 2007, 23, 403-407.

[129] Lavrik I.N., Golks A., Krammer P.H. Caspases: pharmacological manipulation of cell death. J Clin Invest. 2005, 115, 2665-2672.

[130] Cohen G.M. Caspases: the executioners of apoptosis. Biochem J. 1997, 326, 1-16.

[131] Susin S.A., Zamzami N., Castedo M., Daugas E., Wang H.G., Geley S., Fassy F., Reed J.C., Kroemer G. The central executioner of apoptosis: multiple links between protease activation and mitochondria in Fas/Apo-1/CD95- and ceramide - induced apoptosis. J Exp Med. 1997, 186, 25-37.

[132] Wolf B.B., Green D.R. Suicidal tendencies: apoptotic cell death by caspase family proteinases. J Biol Chem. 1999, 274, 20049-20052.

5

Cytokines in Systemic Sclerosis: Focus on IL-17

Julie Baraut[1], Dominique Farge[1,2], Elena Ivan-Grigore[1], Franck Verrecchia[3] and Laurence Michel[1]
[1]*Inserm U 976, Hôpital Saint-Louis, Paris,*
[2]*Service de Médecine Interne, Hôpital Saint-Louis, Paris,*
[3]*Inserm U 957, Laboratoire EA-3822, Université de Nantes, Nantes, France*

1. Introduction

Systemic sclerosis (SSc) is an autoimmune disease characterized by progressive sclerosis of the skin and internal organ dysfunction. Cytokine production and release are key events in SSc pathogenesis as they are involved in T and B cell activation leading to inflammation, auto-antibodies production, microvascular damage and fibrosis (Katsumoto et al. 2011). The Th1/Th2/Th17/Treg balance is one of the hallmarks of SSc pathogenesis, as the Th2 and Th17 cytokines response leads to tissue fibrosis, whereas Th1 and Th17 cytokines promote inflammation in SSc patients. In our previous review, we analyzed the relationship between cytokine release and SSc pathogenesis, based on experimental and clinical data. We concluded that circulating or in situ cytokine levels could be assessed as diagnostic and prognostic markers in SSc patients (Baraut et al. 2010).

The precise pathogenesis of SSc is still poorly understood. The use of microarray technology showed significant differences of gene patterns in skin biopsies from diffuse scleroderma (dSSc) and limited scleroderma (lSSc) patients, which also differed from normal controls (Milano et al. 2008). An immune signaling cluster was evidenced, suggestive for a role of B and T cells in SSc pathogenesis. Interleukin IL-1α, IL-4, tumor necrosis factor-α (TNF- α), connective tissue growth factor (CTGF), and transforming growth factor-β (TGF-β) have been identified as some relevant genes related to SSc disease. More recently, major contributions were made by experiments using genome-wide screening technology, which identified specific nucleotide polymorphisms (SNPs) in relevant genes related to SSc disease, including genes coding for cytokines and growth factors (Agarwal et al. 2008). The first genome-wide association study (GWAS), performed in Korean patients and confirmed in US Caucasians population, indicated that specific SNPs of HLA-DPB1 and/or DPB2 were strongly associated with SSc patients who had anti-DNA topoisomerase I or anticentromere autoantibodies (X. Zhou et al. 2009). More recently, a larger GWAS identified a new susceptibility locus for SSc susceptibility, previously found in systemic lupus erythematosus, at CD247 (T cell receptor T3 zeta chain). The role of Major Histocompatibility complex (MHC), Interferon regulatory factor 5 (IRF5) and STAT4 gene regions as SSc genetic risk factors has also been confirmed in this recent GWAS study (Radstake et al. 2010). GWAS approaches have identified multiple genetic markers related to innate and adaptive immunity as SSc susceptibility, such as HLA class II, STAT-4, IRF5, B cell scaffold protein BANK1, B lymphocyte kinase (BLK), Tumor necrosis factor ligand super-family member 4 (TNFSF4) and CD247 genes (Romano et al. 2011). However no GWAS have been preformed to clarify the role of genes involved in vascular and fibrotic processes in SSc susceptibility.

2. Th17 lineage differentiation

The identification of a new subset of inflammatory T cells distinct from Th1 and Th2 cells, so-called Th17 T cells, secreting interleukin IL-17A/F, IL-21 and IL-22, which play a major role in inflammation, has significantly improved our understanding of autoimmune diseases. Th17 cell differentiation can be induced by the combination of TGF-β and IL-6 or IL-21 (Dong 2008). IL-1 also plays a crucial role in early Th17 cell differentiation (Chung et al. 2009). Moreover, development and propagation of the Th17 lineage requires IL-1, IL-6, IL-23, and TGF-β stimulation, whereas Th17 differentiation is inhibited by IFN-γ and IL-4 (Harrington et al. 2005). The pro-inflammatory cytokine IL-23 is involved in Th17-mediated immune pathology since IL-23-deficient (p19−/−) mice contain very few Th17 cells and are protected from autoimmune diseases such as experimental autoimmune encephalomyelitis (EAE) and collagen-induced arthritis. However IL-23 is not required for the differentiation of Th17 from naïve CD4 T cells. Several transcription factors have been shown as critical regulators of Th17 cell differentiation (Dong 2011). STAT3 has been reported to be a crucial component of IL-6 and IL-21-mediated Th17-cell regulation. Moreover, STAT3 deficiency greatly decreased the expression of RORγt and RORα, transcriptions factors that drives Th17-cell lineage differentiation. RORγt and RORα overexpression are induced by TGFβ or IL-6 and promote Th17-cell differentiation. Both transcription factors RORγt and RORα have a synergistic effect in promoting Th17-cell differentiation and have similar and redundant functions. Furthermore, Smad2 was reported by several groups to positively regulate Th17 cell differentiation and Th17 immune response *in vivo* during pathogen infection or in autoimmune disease (Malhotra et al. 2010) (Martinez et al. 2010) (Takimoto et al. 2010). Smad2 might be a co-factor for RORγt to mediate the expression of Th17-specific genes (Martinez et al. 2010). In addition to the ROR, STAT and Smad factors, interferon-regulatory factor 4 (IRF4) was recently shown to be essential for Th17-cell differentiation upstream of RORγt (Brüstle et al. 2007). Other transcription factors such as the aryl hydrocarbon receptor (AHR), Batf (member of AP-1 transcription factor family), IκBζ (encoded by the Nfkbiz gene) have recently been shown to be required for Th17 cell development (Dong 2011).

Differentiation of Th17 and regulatory T cells, both of which depend on TGF-β, shares a reciprocal regulation. In relation with tolerance induction, TGF-β is able to increase Foxp3 levels and reduces IL-23R expression shifting the differentiation of Th cells from Th17 towards regulatory T cells (L. Zhou et al. 2008). Foxp3 interacts with RORs and recruits histone deacetylases to Th17-specific genes, thus inhibiting the transcriptional activity of RORγt genes (X. O. Yang et al. 2008). Although Foxp3 has a strong inhibitory role in Th17 differentiation, IL-6 has been found to down-regulate Foxp3 expression in TGFβ-induced and thymically derived Treg cells and together with IL-1, to upregulate Th17-specific gene expression (X. O. Yang et al. 2008) (L. Xu et al. 2007).

In addition to Th17 cells, a wide variety of T cells also produce IL-17A and IL-17F: cytotoxic CD8+ T cells (Tc17), distinct populations of γδT (γδ-17) cells, NKT (NKT-17) cells, neutrophils, monocytes and lymphoid tissue inducer (LTi)-like cells (Iwakura et al. 2011).
NKT-17 and γδ-17 cells rapidly produce IL-17A and IL-17F in response to pro-inflammatory cytokine stimulation and may therefore provide an essential initial source of these two cytokines. In contrast to naive $CD4^+$ and $CD8^+$ T cells, IL-23 and IL-1 can directly induce γδ-17 cell development in the absence of IL-6 and TCR ligation because they constitutively express IL-23R, IL-1R, and RORγt.
Th17 which is a distinct lineage of T cells bridging the innate and adaptive immunity, is characterized by expression of the transcription factors RORγt and RORα, as well as the surface markers CCR4, CCR6 and IL-23R, the production of the potent proinflammatory molecules IL-17, IL-17F, IL-21, IL-22, IL-26 and G-CSF as well as the chemokine CCL20. However, the mechanisms underlying the generation of these cells *in vivo* remain incomplete.

3. Th17 involvement in inflammation and fibrosis

Th17 effectors, IL-17A/F, IL-21 and IL-22, encompass both pro-inflammatory and pro-fibrotic characteristics, suggesting that this cell type may act as an intermediate between the Th1 and Th2 lineages. Indeed, IL-17 has been shown to enhance the secretion of the pro-inflammatory and pro-fibrotic cytokines IL-6 and IL-8 from fibroblasts (Fossiez et al. 1996). Both IL-17 and IL-22 are mainly produced by Th17 cells and promote production of antimicrobial peptides (Liang et al. 2006) constituting thereby a link between innate and adaptive responses (Stockinger et al. 2007).
Several studies have shown implication of Th17 cytokines in rheumatoid arthritis, asthma, psoriasis, multiple sclerosis, systemic lupus erythematous, inflammatory bowel disease, graft versus host (GVH), autoimmune diabetes, Sjogren's syndrome, autoimmune thyroid diseases and thrombocytopenia (Stockinger & Veldhoen 2007) (Hemdan et al. 2010). Th17 cells have been implicated as the pivotal driving force of autoimmune inflammation in several animal models of human autoimmune diseases, including autoimmune colitis (Elson et al. 2007), experimental autoimmune encephalomyelitis (Langrish et al. 2005), collagen-induced arthritis (CIA) (Nakae et al. 2003), and rat adjuvant-induced arthritis (AIA) (Bush et al. 2002).
It has been demonstrated that IL-17A and IL-17F contribute to rheumatoid arthritis (RA) pathogenesis by inducing specific expression patterns in RA synovial fibroblasts (Fossiez et al. 1996). They enhance their response by stabilizing mRNA of IL-6 and IL-8 cytokines (Hot & P. Miossec 2011) and enhancing IL-17RA and IL-17RC receptor expression (Zrioual et al. 2008) in the presence of TNFα. They contribute to the inflammatory cell accumulation by increasing migration, chemokine gene expression (CXCL12 and its receptor CXCR4, CCL20) and invasiveness of synoviocytes (K.-W. Kim et al. 2007) (Hirota et al. 2007). Moreover, they induce up-regulation of RANKL, an important positive regulator of osteoclastogenesis (Kelchtermans et al. 2009). They contribute to disease chronicity by inhibiting synoviocyte apoptosis (Toh et al. 2010). Finally, they enhance metalloprotease secretion, such as MMP-1, -2, -9 and -13 leading to cartilage damage (Moran et al. 2009). A recent study demonstrated that Th17 cells mediate inflammation at very early stages of RA development and progression (Leipe et al. 2010). They showed an impaired inhibition of Th17 cell development in RA leading to increased frequencies of Th17 cells together with enhanced production of IL-17.

Recently, a role of IL-17 in SSc pathogenesis has been shown. First, Kurasama et al. demonstrated that IL-17 is overproduced by T cells from the peripheral blood and fibrotic lesions of the skin and lungs in SSc patients (Kurasawa et al. 2000). They reported that IL-17 also enhances the proliferation of fibroblasts and induces the expression of adhesion molecules and IL-1 production in endothelial cells *in vitro*, while no collagen stimulation was observed. This study also demonstrated that IL-17 overproduction was involved in the early stage of SSc pathogenesis. Consistent with this report, another study showed that IL-17 production was transiently increased in the earlier phase of the disease (Murata et al. 2008). More recently, Radstake et al. described increase levels of activated $CD4^+$ cells in SSc patients compared to healthy controls and $CD4^+$ lymphocytes (activated or not) highly expressed the IL23R, which was associated with a higher IL-17 expression. They also observed increased levels of IL-6, IL-23 and IL-1α cytokines in SSc patients, which all induced IL-17 production (Radstake et al. 2009). Furthermore, IL-21 cytokine, which is mainly produced by Th17 and NK cells, potentiates Th17 inflammatory response via stimulation of IL-23 receptor expression and Treg inhibition. IL-21 can also regulate the Th1/Th2 response and Ig production (Wurster et al. 2002). It has been demonstrated that cell adhesions molecules such as L-selectin and ICAM-1 were able to regulate Th2 and Th17 cell accumulation into the skin and lung, leading to the development of fibrosis, whereas P-selectin, E-selectin, and PSGL-1 regulated Th1 cell infiltration, resulting in the inhibition of fibrosis (Yoshizaki et al. 2010).

4. IL-17 and auto-immunity

Distinct from its pro-inflammatory effects, IL-17 promotes autoimmune disease by enhancing formation of spontaneous germinal centers (GCs), as shown by autoimmune BXD2 recombinant inbred mouse strain which spontaneously develop glomerulonephritis and erosive arthritis. These mice express more IL-17 than wild-type counterparts and show spontaneous development of GCs by retaining B cells and promoting CD4 T-cell and B-cell interactions, resulting in increased autoimmune antibodies (Hsu et al. 2008). Furthermore, long-lasting apoptosis-resistant Th17 cells activate B cells and their immunoglobulin production mediated by IL-21.

Effects of IL-17 on B-cell activation and antibody production have been also described recently. Milovanovic and colleagues' study showed that IL-17A enhances IgE production (Milovanovic et al. 2010). Indeed, depletion of Th17 cells *in vitro* from allergic patients' blood cells induced a decrease in IgE production; addition of IL-17A in the depleted cultures reversed IgE reduction. In this study, PBMC cultures were stimulated with IL-17 + IL-4, this leading to memory B-cell activation, IgE class switching and differentiation into plasma cells.

Interestingly, a novel population of CD4 memory T cells (Th17/Th2) that produce both IL-17 and IL-4 has recently been described (Cosmi et al. 2010). IL-17 and IL-4-coproducing CD4 T cells were increased in the circulation of patients with severe asthma. This could explain the relationship between Th17 cells and increased IgE levels observed in this disease.

Moreover, the gene encoding for IL-23 receptor has been identified as a susceptibility gene for SSc development, and IL-23R polymorphisms are associated with anti-topoisomerase-I positivity and lower frequency of pulmonary hypertension (Agarwal et al. 2009).

5. IL-17 and tolerance

Th17 and Treg differentiations are interconnected as previously introduced upper. Indeed, naïve T cells can differentiate into Treg cells in response to TGF-β, whereas in the presence of TGF-β plus IL-6/IL-21, they will differentiate into Th17 lineage (Bettelli et al. 2006). Treg and Th17 cells are reciprocally regulated via the induction of the transcription factors Foxp3 and RORγt, respectively, together in the presence of low or high levels of IL-6. The increase in IL-6 production inhibits Th1 and Treg cells and with low TGF-β levels promotes differentiation of Th17 cells with a regulatory function. They still need support of IL-23 to attain their full effectors' potency with capacity to produce IL-22, CXC chemokines, antimicrobial peptides and IL-21. The present literature clearly indicates that IL-6 and IL-21 play a major role in dictating how the immune response will be dominated by pro-inflammatory Th17 cells or by protective Treg.

6. IL-17 measurement in SSc serum before and after HSCT

Autologous hematopoietic stem cell transplantation (HSCT) has been shown as a promising treatment modality for severe and refractory autoimmune disorders, especially in diffuse systemic sclerosis (Farge et al. 2002). Our data and others demonstrate that HSCT induced a significant, progressive and sustained reduction of the modified Rodnan skin score (mRSS) throughout follow-up, 4 years (M48) after HSCT (Vonk et al. 2008). In this context, we analysed the IL-17 profile before and up to 4 years after HSCT and its potential correlation with skin involvement in patients treated for diffuse systemic cutaneous sclerosis (SSc). Our results showed that IL-17 levels were significantly higher in SSc compared to control sera from healthy donors (106.7±33.7pg/ml (n=16) *vs* 24.2±8.6pg/ml (n=6), $p<0.05$) (Fig.1). IL-17 levels observed in SSc patients were similar to those observed in psoriasis patients (137.8±70.5/ml (n=3)). In regards to HSCT follow-up, serum IL-17 levels were measured at 6, 12, 24, 36, 48 months after HSCT in SSc patients. As compared to initial levels, IL-17 levels were reduced at M6 (39.3±17.6pg/ml), but not significantly because of the wide-range of inter-individual variations (Fig.2). A progressive recovery was observed throughout follow up to 183.9±63.7pg/ml 4 years (M48) after HSCT (Fig.2). This observation confirmed the involvement of IL-17 in the pathogenesis of SSc and the efficacy of HSCT to down-regulate IL-17 initially levels. The increase observed after 6 months after HSCT cannot be involved in the fibrotic process since we observed reduction of Rodnan skin score throughout follow-up. More patients treated by HSCT must be further investigated during long-term follow-up to conclude about IL-17 involvement and cellular origin of this cytokine in the immune reconstitution. Our previous report showed that 4 years after HSCT, pro-fibrotic (VEGF, MCP1) and Th2 (IL-6, IL-8,) cytokines were significantly decreased and associated with the progressive and sustained reduction of the Rodnan skin score (Michel et al. 2011 submitted). That cytokine changes coincided with increasing numbers of reemerging CD3+ CD4+ T cells and memory CD4+CD45RA+RO-CD4+ T cells in SSc patients. It might be suggested that IL-17 progressive increase observed after HSCT could be due to an active and efficient immune reconstitution.

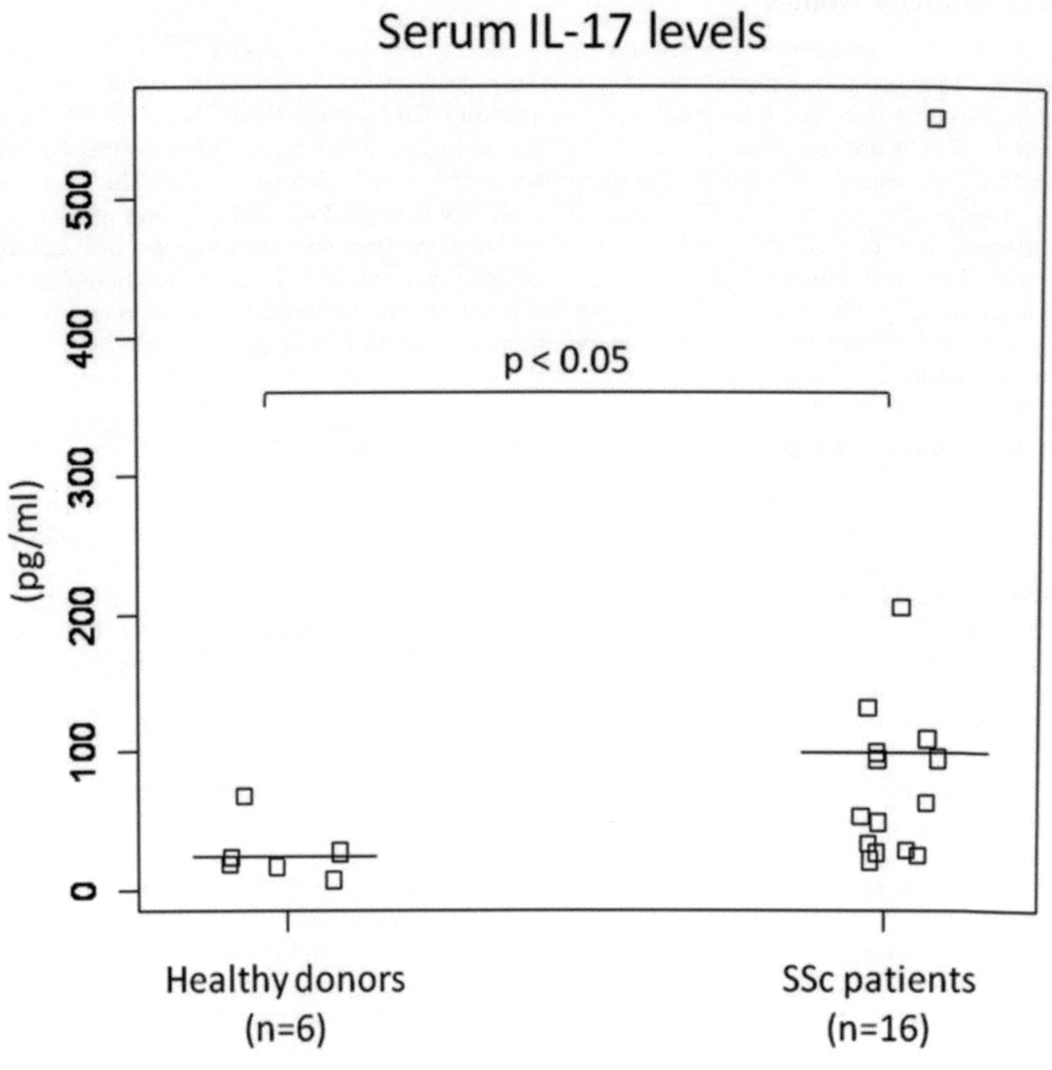

Fig. 1. Serum levels of interleukin 17 (IL-17) in patients with systemic sclerosis (SSc) and healthy donors

Serum levels of IL-17 were determined by a specific ELISA (R&D Systems Inc., Minneapolis, MN, USA) in patients with systemic sclerosis (SSc) and healthy donors. Data are presented as dot plots and the lines indicate the mean values. IL-17 levels are expressed in pg/ml.

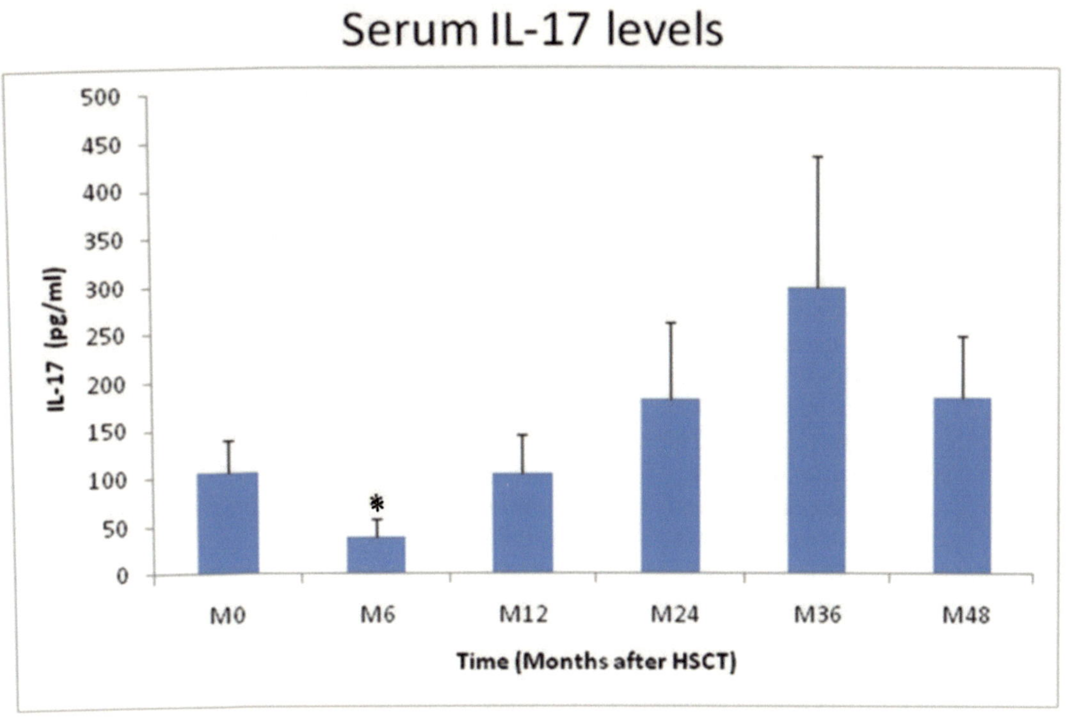

Fig. 2. Serum interleukin 17 (IL-17) levels in SSc patients after HSCT

Serum interleukin 17 (IL-17) levels at M0 and following HSCT (M: month) in 6 patients with systemic sclerosis (SSc). Mean (±SD) levels of IL-17 detected in the serum by ELISA assay are expressed in pg/ml.
*$p<0.05$, significant difference between mean levels at M6 compared with basal level detected at M0.

7. Conclusion

Th17 cells have been implicated as the pivotal driving force of autoimmune inflammation and fibrosis in several animal models and autoimmune diseases. Several studies showed that circulating and *in situ* IL-17 levels are up regulated in SSc patients. It is well known that IL-17 plays a major role in the pathogenesis of SSc through its involvement in the inflammation process, the fibrosis and the auto-antibody production, as confirmed by our present data.

8. References

Agarwal, S.K., Gourh, P., et al., 2009. Association of interleukin 23 receptor polymorphisms with anti-topoisomerase-I positivity and pulmonary hypertension in systemic sclerosis. *The Journal of Rheumatology*, 36(12), p.2715-2723.

Agarwal, S.K., Tan, F.K. & Arnett, F.C., 2008. Genetics and genomic studies in scleroderma (systemic sclerosis). *Rheumatic Diseases Clinics of North America*, 34(1), p.17-40; v.

Baraut, J. et al., 2010. Relationship between cytokine profiles and clinical outcomes in patients with systemic sclerosis. *Autoimmunity Reviews*, 10(2), p.65-73.

Bettelli, E. et al., 2006. Reciprocal developmental pathways for the generation of pathogenic effector TH17 and regulatory T cells. *Nature*, 441(7090), p.235-238.

Brüstle, A. et al., 2007. The development of inflammatory T(H)-17 cells requires interferon-regulatory factor 4. *Nature Immunology*, 8(9), p.958-966.

Bush, K.A. et al., 2002. Reduction of joint inflammation and bone erosion in rat adjuvant arthritis by treatment with interleukin-17 receptor IgG1 Fc fusion protein. *Arthritis and Rheumatism*, 46(3), p.802-805.

Chung, Y. et al., 2009. Critical regulation of early Th17 cell differentiation by interleukin-1 signaling. *Immunity*, 30(4), p.576-587.

Cosmi, L. et al., 2010. Identification of a novel subset of human circulating memory CD4(+) T cells that produce both IL-17A and IL-4. *The Journal of Allergy and Clinical Immunology*, 125(1), p.222-230.e1-4.

Dong, C., 2011. Genetic controls of Th17 cell differentiation and plasticity. , 43(1), p.1-6.

Dong, C., 2008. Regulation and pro-inflammatory function of interleukin-17 family cytokines. *Immunological Reviews*, 226, p.80-86.

Elson, C.O. et al., 2007. Monoclonal anti-interleukin 23 reverses active colitis in a T cell-mediated model in mice. *Gastroenterology*, 132(7), p.2359-2370.

Farge, Dominique et al., 2002. Autologous bone marrow transplantation in the treatment of refractory systemic sclerosis: early results from a French multicentre phase I-II study. *British Journal of Haematology*, 119(3), p.726-739.

Fossiez, F. et al., 1996. T cell interleukin-17 induces stromal cells to produce proinflammatory and hematopoietic cytokines. *The Journal of Experimental Medicine*, 183(6), p.2593-2603.

Harrington, L.E. et al., 2005. Interleukin 17-producing CD4+ effector T cells develop via a lineage distinct from the T helper type 1 and 2 lineages. *Nature Immunology*, 6(11), p.1123-1132.

Hemdan, N.Y.A. et al., 2010. Interleukin-17-producing T helper cells in autoimmunity. *Autoimmunity Reviews*, 9(11), p.785-792.

Hirota, K. et al., 2007. Preferential recruitment of CCR6-expressing Th17 cells to inflamed joints via CCL20 in rheumatoid arthritis and its animal model. *The Journal of Experimental Medicine*, 204(12), p.2803-2812.

Hot, A. & Miossec, P., 2011. Effects of interleukin (IL)-17A and IL-17F in human rheumatoid arthritis synoviocytes. *Annals of the Rheumatic Diseases*, 70(5), p.727-732.

Hsu, H.-C. et al., 2008. Interleukin 17-producing T helper cells and interleukin 17 orchestrate autoreactive germinal center development in autoimmune BXD2 mice. *Nature Immunology*, 9(2), p.166-175.

Iwakura, Y. et al., 2011. Functional specialization of interleukin-17 family members. *Immunity*, 34(2), p.149-162.

Katsumoto, T.R., Whitfield, M.L. & Connolly, M.K., 2011. The pathogenesis of systemic sclerosis. *Annual Review of Pathology*, 6, p.509-537.

Kelchtermans, H. et al., 2009. Effector mechanisms of interleukin-17 in collagen-induced arthritis in the absence of interferon-gamma and counteraction by interferon-gamma. *Arthritis Research & Therapy*, 11(4), p.R122.

Kim, K.-W. et al., 2007. Up-regulation of stromal cell-derived factor 1 (CXCL12) production in rheumatoid synovial fibroblasts through interactions with T lymphocytes: role of interleukin-17 and CD40L-CD40 interaction. *Arthritis and Rheumatism*, 56(4), p.1076-1086.

Kurasawa, K. et al., 2000. Increased interleukin-17 production in patients with systemic sclerosis. *Arthritis and Rheumatism*, 43(11), p.2455-2463.

Langrish, C.L. et al., 2005. IL-23 drives a pathogenic T cell population that induces autoimmune inflammation. *The Journal of Experimental Medicine*, 201(2), p.233-240.

Leipe, J. et al., 2010. Role of Th17 cells in human autoimmune arthritis. *Arthritis and Rheumatism*, 62(10), p.2876-2885.

Liang, S.C. et al., 2006. Interleukin (IL)-22 and IL-17 are coexpressed by Th17 cells and cooperatively enhance expression of antimicrobial peptides. *The Journal of Experimental Medicine*, 203(10), p.2271-2279.

Malhotra, N., Robertson, E. & Kang, J., 2010. SMAD2 is essential for TGF beta-mediated Th17 cell generation. *The Journal of Biological Chemistry*, 285(38), p.29044-29048.

Martinez, G.J. et al., 2010. Smad2 positively regulates the generation of Th17 cells. *The Journal of Biological Chemistry*, 285(38), p.29039-29043.

Milano, A. et al., 2008. Molecular Subsets in the Gene Expression Signatures of Scleroderma Skin G. Butler, éd. *PLoS ONE*, 3(7), p.e2696.

Milovanovic, M. et al., 2010. Interleukin-17A promotes IgE production in human B cells. *The Journal of Investigative Dermatology*, 130(11), p.2621-2628.

Moran, E.M. et al., 2009. Human rheumatoid arthritis tissue production of IL-17A drives matrix and cartilage degradation: synergy with tumour necrosis factor-alpha, Oncostatin M and response to biologic therapies. *Arthritis Research & Therapy*, 11(4), p.R113.

Murata, M. et al., 2008. Clinical association of serum interleukin-17 levels in systemic sclerosis: is systemic sclerosis a Th17 disease? *Journal of Dermatological Science*, 50(3), p.240-242.

Nakae, S. et al., 2003. Suppression of immune induction of collagen-induced arthritis in IL-17-deficient mice. *Journal of Immunology (Baltimore, Md.: 1950)*, 171(11), p.6173-6177.

Radstake, T.R.D.J. et al., 2009. The pronounced Th17 profile in systemic sclerosis (SSc) together with intracellular expression of TGFbeta and IFNgamma distinguishes SSc phenotypes. *PloS One*, 4(6), p.e5903.

Radstake, T.R.D.J. et al., 2010. Genome-wide association study of systemic sclerosis identifies CD247 as a new susceptibility locus. *Nature Genetics*, 42(5), p.426-429.

Romano, E. et al., 2011. The genetics of systemic sclerosis: an update. *Clinical and Experimental Rheumatology*, 29(2 Suppl 65), p.S75-86.

Stockinger, B. & Veldhoen, M., 2007. Differentiation and function of Th17 T cells. *Current Opinion in Immunology*, 19(3), p.281-286.

Stockinger, B., Veldhoen, M. & Martin, B., 2007. Th17 T cells: linking innate and adaptive immunity. *Seminars in Immunology*, 19(6), p.353-361.

Takimoto, T. et al., 2010. Smad2 and Smad3 are redundantly essential for the TGF-beta-mediated regulation of regulatory T plasticity and Th1 development. *Journal of Immunology (Baltimore, Md.: 1950)*, 185(2), p.842-855.

Toh, M.-L. et al., 2010. Role of interleukin 17 in arthritis chronicity through survival of synoviocytes via regulation of synoviolin expression. *PloS One*, 5(10), p.e13416.

Vonk, M.C. et al., 2008. Long-term follow-up results after autologous haematopoietic stem cell transplantation for severe systemic sclerosis. *Annals of the Rheumatic Diseases*, 67(1), p.98-104.

Wurster, A.L. et al., 2002. Interleukin 21 Is a T Helper (Th) Cell 2 Cytokine that Specifically Inhibits the Differentiation of Naive Th Cells into Interferon {gamma}-producing Th1 Cells. *J. Exp. Med.*, 196(7), p.969-977.

Xu, L. et al., 2007. Cutting edge: regulatory T cells induce CD4+CD25-Foxp3- T cells or are self-induced to become Th17 cells in the absence of exogenous TGF-beta. *Journal of Immunology (Baltimore, Md.: 1950)*, 178(11), p.6725-6729.

Yang, X.O. et al., 2008. T helper 17 lineage differentiation is programmed by orphan nuclear receptors ROR alpha and ROR gamma. *Immunity*, 28(1), p.29-39.

Yoshizaki, A. et al., 2010. Cell adhesion molecules regulate fibrotic process via Th1/Th2/Th17 cell balance in a bleomycin-induced scleroderma model. *Journal of Immunology (Baltimore, Md.: 1950)*, 185(4), p.2502-2515.

Zhou, L. et al., 2008. TGF-beta-induced Foxp3 inhibits T(H)17 cell differentiation by antagonizing RORgammat function. *Nature*, 453(7192), p.236-240.

Zhou, X. et al., 2009. HLA-DPB1 and DPB2 are genetic loci for systemic sclerosis: a genome-wide association study in Koreans with replication in North Americans. *Arthritis and Rheumatism*, 60(12), p.3807-3814.

Zrioual, S. et al., 2008. IL-17RA and IL-17RC receptors are essential for IL-17A-induced ELR+ CXC chemokine expression in synoviocytes and are overexpressed in rheumatoid blood. *Journal of Immunology (Baltimore, Md.: 1950)*, 180(1), p.655-663.

6

Biological Ageing Research in Systemic Sclerosis: Time to Grow up?

J.C.A. Broen[1,2], L. McGlynn[2], Timothy Radstake[1,3] and P.G. Shiels[2]
[1]Department of Rheumatology, Radboud University Medical Center, Nijmegen,
[2]University of Glasgow, MVLS, Glasgow,
[3]The Scleroderma Center, Boston University School of Medicine, Massachusetts,
[1]The Netherlands
[2]United Kingdom
[3]U.S.A.

1. Introduction

Systemic Sclerosis (SSc) is an autoimmune disease that is typified by several characteristic hallmarks such as vasculopathy, immune activation and extensive fibrosis of the skin and inner organs (1). Although the disease has an overwhelming effect on morbidity and mortality, a cure or even a well defined pathogenic chain of events remains to be discovered. SSc is quite a rare disease (prevalence between 3 and 24 per 100,000 persons) and as a consequence, it has taken a relatively long time to define well-recognised classification criteria. This initially hindered detailed research into the pathogenesis of this debilitating disease (2-7). However, during the last 20 years research has intensified and several significant leaps forward have been made, assessing susceptibility risk either via epidemiologic/environmental or genetic research. SSc susceptibility disease does not show typical Mendelian heritability, but appears multi-factorial, with an onset later in life. This implies that the effects of many small genetic variations may combine over time to precipitate the disease in a SSc susceptible individual. Recently, this dogma was further underscored by a genome wide association study in SSc, showing that there was not one single genetic factor posing enough risk to be fully accountable for SSc development (8). However, investigations of interaction networks composed of multiple genetic risk variants, which together culminate in a higher disease risk, are just starting in this field (9-10).
Research focusing on environmental factors has initially yielded some interesting results. Environmental risk factors range from exposure to solvents and silicone breast implants, as well as CMV and parvo B19 virus infection (11,12). Although interesting, these results remain not well established, due to the lack of replication or small cohort size (11). Silica exposure is an exception and seems to be a rather reproducible risk factor among multiple small cohorts and case-series. This even led to the incorporation of SSc in insurance fees for silica workers in some countries (11). Next to these associations, a few studies failed to show an association between silica and SSc risk. A recently published and highly anticipated meta-analysis on this matter was severely hampered by heterogeneity in the methods used by the separate studies (13).

When we overview the results from these two fields of interest in SSc research, it becomes clear that the risk for developing SSc is highly unlikely to be fully explained by genetic factors on the one hand, but that the field of epidemiology failed to identify clear environmental factors on the other hand. Hence, these observations are suggestive for the presence of more subtle processes that may be involved in determining disease on a genetically susceptible background. Since SSc rarely develops at very young age, it is logical to suppose that these processes may take place in the temporal dimension. More specifically, ageing at the level of cells, tissues and organs, i.e. biological as opposed to chronological ageing, might have an impact on development of the disease and has been increasingly implicated in SSc pathogenesis over the last few years. This review aims at critically describing findings coming forth from this area of research and attempts to place them in a hypothetical framework with regard to SSc pathogenesis.

2. What is biological ageing, how is it defined and how is it measured

Biological ageing is ageing at the level of a cell, tissue or organ and by extrapolation the whole organism. It need not necessarily equate with the chronological age of the individual. Indeed, it can be used to explain inter-individual variation in the rate of ageing between individuals of the same chronological age. Extrapolation of cellular ageing to the level of the tissue or organ, or the whole organism, is not straightforward. To do so, one must take account of the number of senescent cells (generated by both replicative senescence and stress or aberrant signaling-induced senescence (STASIS)), their location and similarly the number and location of cells lost through insult, in each respective organ or tissue, to gauge properly the effect on its functional capacity. Typically, functional capacity would be expected to decline with increasing biological age. The rate of biological ageing is influenced by the levels of oxidative insult at a cellular level, by lifestyle, socio-economic factors and environmental factors.

3. Telomeres

Telomeres are specialized nucleoprotein complexes at the end of eukaryotic chromosomes. They comprise tandem TTAGGG repeat arrays bound to a variety of proteins with roles in chromosomal protection, nuclear attachment and replication. Telomeres function to cap the chromosome, preventing chromosomal fusions and the recognition of the chromosome end as a DNA break. Telomeres facilitate chromosomal attachment within the correct sub-cellular compartment and have a critical role in DNA replication. The proteinaceous component of the telomere helps maintaining its structural integrity and functions in sensing, signalling and repair of DNA damage (14). The length of telomeric DNA repeats shortens during the ageing of cultured somatic cells (e.g. fibroblasts, peripheral blood lymphocytes and colon epithelia), but the rate of shortening is also under both polygenic and environmental influences (15,16). As a consequence, telomere length reflects the "miles on the clock" of a given individual or cell type. The characteristic telomeric repeats typically end in a 3' single guanine strand overhang (17). This is folded back into a double loop structure, comprising a large telomeric loop (the T loop) with the single stranded repeat invading the adjacent double stranded DNA helix to form a second loop, called the displacement, or D loop. This loop is stabilized by, and dependent on, a cluster of proteins called the shelterin complex, which allows cells to distinguish telomeres from sites of DNA damage. (18).

Of interest in this respect, is another, non shelterin, telomeric protein, the Werner syndrome protein (WRN) protein, which is involved inthe maintenance of telomeric stability (19,20). Mutations in the WRN gene cause the progeroid condition Werner syndrome. Notably, this syndrome is macroscopically quite similar to SSc, with features of scleroderma like skin changes, calcinosis cutis and ulcera and therefore is advocated to be entitled a place in the differential diagnosis when considering SSc (21-23). However, the syndrome has also many features, such as hyperglycemia and osteoporosis that are atypical for SSc and Werner's is virtually never accompanied by Raynaud's phenomenom or the typical SSc related auto-antibodies (23).

Increased chromosomal damage has been repeatedly reported in SSc lymphocytes as well as fibroblasts, (24-29). Most authors advocate that such damage is due to a higher amount of oxidative damage, caused by the production of reactive oxygen species (ROS) in the SSc inflammatory state (24, 25). In addition, SSc fibroblasts produce more ROS than their healthy counterparts. It is reasonable to expect that in the presence of such elevated levels of ROS, that telomere biology would be implicated in the chromosomal abberances observed in SSc.

An initial study investigated telomere lengths of peripheral blood leukocytes (PBLs) and fibroblasts from 43 SSc patients, 182 SSc family members and 96 age-matched controls restriction fragment length polymorphism (RFLP) and chemiluminescent labelled probes. They observed an average loss of telomeric DNA in PBLs from SSc patients and their family members of 3 kb compared to the controls. This loss withstood correction for age and disease duration. Of interest, although telomeres in SSc fibroblasts were shorter overall compared to healthy control fibroblasts, this difference was not significant. The investigators did not observe an association with antibody profiles and telomere shortening. Furthermore, family members of SSc patients often had shorter telomeres compared to the patients. Two things can be distilled from this observation. Firstly, it seems unlikely that the telomeres shorten as a consequence of the disease, but that shorter telomeres are a risk factor for SSc themselves, or a secondary effect from another risk factor. Secondly, following from the previous hypthesis, this risk factor might very well be a genetic one, considering the familial occurrence of the shortened telomeres regardless of age (30).

Another study addressing telomere length in SSc focused solely on females with the lcSSc phenotype. Forty-three lcSSc patients with an age ranging from 37 to 80 years were included. Terminal restriction fragment (TRF) analyses were used to determine telomere lengths in this study. Regression analysis showed significantly longer mean TRF lengths in lcSSc patients compared to their age-matched healthy counterparts. Moreover, these telomeres did not show any attrition, usually observed with ageing. When the authors analyzed the results by defined age groups, the difference between the lcSSc and control telomere lengths was only significant beyond the fifth decade. Below 50 years of age, no difference was observed between healthy females and females with lcSSc. Noteworthy, patients using non-steroid anti-inflammatory drugs (n=3) were observed to have longer telomeres, than those not on NSAIDs (n=17) (31). It is noteworthy that using Southern blotting to determine terminal restriction fragment lengths also includes detection of subtelomeric region sequences which are known to show interindividual variation. Consequently, these observations may indicate a subtelomeric component in lcSSc and masking TTAGGG repeat attrition, simply as a matter of methodology.

Until now, literature addressing the role of telomeres in SSc appears conflicting, but this may be due to the different clinical subsets of SSc investigated by these studies and or methodological differences (see above). In this aspect it is important to note that each single telomeric repeat is a potential topoisomerase cleavage site (32). Since anti-topoisomerase antibody (ATA) positive patients are usually not of the lcSSc subset but from the dcSSc subset, it is tempting to speculate that the presence of these antibodies contributes to the differences between the studies. This is likely considering the first study included 40% patients with dcSSc. Although the study states no differences were observed with the antibody status of these patients, the authors do not provide numbers or data on this matter. When considering the size of both these studies, it is yet unlikely that they harbour enough power to provide a conclusive answer on the involvement of ATA+ in telomere shortening. A second point of consideration is the dissimilar methodology used in both studies. Both studies used different percentage gels affecting resolution; this is partially reflected by the differences in variation of the mean TRF, which was remarkably larger in the initial study. Considering the currently increasing amount of discrepancies coming forth from the use of diverse methodologies in telomere measurements, a study with a sufficient number of fully clinically characterized patients, analyzed by a single method, is essential to define the exact impact of different SSc clinical features on telomere length (33).

4. Telomerase

Telomerase is a holo-enzyme able to synthesize novel telomeric DNA. Typically, in the absence of telomerase activity (or of a second mechanism-alternative lengthening of telomeres-ALT), telomeres in somatic cells will gradually shorten resulting in cell growth arrest and eventual apoptosis. Telomerase activity is able to circumvent these processes by adding new TTAGGG repeats, thus enlarging the cells proliferative lifespan and combating the cellular ageing process (14). Telomerase has been a target of investigation in SSc several times, although each of the respective studies focused on different aspects of telomerase biology. A synopsis of these studies is presented below.

One study investigating the role of telomerase in SSc hypothesized that telomerase activation may participate in activation and proliferation of circulating lymphocytes. This was based on a study in rheumatoid arthritis (RA) and pigmented villonodular synovitis (PVS) showing that telomerase activity is present at a high level in synovial infiltrating lymphocytes obtained from patients with RA, indicating that telomerase activation may be involved in lymphocyte activation and proliferation in RA (34). To address the role of telomerase activity, peripheral blood mononuclear cells from 9 female SSc patients and 10 healthy age-matched females were obtained and subjected to the telomeric repeat amplification protocol. Next to this, PBLs from SLE, Sjogren syndrome (SS) and mixed connective tissue disease (MCTD) were included. Telomerase activity was detected in 64.7% of SLE patients, 63.6% of MCTD, 54.5% of SS, and 44.4% of SSc. Telomerase activity in SSc was not significantly different from the activity observed in the controls, although it has to be noted that high telomerase activity was detected in some patients with this disease. However, a significant difference was observed in PBLs from patients with SLE, MCTD, and SS. Although of interest, this study is not conclusive considering the very small number of SSc patients included (35).

In SSc, the observation was made that SSc fibroblasts had a longer longevity and were less likely to go into apoptosis than fibroblasts from healthy controls (36). From this perspective, the hypothesis was put forward that SSc fibroblasts have higher telomerase activity compared to fibroblasts from their healthy counterparts. To address this issue indirectly, a study investigated the presence of a polymorphism at position 514 in the telomerase gene in 53 patients with SSc and 98 healthy controls restriction fragment length analysis. The investigators found a significant higher presence of the *514 AA* genotype in SSc. Again, these results are interesting, but the very small sample size and the lack of clearness of any functional implication of this polymorphism renders any firm conclusions vain (37). Notably, somatic cells such as fibroblasts express negligible levels of telomerase, so that a hypothesis based on differential telomerase activity between healthy and diseased cells, is highly questionable.

A further cross-sectional study aimed at evaluating telomerase activity in various connective tissue diseases was similarly hampered by lack of power (38). This used 19 patients with SSc, 15 with SLE, 10 with RA and 14 with SS. Twenty-nine healthy subjects were also included. Human telomerase-specific reverse transcriptase (hTERT) was measured in PBLs, using RT-PCR. The highest values were observed subsequently in RA, SLE and SS. Whereas RA was the only disease with significantly higher telomerase expression than controls; SSc PBLs displayed significantly lower expression compared to controls.

To place this observation in the proper perspective, additional features have to be considered. The mean age of the SSc patients was not the highest of the tested groups, making an effect of age on telomerase activity unlikely. In their discussion the authors put their findings in the light of the study by *Artlett et al.* describing significantly shorter telomeres in SSc PBLs (reviewed above). They advocated that the shorter telomeres in SSc might be caused by lower telomerase activity. This is not intuitive from the point of view of telomere biology, where disease stress may simply result in increased telomeric attrition and replicative senescence. None of the studies above have tested for this, even by simply looking at senescence associated cell surface markers on PBLs (39). Another pivotal observation is that nearly half of the SSc patients included in this study received cyclophosphamide treatment, which has been suggested to influence telomerase activity (40). Unfortunately, the authors do not provide a comparison between the SSc patients with and without cyclophosphamide treatment, which would have certainly been helpful to rule out this possible bias.

Also of note, is that the initial hypothesis of higher telomerase activity in SSc fibroblasts recently inspired researchers to isolate high collagen-producing fibroblasts from SSc biopsies and extend their lifespan with hTERT immortalization by lentiviral infection. This was done to the purpose of creating long living SSc fibroblast cell lines to better study and phenotype the characteristics of the SSc fibroblast in a consistent model (41). Such cell lines , while useful research tools, are blunt instruments, and negate primary telomere based damage response mechanisms that may be subverted by the disease, as they artificially immortalise the fibroblasts and bypass damage responses, as a consequence. It will be interesting to evaluate such cell lines for levels of DNA damage and chromosomal abnormalities with increasing passage in culture, in order to try to disentangle these from disease specific changes. A further criticism of such an approach is that it negates the contribution of any epigenetic driver of the disease state which may affect telomere biology and hence cellular life span.

5. Impaired cytological senescence in SSc

Immune senescence describes the ageing of the immune system and is rather than a chronological ageing process a biological ageing process. The most well defined findings in this field surround the involution of the thymus. This process starts after puberty, continues during ageing and ultimately results in partial failure of T cell receptor expression and a decrease in production of CD4+ and CD8+ cells. This ultimately results in a larger T memory cell pool. Both CD4+ and CD8+ cells lose CD28 expression. Intriguingly, CD28- T cells are less prone to apoptosis, autoreactive and profoundly interferon gamma (IFNg) producing. Among others, defective Fas signalling also plays an important role in the maintenance of thymus function. In addition, interleukin 2 (IL-2) production and response of aged people declines. A recent study showed that patients with SSc, during their lifespan, undergo a progressive expansion of the naive CD4+ T cell subset. This could be addressed to an age-inappropriate peripheral distribution of naive CD4+ T cells. It was regarded as age-inappropriate because, in contrast to healthy controls, the distribution of naive cells increased with age in SSc patients. Intriguingly, this is also in sharp contrast to RA, where the high levels of T cell activation and apoptosis ultimately produce a larger memory subset pool in disadvantage of the naive T cell pool (42). As described above, thymus involution seems to play an important role in maintaining the T cell pool. To investigate the role of thymus involution in the observed differences in T cell populations, the proportion of recent thymus emigrants by analysis of CD31 expression has been investigated. This has led to the observation that there was no correlation with decrease of recent thymus emigrants in the peripheral blood in inactive and the lcSSc forms of the disease, but not in patients with the diffuse and active disease. This indicates that in the lcSSc and inactive disease subsets, the physiological ageing related decrease in thymic T cells is evaded. However, there seems to be more at play than just an increase in thymically produced cells, since the observed increase in CD31 cells did not correlate significantly with the total number of CD4+ T cells. Based on this finding, it has been hypothesized that peripheral mechanisms must be involved as well to explain the increased frequencies of naive CD4+ T cells discovered in SSc patients. Several explanations have been proposed for these observations, including persistent in vivo antigenic stimulation and cytokine production. Of interest however is the finding that higher sFAS and Bcl-2 levels were detected in the SSc patients included in this study, possibly contributing to the difference in T cell homeostasis (43). As mentioned above, defective FAS functioning is implicated in conserving thymic function and has been involved on a functional and genetic level in SSc previously, more specifically in lcSSc patients, which fit with the lcSSc specific observations made in this study (44,45).

Following injury, epithelial cells undergo an epithelial–mesenchymal transition (EMT), in which they start migrating over the wound site and begin proliferating to replace lost cells. In this respect, it is important to note that most cells exhibit a finite ability to replicate, termed the Hayflick limit (46). Based on this, it has been proposed that repeated eptithelial injury can lead to epithelial cells that enter a state of replicative senescence and can no longer proliferate. At this point a fibroblast response can be initiated as a compensatory mechanism that serves to patch injury site. This, partially hypothetical framework is consistent with an increasing prevalence of SSc in age and with the occurrence of the most aggressive SSc cases being described in late onset disease (47). More importantly, this hypothesis provides a direct connection between the process of ageing and fibrosis. In line with this hypothesis, although targeting endothelial cells, is a recent study addressing the ability of mesenchymal stem cells (MSCs) to differentiate into endothelial cells in SSc. This process is of interest in SSc, since endothelial damage has been strongly implicated in its characteristic vasculopathy. A recent study investigated the ability of MSCs derived from 7 SSc patients and 15 healthy controls to differentiate into endothelial cells. The cells were cultured in endothelial-specific medium, and subsequently the endothelial-like MSC phenotype was characterized by surface expression of vascular endothelial growth factor receptors. In addition, the authors investigated cellular senescence of these cells by measuring the telomerase activity in MSCs from SSc patients and controls. Intriguingly, telomerase activity in MSCs from SSc patients was significantly reduced as compared with that in MSCs from the controls. This observation is counterintuitive to previous hypotheses relating to higher telomerase activity in disease SSc. MSC's are a telomerase positive cell type. A lack of or a decrease in telomerase activity in these cells is indicative of a reduced proliferative repair capacity. This significant difference between SSc and control MScs disappeared after full endothelial differentiation. At this point, both subsets displayed decreased activity, with a stronger decrease in endothelial like MSCs from SSc patients as compared with those from controls. The authors propose that this reflects early senescence and that it is caused by an increased number of pathologic stimuli and events encountered by these cells during their lifespan in the SSc patients (48). It is also consistent with aberrant telomere biology in SSc and a reduced damage repair capacity.

6. The X chromosome and age

Perhaps unexpectedly at a first glance, X chromosomal expression alters with age. This is of particular interest in SSc, since this disease predominantly affects females, with ratio's reported as high as 14:1 (2-6). Interestingly, skewing of X chromosome inactivation and X chromosome monosomy, both affecting X chromosomal expression, have been implicated in SSc susceptibility or pathogenesis. These two aspects of biological ageing will be discussed in this paragraph in the context of SSc.

The X-chromosome accommodates 1098 genes (49). Most X-linked genes are present with one copy in males (XY) and two copies in females (XX). To level differences between males and females in X chromosomal gene expression, several species including mammals, evolved dosage compensation mechanisms (50). One of these mechanisms balances expression of the X-linked genes, present as a single copy in males (XY) and as two copies in females (XX), by inactivation of one of the two X-chromosomes in females (50). The human X chromosome goes through several phases of inactivation and reactivation during germ cell development and in the first part of the embryogenesis. In female embryos, imprinted inactivation of the paternal X chromosome is effectuated at the two- to four-cell phase, pursued by random X-inactivation at the blastocyst stage. As a consequence of this, females are functional mosaics for inactivation of the paternal or maternal X-chromosome (51). About 15% from the X chromosomal genes escapes inactivation; this inactivation pattern shows some heterogeneity between females (52). Although inactivation of the X-chromosome is apparent to be permanent for all descendants of a cell, the XCI pattern alters with age. The frequency of skewed XCI in peripheral blood cells increases in elderly compared to younger healthy females. This is thought to be caused by the exhaustion of progenitor cell populations in the bone marrow with ageing, leaving only a few progenitor cells left to produce cells that will reflect the skewed XCI patterns of their progenitors in the periphery (53).

Intriguingly, women with SSc comprise a significantly higher frequency of peripheral blood cells with a skewed XCI pattern compared to healthy women. The same observation has been made in females with auto-immune thyroid disease and juvenile arthritis, but was not observed in systemic lupus erythemathosous and primary biliairy cirrosis (54). Two overlapping Turkish studies postulated that in 195 female SSc patients and 160 female controls skewed XCI patterns were significantly more present; 44.9% of 149 informative patients and in 8% of 124 healthy controls. (55,56). Interestingly, there seemed to be no age related increase in skewed XCI patterns. A recent study replicated the significantly higher percentage of XCI skewing in a cohort of 217 women with SSc and 107 healthy women. More depth was added to this observation by showing that there was no significant difference between skewing patterns of peripheral blood mononuclear cells, plasmacytoid dendritic cells, T cells, B cells, myeloid dendritic cells and monocytes. At sharp contrast with the healthy control population, skewing percentages of X chromosomal inactivation were independent of age in patients with SSc. Furthermore; this study investigated the effect of the skewed XCI on Foxp3 gene expression. Foxp3 plays an important role in T regulatory cell development. Intriguingly, Foxp3 expression was diminished in the patients with SSc exhibiting the most markedly increased skewing, which in turn was associated with less efficient suppressive activity (57).

Females suffering from Turner's syndrome, and are hence harbouring only one X chromosome, are at increased risk for developing autoimmune disease. Based on this observation an effort was undertaken to investigate the presence of X monosomy in peripheral blood leukocytes from 44 females with SSc and 73 age-matched healthy women. Interestingly, monosomy rates in SSc, regardless of its clinical subtype, were significantly higher compared to healthy women. Furthermore, X monosomy rates increased with age and were higher in T and B cells compared to monocytes/macrophages, polymorphonuclear, and natural killer cells. Noteworthy, male cell microchimerism, also advocated to play a role in SSc, was ruled out by excluding the presence of an Y chromosome in these cells (58). These observations together imply that age related X chromosomal changes might play a role in the higher SSc prevalence in females at increasing age.

7. Conclusions

This review aimed to summarize findings related to biological ageing that are involved in SSc susceptibility and pathogenesis. When we overlook the publications in this field it becomes obvious that most of the investigations can be traced back to chromosomal changes, whether it concerns telomere and telomerase associated damage control, or senescence as well as well as altering X chromosomal expression.

The pivotal question in addressing the relevance of the described findings is whether the observed changes in cell senescence, XCI and telomeres/telomerase are caused by a higher turnover of cells, forced by the ongoing inflammatory processes in SSc, or that some of these results are truly involved in initiating or perpetuating SSc. When considering the results describing telomere shortening, increased XCI, X monosomy and early MSC senescence, these results might all flow logically from a higher demand of immune progenitor cells and epithelial/endothelial cells in SSc. This cannot be said about the finding of decreased telomere attrition in lcSSc PBLs and the decreased rate of physiologic thymus function reduction, which seems counterintuitive considering healthy ageing processes and which is different to other autoimmune diseases. These findings are potentially very relevant in pointing towards processes sustaining or initiating the inflammatory status. More specifically, the factors sustaining thymic cell production and telomeric repeat length could be involved in the decreased capability to drive out immune cells based on cell damage or senescence, more prone to be autoreactive. It has to be noted here, that both processes take place predominantly in the lcSSc subset of patients, advocating for full clinical data to be included in future studies. The sustenance of telomeric length in PBLs from lcSSc patients is, based on the published literature, unlikely to come from an increase in telomerase activity, which was found steeply decreased in SSc patients. In this light it is of interest to compare telomere shortening in SSc with other ageing markers, such as CDKN2A, to see whether the shortening is an isolated process, or follows a general, systemic state of increased biologic ageing (33). Notably, although telomeric shortening seems to be influenced by socio-economic factors and events, no ubiquitous socio-economic correlations have been made with SSc so far (2-6, 15, 59).

The involvement of the X chromosome in SSc is also interesting, considering the increased prevalence of SSc in females. In this light it has to be noted that genetic data on X chromosomal genes in SSc are a scarce commodity and were not included in a recent GWAS publication (8). Genetic analysis of the X chromosome might identify genes involved in SSc directly or either indirectly in prompting XCI and X monosomy at an earlier onset than expected by physiological ageing alone.

Finally, when over-viewing the literature in this field it becomes apparent that although very interesting observations have been made, the results described are hampered by small numbers of SSc patients and therefore have to be regarded cautiously. Nevertheless, these observations warrant more research since a strong point can be made for the involvement of age related phenomena in SSc. Therefore, a large study with well characterized SSc patients addressing current controversies in telomere and telomerase functioning, as well as further corroboration of EMT response aberrances is currently highly anticipated.

8. References

[1] Varga J, Abraham D. Systemic sclerosis: a prototypic multisystem fibrotic disorder. J Clin Invest. 2007 Mar;117(3):557-67.

[2] Roberts-Thomson PJ, Jones M, Hakendorf P, Kencana Dharmapatni AA, Walker JG, MacFarlane JG, Smith MD, Ahern MJ. Scleroderma in South Australia: epidemiological observations of possible pathogenic significance. Intern Med J. 2001 May-Jun;31(4):220-9.

[3] Mayes MD, Lacey JV Jr, Beebe-Dimmer J, Gillespie BW, Cooper B, Laing TJ, Schottenfeld D. Prevalence, incidence, survival, and disease characteristics of systemic sclerosis in a large US population. Arthritis Rheum. 2003 Aug;48(8):2246-55.

[4] Chifflot H, Fautrel B, Sordet C, Chatelus E, Sibilia J. Incidence and prevalence of systemic sclerosis: a systematic literature review. Semin Arthritis Rheum. 2008 Feb;37(4):223-35. Epub 2007 Aug 9.

[5] Arias-Nuñez MC, Llorca J, Vazquez-Rodriguez TR, Gomez-Acebo I, Miranda-Filloy JA, Martin J, Gonzalez-Juanatey C, Gonzalez-Gay MA. Systemic sclerosis in northwestern Spain: a 19-year epidemiologic study. Medicine (Baltimore). 2008 Sep;87(5):272-80.

[6] Tamaki T, Mori S, Takehara K. Epidemiological study of patients with systemic sclerosis in Tokyo. Arch Dermatol Res. 1991;283(6):366-71.

[7] Subcommittee for scleroderma criteria of the American Rheumatism Association Diagnostic and Therapeutic Criteria Committee. Preliminary criteria for the classification of systemic sclerosis (scleroderma). Arthritis Rheum. 23(5), 581-590 (1980).

[8] Radstake TR, Gorlova O, Rueda B, Martin JE, Alizadeh BZ, Palomino-Morales R, Coenen MJ, Vonk MC, Voskuyl AE, Schuerwegh AJ, Broen JC, van Riel PL, van 't Slot R, Italiaander A, Ophoff RA, Riemekasten G, Hunzelmann N, Simeon CP, Ortego-Centeno N, González-Gay MA, González-Escribano MF; Spanish Scleroderma Group, Airo P, van Laar J, Herrick A, Worthington J, Hesselstrand R, Smith V, de Keyser F, Houssiau F, Chee MM, Madhok R, Shiels P, Westhovens R, Kreuter A, Kiener H, de Baere E, Witte T, Padykov L, Klareskog L, Beretta L, Scorza R, Lie BA, Hoffmann-Vold AM, Carreira P, Varga J, Hinchcliff M, Gregersen PK, Lee AT, Ying J, Han Y, Weng SF, Amos CI, Wigley FM, Hummers L, Nelson JL, Agarwal SK, Assassi S, Gourh P, Tan FK, Koeleman BP, Arnett FC, Martin J, Mayes MD. Genome-wide association study of systemic sclerosis identifies CD247 as a new susceptibility locus. Nat Genet. 2010 May;42(5):426-9. Epub 2010 Apr 11.

[9] Dieudé P, Wipff J, Guedj M, Ruiz B, Melchers I, Hachulla E, Riemekasten G, Diot E, Hunzelmann N, Sibilia J, Tiev K, Mouthon L, Cracowski JL, Carpentier PH, Distler J, Amoura Z, Tarner I, Avouac J, Meyer O, Kahan A, Boileau C, Allanore Y. BANK1 is a genetic risk factor for diffuse cutaneous systemic sclerosis and has additive effects with IRF5 and STAT4. Arthritis Rheum. 2009 Nov;60(11):3447-54.

[10] Beretta L, Santaniello A, Mayo M, Cappiello F, Marchini M, Scorza R. A 3-factor epistatic model predicts digital ulcers in Italian scleroderma patients. Eur J Intern Med. 2010 Aug;21(4):347-53. Epub 2010 Jun 23.

[11] Ranque B, Mouthon L. Geoepidemiology of systemic sclerosis. Autoimmun Rev. 2010 Mar;9(5):A311-8. Epub 2009 Nov 10.

[12] Radić M, Martinović Kaliterna D, Radić J. Infectious disease as aetiological factor in the pathogenesis of systemic sclerosis. Neth J Med. 2010 Nov;68(11):348-53.

[13] McCormic ZD, Khuder SS, Aryal BK, Ames AL, Khuder SA. Occupational silica exposure as a risk factor for scleroderma: a meta-analysis. Int Arch Occup Environ Health. 2010 Oct;83(7):763-9. Epub 2010 Jan 3.

[14] Lamb KJ, Shiels PG. Telomeres, ageing and oxidation. SEB Exp Biol Ser. 2009;62:117-37.

[15] Carrero JJ, Stenvinkel P, Fellström B, Qureshi AR, Lamb K, Heimbürger O, Bárány P, Radhakrishnan K, Lindholm B, Soveri I, Nordfors L, Shiels PG. Telomere attrition is associated with inflammation, low fetuin-A levels and high mortality in prevalent haemodialysis patients. J Intern Med. 2008 Mar;263(3):302-12. Epub 2007 Dec 7.

[16] Simpson RJ, Cosgrove C, Chee MM, McFarlin BK, Bartlett DB, Spielmann G, O'Connor DP, Pircher H, Shiels PG. Senescent phenotypes and telomere lengths of peripheral

blood T-cells mobilized by acute exercise in humans. Exerc Immunol Rev. 2010;16:40-55.

[17] Kanoh J, Ishikawa F. Composition and conservation of the telomeric complex. Cell Mol Life Sci. 2003 Nov;60(11):2295-302.

[18] O'Sullivan RJ, Karlseder J.Telomeres: protecting chromosomes against genome instability.Nat Rev Mol Cell Biol. 2010 Mar;11(3):171-81. Epub 2010 Feb 3.

[19] Liu FJ, Barchowsky A, Opresko PL.The Werner syndrome protein suppresses telomeric instability caused by chromium (VI) induced DNA replication stress.PLoS One. 2010 Jun 16;5(6):e11152.

[20] Reddy S, Li B, Comai L.Processing of human telomeres by the Werner syndrome protein.Cell Cycle. 2010 Aug 15;9(16):3137-8. Epub 2010 Aug 9. No abstract available.

[21] Bes C, Vardi S, Güven M, Soy M. Werner's syndrome: a quite rare disease for differential diagnosis of scleroderma. Rheumatol Int. 2010 Mar;30(5):695-8. Epub 2009 Jun 3.

[22] Khraishi M, Howard B, Little H.A patient with Werner's syndrome and osteosarcoma presenting as scleroderma.J Rheumatol. 1992 May;19(5):810-3.

[23] Foti R, Leonardi R, Rondinone R, Di Gangi M, Leonetti C, Canova M, Doria A.Scleroderma-like disorders. Autoimmun Rev. 2008 Feb;7(4):331-9. Epub 2008 Jan 11.

[24] Migliore L, Bevilacqua C, Scarpato R. Cytogenetic study and FISH analysis in lymphocytes of systemic lupus erythematosus (SLE) and systemic sclerosis (SS) patients. Mutagenesis 1999;14:227–31.

[25] Martins EP, Fuzzi HT, Kayser C, Alarcon RT, Rocha MG, Chauffaille ML, Andrade LE.Increased chromosome damage in systemic sclerosis skin fibroblasts.Scand J Rheumatol. 2010;39(5):398-401.

[26] Housset E, Emerit I, Baulon A, de Grouchy YJ. Anomalies chromosomiques dans la sclérodermie: etude de 10 malades. Cr Acad Sci Paris 1969;296:413–16.

[27] Wolff DJ, Needleman BW, Wasserman SS, Schwartz S. Spontaneous and clastogen induced chromosomal breakage in scleroderma. J Rheumatol 1991;18:837–40.

[28] Pan SF, Rodnan GP, Deutsch M, Wald N. Chromosomal abnormalities in progressive systemic sclerosis (scleroderma) with consideration of radiation effects. J Lab Med 1975;86:300–8.

[29] Porciello G, Scarpato R, Ferri C, Storino F, Cagetti F, Morozzi G, Spontaneous chromosome damage (micronuclei) in systemic sclerosis and Raynaud's phenomenon. J Rheumatol 2003;30:1244–7.

[30] Artlett CM, Black CM, Briggs DC, Stevens CO, Welsh KI. Telomere reduction in scleroderma patients: a possible cause for chromosomal instability. Br J Rheumatol. 1996 Aug;35(8):732-7.

[31] MacIntyre A, Brouilette SW, Lamb K, Radhakrishnan K, McGlynn L, Chee MM, Parkinson EK, Freeman D, Madhok R, Shiels PG. Association of increased telomere lengths in limited scleroderma, with a lack of age-related telomere erosion. Ann Rheum Dis. 2008 Dec;67(12):1780-2. Epub 2008 Jul 28.

[32] Kang MR, Muller MT, Chung IK. Telomeric DNA damage by topoisomerase I. A possible mechanism for cell killing by camptothecin. J Biol Chem. 2004 Mar 26;279(13):12535-41. Epub 2004 Jan 16.

[33] Shiels PG. Improving precision in investigating aging: why telomeres can cause problems. J Gerontol A Biol Sci Med Sci. 2010 Aug;65(8):789-91. Epub 2010 Jun 10.

[34] Georgin-Lavialle S, Aouba A, Mouthon L, Londono-Vallejo JA, Lepelletier Y, Gabet AS, Hermine O.The telomere/telomerase system in autoimmune and systemic immune-mediated diseases. Autoimmun Rev. 2010 Aug;9(10):646-51. Epub 2010 May 6.

[35] Katayama Y, Kohriyama K. Telomerase activity in peripheral blood mononuclear cells of systemic connective tissue diseases. J Rheumatol. 2001 Feb;28(2):288-91.

[36] Jelaska A, Korn JH. Role of apoptosis and transforming growth factor beta1 in fibroblast selection and activation in systemic sclerosis. Arthritis Rheum. 2000 Oct;43(10):2230-9.

[37] Ohtsuka T, Yamakage A, Yamazaki S. The polymorphism of telomerase RNA component gene in patients with systemic sclerosis. Br J Dermatol. 2002 Aug;147(2):250-4.

[38] Tarhan F, Vural F, Kosova B, Aksu K, Cogulu O, Keser G, Gündüz C, Tombuloglu M, Oder G, Karaca E, Doganavsargil E. Telomerase activity in connective tissue diseases: elevated in rheumatoid arthritis, but markedly decreased in systemic sclerosis. Rheumatol Int. 2008 Apr;28(6):579-83. Epub 2007 Oct 16.

[39] Simpson RJ, Guy K. Coupling aging immunity with a sedentary lifestyle: has the damage already been done?--a mini-review. Gerontology. 2010;56(5):449-58. Epub 2009 Dec 19.

[40] Kiyozuka Y, Yamamoto D, Yang J, Uemura Y, Senzaki H, Adachi S, Tsubura A. Correlation of chemosensitivity to anticancer drugs and telomere length, telomerase activity and telomerase RNA expression in human ovarian cancer cells. Anticancer Res. 2000 Jan-Feb;20(1A):203-12.

[41] Kapanadze B, Morris E, Smith E, Trojanowska M.Establishment and characterization of scleroderma fibroblast clonal cell lines by introduction of the hTERT gene. J Cell Mol Med. 2010 May;14(5):1156-65. Epub 2009 May 11.

[42] Larbi A, Pawelec G, Wong SC, Goldeck D, Tai JJ, Fulop T. Impact of age on T cell signaling: A general defect or specific alterations? Ageing Res Rev. 2011 Jul;10(3):370-8. Epub 2010 Oct 8.

[43] Giovannetti A, Rosato E, Renzi C, Maselli A, Gambardella L, Giammarioli AM, Palange P, Paoletti P, Pisarri S, Salsano F, Malorni W, Pierdominici M. Analyses of T cell phenotype and function reveal an altered T cell homeostasis in systemic sclerosis. Correlations with disease severity and phenotypes. Clin Immunol. 2010 Oct;137(1):122-33. Epub 2010 Jun 26.

[44] Broen J, Gourh P, Rueda B, Coenen M, Mayes M, Martin J, Arnett FC, Radstake TR; European Consortium on Systemic Sclerosis Genetics. The FAS -670A>G polymorphism influences susceptibility to systemic sclerosis phenotypes. Arthritis Rheum. 2009 Dec;60(12):3815-20.

[45] Cipriani P, Fulminis A, Pingiotti E, Marrelli A, Liakouli V, Perricone R, Pignone A, Matucci-Cerinic M, Giacomelli R. Resistance to apoptosis in circulating alpha/beta and gamma/delta T lymphocytes from patients with systemic sclerosis. J Rheumatol. 2006 Oct;33(10):2003-14.

[46] Hayflick L, Moorehead PS. The serial cultivation of human diploid cell strains. Exp Cell Res. 1961 Dec;25:585-621. No abstract available.

[47] Hügle T, Schuetz P, Daikeler T, Tyndall A, Matucci-Cerinic M, Walker UA, van Laar JM; EUSTAR members. Late-onset systemic sclerosis--a systematic survey of the EULAR scleroderma trials and research group database. Rheumatology (Oxford). 2011 Jan;50(1):161-5. Epub 2010 Sep 30.

[48] Cipriani P, Guiducci S, Miniati I, Cinelli M, Urbani S, Marrelli A, Dolo V, Pavan A, Saccardi R, Tyndall A, Giacomelli R, Cerinic MM. Impairment of endothelial cell differentiation from bone marrow-derived mesenchymal stem cells: new insight into the pathogenesis of systemic sclerosis. Arthritis Rheum. 2007 Jun;56(6):1994-2004.

[49] Ross MT, Bentley DR, Tyler-Smith C. The sequences of the human sex chromosomes. Curr Opin Genet Dev. 2006 Jun;16(3):213-8. Epub 2006 May 2.

[50] Graves JA, Disteche CM, Toder R. Gene dosage in the evolution and function of mammalian sex chromosomes. Cytogenet Cell Genet. 1998;80(1-4):94-103.

[51] Lyon MF. Gene action in the X-chromosome of the mouse (Mus musculus L.). Nature. 1961 Apr 22;190:372-3.

[52] Carrel L, Willard HF. X-inactivation profile reveals extensive variability in X-linked gene expression in females. Nature. 2005 Mar 17;434(7031):400-4.

[53] Kristiansen M, Knudsen GP, Bathum L, Naumova AK, Sørensen TI, Brix TH, Svendsen AJ, Christensen K, Kyvik KO, Ørstavik KH. Twin study of genetic and aging effects on X chromosome inactivation. Eur J Hum Genet. 2005 May;13(5):599-606.

[54] Invernizzi P, Pasini S, Selmi C, Gershwin ME, Podda M. Female predominance and X chromosome defects in autoimmune diseases. J Autoimmun. 2009 Aug;33(1):12-6. Epub 2009 Apr 7.

[55] Ozbalkan Z, Bagişlar S, Kiraz S, Akyerli CB, Ozer HT, Yavuz S, Birlik AM, Calgüneri M, Ozçelik T. Skewed X chromosome inactivation in blood cells of women with scleroderma. Arthritis Rheum. 2005 May;52(5):1564-70.

[56] Uz E, Loubiere LS, Gadi VK, Ozbalkan Z, Stewart J, Nelson JL, Ozcelik T. Skewed X-chromosome inactivation in scleroderma. Clin Rev Allergy Immunol. 2008 Jun;34(3):352-5.

[57] Broen JC, Wolvers-Tettero IL, Geurts-van Bon L, Vonk MC, Coenen MJ, Lafyatis R, Radstake TR, Langerak AW. Skewed X chromosomal inactivation impacts T regulatory cell function in systemic sclerosis. Ann Rheum Dis. 2010 Dec;69(12):2213-6. Epub 2010 Aug 10.

[58] Invernizzi P, Miozzo M, Selmi C, Persani L, Battezzati PM, Zuin M, Lucchi S, Meroni PL, Marasini B, Zeni S, Watnik M, Grati FR, Simoni G, Gershwin ME, Podda M. X chromosome monosomy: a common mechanism for autoimmune diseases. J Immunol. 2005 Jul 1;175(1):575-8.

[59] Cherkas LF, Aviv A, Valdes AM, Hunkin JL, Gardner JP, Surdulescu GL, Kimura M, Spector TD. The effects of social status on biological aging as measured by white-blood-cell telomere length. Aging Cell. 2006 Oct;5(5):361-5.

7

Fibrocytes in Scleroderma Lung Fibrosis

Ronald Reilkoff, Aditi Mathur and Erica Herzog
Yale University School of Medicine
United States

1. Introduction

Systemic sclerosis (SSc) or "Scleroderma" is a disease characterized by cutaneous and visceral fibrosis that affects both the skin and internal organs. The worldwide prevalence ranges from 50-300 cases per million (Chifflot et al., 2008) and much of the morbidity in this population results from pulmonary complications. In fact, nearly 70% of scleroderma patients show some form of lung disease. Of the two forms of lung involvement, pulmonary arterial hypertension and interstitial lung disease, the latter has emerged as the greatest cause of death in these patients. The lungs of patients with scleroderma associated interstitial lung disease (SSc-ILD) exhibit replacement of the normal lung architecture with inflamed and fibrotic tissue that cannot participate in gas exchange. While approximately 42% of patients with SSc-ILD die of disease progression within ten years of diagnosis (Steen & Medsger, 2007) evidence is emerging that some patients progress slowly and in some cases spontaneously improve while others follow an accelerated clinical course (Goh et al., 2008). There is currently no way to predict which patients will progress rapidly and require more intensive therapy (Daoussis et al., 2010 ; Swigris et al., 2006; Tashkin et al., 2006) and/or referral for lung transplantation (D'Ovidio et al., 2005a; D'Ovidio et al., 2005b); and which patients will follow a more indolent course requiring less intense follow up. Therefore the development of a clinically predictive measure of pathologic progression would benefit physicians caring for patients with this disease. The ideal biomarker would be present in easily accessible clinical specimens, would be a potential contributor to disease development, and would be easily studied in murine models of disease. For this reason, peripheral blood fibrocytes have emerged as an exciting new area of study in the field of Scleroderma (Gan et al., 2011; Mathai et al., 2010; Peng et al., 2011 ; Tourkina et al.,2011; Reilkoff et al., 2011).

2. Fibrocytes

Fibrocytes are blood borne collagen-producing cells that were initially described in 1994. Since then, they have been associated with a broad range of fibrosing disorders including autoimmune illnesses and chronic inflammatory diseases. In some of these diseases, high circulating levels correlate with poor outcomes. In addition to extracellular matrix (ECM) synthesis, fibrocytes display other functions including antigen presentation and the secretion of pro-fibrotic and pro-angiogenic factors.

2.1 Disease associations

Identified by their co-expression of leukocyte markers such as CD45, extracellular matrix proteins such as Collagen-1α and in some cases markers expressed by progenitor cells such as CD34 (Bucala et al., 1994), fibrocytes are easily detected via flow cytometric and in vitro culture techniques. These approaches demonstrate that abnormalities in peripheral blood fibrocytes exist in diverse forms of autoimmune disease such as rheumatoid arthritis (Galligan et al., 2010), autoimmune thyroiditis (Douglas et al., 2009), amyopathic antisynthetase syndrome (Peng et al., 2011), and scleroderma (Gan et al., 2011 ; Mathai et al., 2010). Elevations in peripheral blood fibrocytes are seen in chronic inflammatory disorders not traditionally associated with autoimmunity such as idiopathic pulmonary fibrosis (Mehrad et al., 2007; Mehrad et al., 2009; Moeller et al., 2009), asthma (Schmidt et al., 2003; Nihlberg et al., 2006; Wang et al., 2008), nephrogenic systemic fibrosis (Vakil et al., 2009), cardiovascular disease (Falk, 2006), pulmonary hypertension (Nikam et al., 2011), and even normal aging (Mathai et al., 2010). Thus it is not surprising that the role fibrocytes play in tissue repair and remodeling is a developing area of interest in the study of fibrosis and autoimmunity.

2.2 Identification of fibrocytes in the circulation

Flow cytometry identifies fibrocytes from the circulation or tissue using the combination of characteristic cell surface marker expression with intracellular staining for collagens or extracellular matrix components. Human fibrocytes express hematopoietic markers such as CD45 (Bucala et al., 1994), Leukocyte specific protein-1 (Yang et al., 2002), as well as markers of adhesion and motility (Pilling et al., 2009), chemokine receptors such as CXCR4 (Mehrad et al., 2007), proteins important in host defense and scavenger receptors (Pilling et al., 2009), antigen presentation (Chesney et al., 1997), and cell surface enzymes such as CD10 and CD13 (Pilling et al., 2009). Fibrocytes typically lack markers of lymphocytes (Bellini & Mattoli, 2007; Pilling et al., 2009). Circulating and cultured fibrocytes also express CD34 (Bucala et al., 1994), a motility protein that allows fibrocytes to be distinguished from other collagen-containing cell types such as fibroblasts and macrophages (Reilkoff et al., 2011). However, because CD34 is frequently lost upon entry into target tissue (Peng et al., 2011; Phillips et al., 2004) its absence does not rule out a cell as being a fibrocyte. Fibrocytes also produce a wide array of ECM components (Bianchetti et al., 2011; Bellini & Mattoli, 2007; Pilling et al., 2009). A listing of fibrocyte markers is shown in Table 1.

2.3 Differentiation and homing

Insight into potential fibrocyte functions may be gleaned from an understanding of the factors promoting their differentiation and recruitment. Fibrocytes differentiate from a precursor population within the CD14+ monocyte fraction of peripheral blood (Abe et al., 2001). The monocyte to fibrocyte transition, which is increased by enrichment for CD11b(+) CD115(+) Gr1(+) expressing monocytes, is promoted by direct contact with activated CD4+ lymphocytes via an mTOR-PI3 kinase dependent pathway (Niedermeier et al., 2009). Other studies have determined that the fibrocyte precursor expresses components of the Fcγ receptor (Pilling et al., 2003). Inhibition of this receptor with the short pentraxin protein serum Amyloid P reduces fibrocyte outgrowth in human (Pilling et al., 2003; Pilling et al., 2006) and rodent samples (Murray et al., 2011; Pilling et al., 2007). This effect appears to be mediated via an ITIM-dependent mechanism (Castano et al., 2009). The monocyte to fibrocyte transition is inhibited by exposure to T_H1 cytokines (IFNγ, TNF, and IL-12); and is augmented by T_H2 cytokines (IL-4 and IL-13) (Shao et al., 2008). Fibrocyte differentiation is further stimulated by TGF-β1, and via engagement of the β1 integrin subunit (Bianchetti et al., 2011 ; Gan et al., 2011 ; Nikam et al., 2011).

Murine modeling demonstrates that certain chemokine receptors such as CCR2, CCR7, and CXCR4 promote fibrocyte recruitment to diseased tissue (Phillips et al., 2004; Moore et al., 2006; Sakai et al., 2006). Thus it is particularly relevant that human fibrocytes express the chemokine receptors CCR3 (eotaxin receptor) and CCR5 (MCP-1 receptor). Human fibrocytes also express Semaphorin 7a (Quan et al., 2004), a GPI-anchored membrane protein with important immunomodulatory effects (Czopik et al., 2006; Suzuki et al., 2007). Our own work in scleroderma patients demonstrates an association between fibrocytes serum concentrations of soluble factors such as TNF, IL-10, MCP-1 and IL-1 receptor antagonist (IL-1Ra), suggesting that fibrocytes may be mobilized into the circulation in response to one or more of these factors. Similarly, idiopathic pulmonary fibrosis (IPF) patients demonstrate high levels of CXCL12 in their blood and lungs, which is the cognate ligand for CXCR4, and these levels correlate with circulating fibrocyte concentrations (Mehrad et al., 2007). When viewed in combination, this array of stimulatory factors suggests that fibrocytes are recruited to injured tissue where they may play a role in the healing processes by via both immunomodulatory and ECM-producing effects.

2.4 Immunologic function

One school of thought posits that the ultimate phenotype of fibrocytes is the activated myofibroblast (Abe et al., 2001; Phillips et al., 2004; Quan et al., 2004; Gomperts & Strieter, 2007). This hypothesis is based on several studies demonstrating cultured fibrocytes respond to TGF-β1 by expressing α-SMA and contracting collagen gels *in vitro* (Abe et al., 2001; Phillips et al., 2004; Quan et al., 2004; Gomperts & Strieter, 2007). However, because *in vivo* studies using bone marrow chimeras show only minimal contributions of fibrocytes to α-SMA production in some models (Hashimoto et al., 2004; Kisseleva et al., 2006; Lin et al., 2008), this feature of fibrocytes may not dominate in tissue remodeling responses. When viewed in this light, it is particularly important to examine the immunomodulatory functions that fibrocytes are known to possess.

Type of Marker	Level of Expression	Reference
Adhesion and Motility		
CD9, CD11a, CD11b, CD11c, CD43, CD164, Mac2, LSP-1	Moderate	(Galligan et al., 2011; Bucala et al., 1994; Yang et al., 2002; Pilling et al., 2009)
CD34	Low	(Mathai et al., 2010; Bucala et al., 1994; Barth et al., 2002)
CD29, CD44, CD81, ICAM-1, CD49 complex, CD81	Low	(Mathai et al., 2010; Nikam et al., 2011; Bucala et al., 1994; Pilling et al., 2009)

Type of Marker	Level of Expression	Reference
Cell Surface Enzymes		
CD10, CD172a	Low	(Bucala et al., 1994)
CD13, Prolyl-4-hydroxylase	Low	
FAP	Low	
Scavenging receptors and host defense		
CD14, CD68, CD163, CD206, CD209, CD35, CD36	Variable	(Bucala et al., 1994)
Fcγ receptors		
CD16, CD32a, CD32b, CD32c	Moderate	(Bucala et al., 1994)
Chemokine receptors		
CCR2, CCR5, CCR4, CCR7, CCR9, CXCR1, CXCR4, CXC3R1	Moderate	(Mehrad et al., 2007; Pilling et al., 2009)
Antigen Presentation		
CD80, CD86, MHCI, MCHII	Low	(Chesney et al., 1997)
Extracellular matrix		
Collagen-I/III/IV, vimentin, tenascin	Low	(Bucala et al., 1994; Schmidt et al., 2003; Pilling et al., 2009)
Fibronectin, α-SMA	Variable	(Bianchetti et al., 2011; Bucala et al., 1994; Schmidt et al., 2003; Pilling et al., 2009)
Collagen V	Moderate	(Bianchetti et al., 2011)
Glycosaminoglycans		
Perlecan, Veriscan, Hyaluronan	Moderate	(Bianchetti et al., 2011)
Decorin	Low	
Miscellaneous		
Semaphorin 7a	Low	(Mathai et al., 2010)
CD115	None	(Pilling et al., 2009)
Thy1.1	Low	(Douglas et al., 2009)
CD105	Low	(Pilling et al., 2009)

Table 1. Fibrocyte Marker Expression

For example, human fibrocytes respond to Interleukin-1 beta (IL-1β) by increasing secretion of proinflammatory mediators such as Interleukin-6 (IL-6), Interleukin-8 (IL-8), and Chemokine (C-C motif) ligand 21. Porcine fibrocytes respond to innate immune stimulation adopting certain properties of antigen presenting cells via their expression of Major Histocompatibility Complex I and II, CD80 and CD86 (Balmelli et al., 2007). This function is also seen in human fibrocytes (Chesney et al., 1997). In addition to these pro-inflammatory effects, fibrocytes also secrete paracrine factors such as Interleukin-10 (Chesney et al., 1998),

TGF-β1, and platelet-derived growth factor (PDGF), which are expected to dampen inflammation and induce repair and angiogenesis.

This latter function is augmented via their secretion of matrix metalloproteinases (MMPs), vascular endothelial growth factor (VEGF), PDGF-A, hepatocyte growth factor (HGF), granulocyte–macrophage colony stimulating factor (GM-CSF), basic fibroblast growth factor (b-FGF), IL-8 and IL-1β (Hartlapp et al., 2001). Via their expression of Semaphorin 7a, fibrocytes may directly activate macrophages and dendritic cells (Suzuki et al., 2007) and negatively regulate T cell responses (Czopik et al., 2006). This array of functions suggest that fibrocytes are a highly plastic cell population that may significantly promote the aberrant immune response and tissue remodeling seen in scleroderma. In order to further explore the factors promoting fibrocyte accumulation in the blood and lungs of patients with SSc-ILD, we performed the following set of translational studies.

3. Materials and methods

TGFβ1 transgenic mice: All mouse experiments were approved by the Yale School of Medicine Institutional Animal Care and Use Committee. The CC10-tTS-rtTA- TGF-β1 transgenic mice used in this study have been described (Lee et al., 2004). The Sema-7a null mice were provided by Dr. Alex Kolodkin (Johns Hopkins) and have been described previously (Pasterkamp et al., 2003).

Doxycycline Administration: Eight-to-10 week old CC10-tTS-rtTA- TGF-β1 transgene positive (Tg+) or transgene negative (Tg-) mice with the Sema-7a locus null or intact were given doxycycline 0.5mg/ml in their drinking water for up to 2 weeks.

Bone marrow transplantation: Mice were prepared for bone marrow transplantation using 400 cGy total body irradiation. Bone marrow harvest, preparation, and injection were performed as previously described (Herzog et al., 2006).

β1 integrin blocking antibodies: TGF-β1 Tg^+ and Tg^- mice with an intact Sema-7a locus were injected with 125 μg of a neutralizing anti-β1 integrin antibody or isotype control (both from Biolegend) as previously described (Bungartz et al., 2006).

Lung inflammation: Euthanasia and bronchoalveolar lavage were performed as previously described (Lee et al., 2004). Lung inflammation was assessed via bronchoalveolar lavage (BAL) samples as described previously (Lee et al., 2004).

Collagen assessment: Total left lung collagen was measured using the Sircol Assay following the manufacturer's protocol (Biocolour, Ireland).

Flow cytometry for fibrocytes: Flow cytometry was performed as previously described (Mathai et al., 2010).

Histologic analysis: Formalin-fixed and paraffin-embedded lung sections were stained with hematoxylin and eosin to assess gross morphology or Mallory's trichrome stains to visualize collagen deposition.

mRNA analyses: Total RNA was obtained using TRIzol reagent (Invitrogen) according to the manufacturer's instructions. Primers specific for human Sema-7a, β1 integrin subunit, Plexin C1 and GAPDH, and murine β1 integrin subunit, Plexin C1, and β-actin were purchased from Superarray Bioscience. Gene expression levels were quantified using real time RT-PCR (Applied Biosystems), according to the manufacturer's protocols and normalized to GAPDH or β-actin mRNA.

Human cell isolation and culture: All studies were performed with HIC approval and written informed consent at Yale University School of Medicine. Cells were cultured as previously described (Mathai et al., 2010).
TUNEL: TUNEL was performed as previously described (Murray et al., 2011).
Caspase activation: Detection of caspase cleavage and activation using immunohistochemistry was performed as previously described (Lee et al., 2004).
Annexin V: Flow cytometric assessment of annexin V externalization was performed via flow cytometry as previously described (Lee et al., 2004).
Statistics: Normally distributed data were expressed as means ± SEM and assessed for significance by Student's *t* test or ANOVA as appropriate. Data that were not normally distributed were assessed for significance using the Mann-Whitney U test.

4. Results

4.1 Circulating fibrocytes are elevated in SSc-ILD

In order to determine whether fibrocytes are found with increased frequency in the circulation of patients with SSc-ILD, peripheral blood mononuclear cells were obtained from a cohort of patients with SSc-ILD (n=12) and normal controls (n= 27) and assessed for fibrocytes based on the coexpression of CD45 and Pro-Collagen-Iα. This double positive population was seen in both cohorts, and while overall percentages of fibrocytes were not increased in the SSc-ILD subjects, total quantities of collagen producing leukocytes, were increased by 79% in the SSc-ILD cohort compared to controls (Figure 1, $p<0.05$) (Mathai et al., 2010) and reflected impairments in ventilatory function as measured by the percent-predicted forced vital capacity (FVC) (E. Herzog, unpublished data). These cells displayed enriched expression of CD34 and in some cases also expressed CD14, indicating both their multipotent potential as well as their monocytic origin. Since this work was first published these results have been confirmed by at least one other group (Tourkina et al., 2011) indicating the reproducibility of the fibrocyte assay in this patient population.

4.2 Circulating fibrocytes exist in a profibrotic milieu

In order to determine the immunologic milieu in which these fibrocytes exist, further phenotyping of these subjects was performed. Further analysis of circulating monocytes from these individuals found them to be skewed towards an alternatively activated, profibrotic phenotype as evidenced by a propensity to adopt both CD163 expression and CCL18 secretion when stimulated with LPS. Multianalyte ELISA of plasma from these patients demonstrated increased concentrations of profibrotic cytokines and chemokines such as IL10, TNF-a, and IL-1 RA (Mathai et al., 2010). Many of the mediators are commonly associated with alternatively activated macrophages (or "M2") leading to some speculation that fibrocytes may simply represent an intermediate population in the terminal differentiation of profibrotic macrophages (Reilkoff et al., 2011). Another interesting aspect of these data were that similar (though not identical) results were seen in a cohort of aged but otherwise healthy individuals, leading to the speculation that the presence of fibrocytes may represent a previously unrecognized form of immunosenscence in patients with SSc-ILD. The presence of increased fibrocytes in the senescence associated mouse model of accelerated aging supports this hypothesis though further work is required to prove its validity.

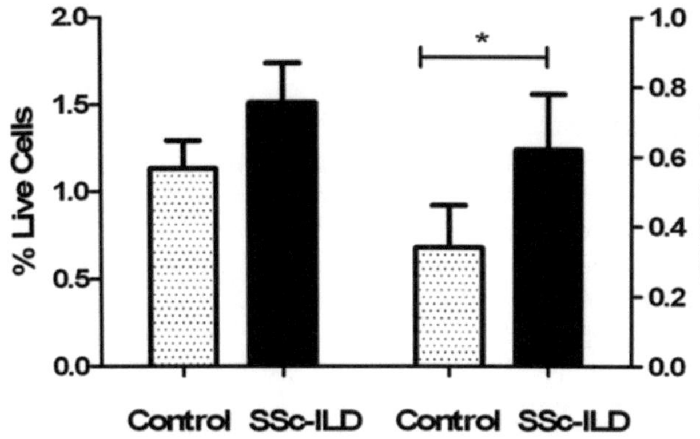

Fig. 1. Comparison of CD45+/pro-Col-Iα$^+$ percentages (left axis) and quantities (right axis) in normal (n=27, gray bar) and SSc-ILD subjects (n=12, black bar). CD45+/pro-Col-Iα$^+$ cell quantities, but not percentages, are increased in SSc-ILD. (Mathai et al., 2010)

4.3 Local apoptosis regulates fibrocyte accumulation

While it has long been noted that fibrocytes arise in the setting of profibrotic stimuli such as TGF-β1, the local factors regulating the monocyte to fibrocyte transition have remained largely unexplored. Several of our recent studies, however, lend insight into these processes. One outstanding question in this area has been the relationship between injury and fibrocytes. A requirement for apoptosis in the intrapulmonary accumulation of fibrocytes was recently explored in a model of lung fibrosis caused by inducible, lung-specific overexpression of the bioactive form of the human TGF-β1 gene. These mice develop an epithelial injury response dominated by apoptosis that peaks at 48 hours following doxycycline administration. Shortly thereafter a dense monocytic infiltrate arises that is predominantly composed of CD206+ M2 macrophages (Murray et al., 2011). These macrophages persist, and are required for the induction of activated myofibroblast development and the induction of a robust accumulation of ECM products and fibrosis that is evident by between 10-14 days of doxycycline exposure. It is not until fibrosis is relatively well established that intrapulmonary fibrocytes appear in this model. Because scleroderma related lung disease is characterized by heightened responsiveness to autocrine TGF-β1 signaling via both canonical and non-canonical pathways (Sargent et al., 2011), this model is an ideal tool to study the pathogenesis of SSc-ILD.

The role of apoptosis in fibrocyte accumulation was tested in this model using a fairly straightforward approach. TGF-β1 mice were randomized to receive systemic injections of the pan-caspase inhibitor Z-VAD/fmk or vehicle control. Reductions in apoptosis were confirmed at 48 hours by comparison of TUNEL staining and caspase 3 activation in Z-VAD/fmk treated TGF-β1 mice. Reductions in lung inflammation and fibrosis were noted at day 14. Fibrocytes, defined via classical flow cytometric criteria by CD45 and Pro-Collagen-Iα co-expression, were reduced by nearly 10-fold at the 14 day time point (Figure 2a, $p<0.001$). The human relevance of these findings was supported by the finding that SSc-ILD lungs contain increased levels of CD45+ collagen-producing cells (Peng et al., 2011), and that these lungs contain increased numbers of TUNEL+ve apoptotic cells. Additionally CD14+ monocytes cultured in the presence of Z/VAD-fmk fail to adopt the spindle-shaped, collagen expressing phenotype that characterizes fibrocytes (Figure 2c,d, $p<0.001$). Thus, from these studies it is reasonable to conclude that fibrocytes arise in response to apoptotic stimuli.

In addition to the information regarding the precise relationship between apoptosis and fibrocytes, these studies also allowed new insight into the relationship between M2 macrophages and fibrocytes. Recent literature has suggested that macrophages are capable of expressing collagen (Pilling et al., 2009) and thus the CD45/Col-Iα signature may not sufficiently differentiate between fibrocytes and alternatively activated (M2) macrophages. Prior studies have demonstrated that alveolar macrophages obtained from patients with SSc-ILD demonstrate a distinct M2 profibrotic phenotype and that alternatively activated macrophages (M2) in part regulate fibrosis (Atamas et al., 2003). Thus it could be argued that the reduction in CD45/Col-Iα cells previously noted could be related to changes in alternatively activated macrophages quantities or rather that M2 macrophages regulate the appearance of CD45/Col-Iα cells. However, in our studies caspase inhibition demonstrated no significant differences in numbers of CD206/MRC positive cells between sham treated and ZVAD treated mice, nor was there a significant difference in M2 related genes CD206/MRC and MSR-1 using quantitative RT-PCR between the two cohorts (Peng et al., 2011). Likewise, in a separate set of studies in which M2 macrophages were removed by intratracheal instillation of liposomal clodronate, removal of M2 macrophages did not affect intrapulmonary fibrocyte content. Curiously, fibrocytes persisted despite profound attenuation of collagen deposition (Murray et al., 2011). When viewed in combination, these studies suggest that fibrocytes and M2 macrophages are regulated independently of each other and that each cell type exert separate, but complementary, effects on TGF-β1 fibrogenesis.

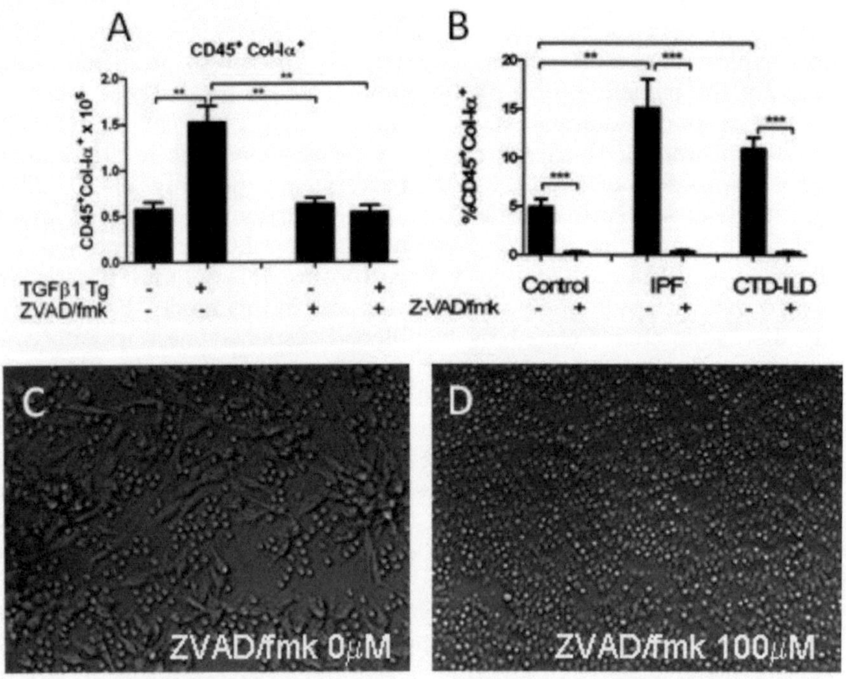

Fig. 2. Caspase inhibition administration attenuates apoptosis and collagen production in cultured human monocytes. (a) Z-VAD/fmk reduces CD45⁺Col-Iα1⁺ cells in TGF-β1 Tg⁺ mice. (b) Treatment with ZVAD/fmk attenuates collagen production in samples from all groups. (c,d) CT-ILD cultured monocytes fail to adopt a spindle shaped phenotype when treated with Z-VAD/fmk. (Peng et al., 2011)

4.4 Role of semaphorin 7a in fibrocyte outgrowth

Previous studies have indicated that fibrocyte biology is induced by exposure to soluble factors such as Th2 cytokines and activation of several chemokine pathways including CXCL12, MCP-1, and CCL21. However, the TGF-β1 specific factors controlling their differentiation has remained less clear. Because SSc-ILD is associated with a unique "signature" of TGF-β1 responsiveness (Sargent et al., 2010) we explored the role of TGF-β1 signaling in fibrocyte accumulation. Because the monocyte-driven effects on fibrosis appear to be SMAD2/3 independent (Murray et al., 2011), we explored noncanonical TGF-β1 pathways in this model. One such pathway is controlled by activation of Semaphorin 7a.

Semaphorins (Semas) are a family of highly conserved, secreted or membrane-associated proteins, expressed on stroma as well as nerve, myeloid and lymphoid cells. Originally discovered as axonal guidance proteins (Pasterkamp et al., 2003), eight classes of Semaphorins have since been discovered with Semas 3-7 subsequently being found to participate in a variety of processes related to organogenesis, angiogenesis, apoptosis, neoplasia and immune regulation (Pasterkamp & Kolodkin, 2003). Semaphorin 7a (Sema 7a), also called CDw108, is a GPI-anchored membrane protein that by signaling through its two main receptors, Plexin C1 and β1 integrin, contributes to inflammation (Suzuki et al., 2007), modulation of T cell function (Czopik et al., 2006), and TGF-β1 induced pulmonary fibrosis (Kang et al., 2007). However, until recently a role for Sema 7a in fibrocyte development had not been explored.

In order to explore this question we crossed TGF-β1 mice with mice harboring null mutations of the Sema 7a gene. In addition to effects on lung fibrosis and remodeling, which had been described previously, we found that fibrosis (quantified via sircol analysis) and fibrocytes were markedly reduced in the TGF-β1 mice that lacked Sema 7a (Figure 3a, $p < 0.001$). These effects were explored further in bone marrow chimera experiments in which TGF-β1 mice were created in which Sema 7a expression was restricted to lung stroma or to bone marrow derived cells. Lung restricted Sema 7a expression in TGF-β1 mice revealed a modest but insignificant reduction in fibrosis and fibrocyte content. However in the TGF-β1 x Sema 7a null cohort of mice where Sema 7a expression was restored on bone marrow derived cells these mice developed increased fibrosis and fibrocytes (Gan et al., 2011). These studies reveal that Sema 7a expressing bone marrow derived cells are sufficient, but not necessary, for the development of fibrosis and fibrocyte accumulation in the TGF-β1 exposed murine lung.

In order to explore the human relevance of these findings we interrogated the relationship between Sema 7a and fibrocyte biology in a second cohort of patients with SSc-ILD. In these studies, enhanced expression of Sema 7a and its two known receptors (β1 integrin and Plexin C1) were detected in peripheral blood mononuclear cells (PBMCs) from patients with SSc-ILD, but not SSc only, indicating that the Sema 7a axis may be unique to patients with interstitial lung involvement. Flow cytometric analysis revealed that the increased expression of Sema 7a appeared to be related to augmented cell surface on fibrocytes and CD19+ lymphocytes. In contrast, Sema 7a receptors β1 integrin and Plexin C1 were located on CD14+ monocytes (Gan et al., 2011). This led to speculation that exogenous ligation of these receptors by Sema 7a (either membrane bound or secreted) controls the monocyte to fibrocyte transition in this patient population.

The validity of this hypothesis was then tested in ex vivo studies of fibrocytes using standard, serum containing conditions. Specifically, monocytes from scleroderma subjects or controls were cultured in the presence or absence of recombinant Sema 7a stimulation for 14 days. These cultures were further exposed to Sema 7a receptor blockade of β1 integrin or Plexin C1. In normal controls, Sema 7a exposure led to enhanced fibrocyte outgrowth, however, in monocytes obtained from individuals with SSc-ILD, stimulation with Sema 7a had little effect on the already markedly enhanced fibrocyte numbers that exist at baseline in these cultures. In both groups these results were attenuated by β1 integrin blockade and enhanced by Plexin C1 blockade (Figure 3 c,d). When viewed in combination it appears that Sema 7a controls the monocyte to fibrocyte transition in a β1 integrin dependent manner that is opposed by Plexin C1 (Gan et al., 2011). Thus, the increased Plexin C1 gene expression seen in the SSc-ILD patients may represent a novel counter-regulatory response and a new target for therapy.

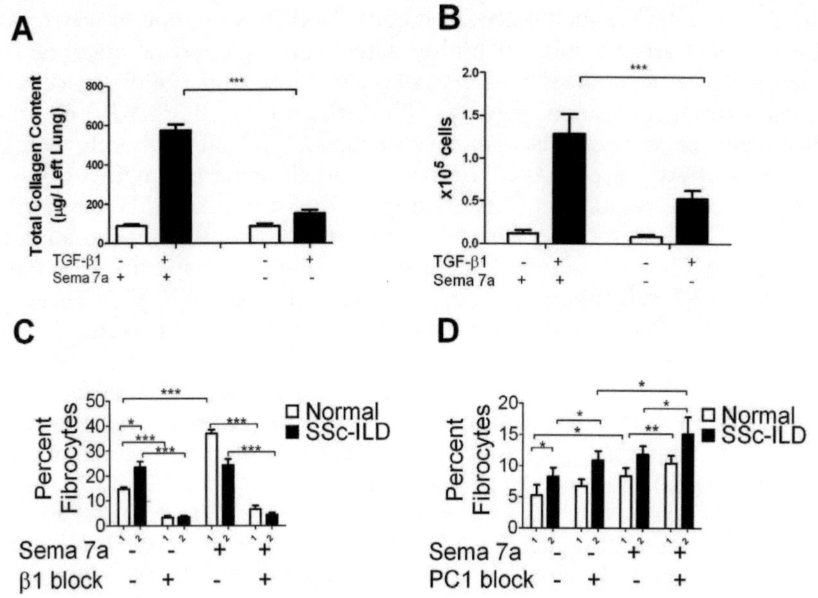

Fig. 3. (a) Total left lung collagen in wild type mice (white bar) and TFG-β1 Tg$^+$ mice (black bar). Left: Sema-7a locus intact. Right: Sema-7a locus deleted. (b) Compared to TGF-β1XWT mice, lungs from TGF-β1XSema-7a null mice contain significantly decreased quantities of CD45$^+$Col-Iα$^+$ cells. White bar: WT. Black bar: TGF-β1 Tg$^+$ mouse. (c) Sema-7a stimulated PBMCs show increased fibrocyte differentiation (white, left comparisons). In contrast, SSc-ILD subjects show increased fibrocyte outgrowth at baseline (black, left comparisons) with no response to exogenous Sema stimulation but pronounced reduction via immunoneutralization of the β1 integrin subunit (right comparisons). (d) Inhibition of Plexin C1 promotes fibrocyte differentiation in Sema-7a stimulated monocytes from control and SSc-ILD subjects as well as in unstimulated SSc-ILD monocytes. (Gan et al., 2011)

5. Conclusion

Fibrocytes have been implicated in a wide array of human autoimmune and inflammatory diseases since their identification 17 years ago. Human and animal studies have confirmed elevated levels of these mesenchymal progenitor cells in blood and tissue during fibrotic disease states. Animal models have also revealed the fibrocytes' complex role in the repair and remodeling of injured tissue, which includes antigen presentation, ECM and cytokine production, promotion of angiogenesis and differentiation to myofibroblasts. Because of their role in the maintenance and homeostasis of connective tissue, they have emerged as a cell of interest in scleroderma, and specifically SSc-ILD. Our work in these patients revealed a significant association between circulating fibrocytes and SSc-ILD. Targeting these cells, and their relationship with such regulatory factors as TGF-β1, apoptosis, and Semaphorin 7a may ultimately lead to the discovery of new biomarkers and perhaps even novel therapeutic targets in SSc-ILD.

6. References

Abe, R., S. C. Donnelly, T. Peng, R. Bucala, and C. N. Metz. 2001. Peripheral blood fibrocytes: differentiation pathway and migration to wound sites. J Immunol 166:7556-7562.

Atamas, S. P., I. G. Luzina, J. Choi, N. Tsymbalyuk, N. H. Carbonetti, I. S. Singh, M. Trojanowska, S. A. Jimenez, and B. White. 2003. Pulmonary and activation-regulated chemokine stimulates collagen production in lung fibroblasts. Am J Respir Cell Mol Biol 29:743-749.

Balmelli, C., M. P. Alves, E. Steiner, D. Zingg, N. Peduto, N. Ruggli, H. Gerber, K. McCullough, and A. Summerfield. 2007. Responsiveness of fibrocytes to toll-like receptor danger signals. Immunobiology 212:693-699.

Barth, P. J., S. Ebrahimsade, A. Hellinger, R. Moll, and A. Ramaswamy. 2002. CD34+ fibrocytes in neoplastic and inflammatory pancreatic lesions. Virchows Arch 440:128-133.

Bellini, A., and S. Mattoli. 2007. The role of the fibrocyte, a bone marrow-derived mesenchymal progenitor, in reactive and reparative fibroses. Lab Invest 87:858-870.

Bianchetti, L., M. Barczyk, J. Cardoso, M. Schmidt, A. Bellini, and S. Mattoli. 2011. Extracellular matrix remodelling properties of human fibrocytes. J Cell Mol Med.

Bucala, R., L. A. Spiegel, J. Chesney, M. Hogan, and A. Cerami. 1994. Circulating fibrocytes define a new leukocyte subpopulation that mediates tissue repair. Mol Med 1:71-81.

Bungartz, G., S. Stiller, M. Bauer, W. Muller, A. Schippers, N. Wagner, R. Fassler, and C. Brakebusch. 2006. Adult murine hematopoiesis can proceed without beta1 and beta7 integrins. Blood 108:1857-1864.

Castano, A. P., S. L. Lin, T. Surowy, B. T. Nowlin, S. A. Turlapati, T. Patel, A. Singh, S. Li, M. L. Lupher, Jr., and J. S. Duffield. 2009. Serum amyloid P inhibits fibrosis through Fc gamma R-dependent monocyte-macrophage regulation in vivo. Sci Transl Med 1:5ra13.

Chesney, J., M. Bacher, A. Bender, and R. Bucala. 1997. The peripheral blood fibrocyte is a potent antigen-presenting cell capable of priming naive T cells in situ. Proc Natl Acad Sci U S A 94:6307-6312.

Chesney, J., C. Metz, A. B. Stavitsky, M. Bacher, and R. Bucala. 1998. Regulated production of type I collagen and inflammatory cytokines by peripheral blood fibrocytes. J Immunol 160:419-425.

Chifflot, H., B. Fautrel, C. Sordet, E. Chatelus, and J. Sibilia. 2008. Incidence and prevalence of systemic sclerosis: a systematic literature review. Semin Arthritis Rheum 37:223-235.

Czopik, A. K., M. S. Bynoe, N. Palm, C. S. Raine, and R. Medzhitov. 2006. Semaphorin 7A is a negative regulator of T cell responses. Immunity 24:591-600.

D'Ovidio, F., M. Mura, M. Tsang, T. K. Waddell, M. A. Hutcheon, L. G. Singer, D. Hadjiliadis, C. Chaparro, C. Gutierrez, A. Pierre, G. Darling, M. Liu, and S. Keshavjee. 2005a. Bile acid aspiration and the development of bronchiolitis obliterans after lung transplantation. J Thorac Cardiovasc Surg 129:1144-1152.

D'Ovidio, F., L. G. Singer, D. Hadjiliadis, A. Pierre, T. K. Waddell, M. de Perrot, M. Hutcheon, L. Miller, G. Darling, and S. Keshavjee. 2005b. Prevalence of gastroesophageal reflux in end-stage lung disease candidates for lung transplant. Ann Thorac Surg 80:1254-1260.

Daoussis, D., S. N. Liossis, A. C. Tsamandas, C. Kalogeropoulou, A. Kazantzi, C. Sirinian, M. Karampetsou, G. Yiannopoulos, and A. P. Andonopoulos. 2010. Experience with rituximab in scleroderma: results from a 1-year, proof-of-principle study. Rheumatology (Oxford) 49:271-280.

Douglas, R. S., N. F. Afifiyan, C. J. Hwang, K. Chong, U. Haider, P. Richards, A. G. Gianoukakis, and T. J. Smith. 2009. Increased generation of fibrocytes in thyroid-associated ophthalmopathy. J Clin Endocrinol Metab 95:430-438.

Falk, E. 2006. Pathogenesis of atherosclerosis. J Am Coll Cardiol 47:C7-12.

Galligan, C. L., K. A. Siminovitch, E. C. Keystone, V. Bykerk, O. D. Perez, and E. N. Fish. 2010. Fibrocyte activation in rheumatoid arthritis. Rheumatology 49:640-651.

Gan, Y., R. Reilkoff, X. Peng, T. Russell, Q. Chen, S. K. Mathai, R. Homer, M. Gulati, J. Siner, J. Elias, R. Bucala, and E. Herzog. 2011. Role of semaphorin 7a signaling in TGF-beta1 induced lung fibrosis and scleroderma-related interstitial lung disease. Arthritis Rheum.

Goh, N. S., S. R. Desai, S. Veeraraghavan, D. M. Hansell, S. J. Copley, T. M. Maher, T. J. Corte, C. R. Sander, J. Ratoff, A. Devaraj, G. Bozovic, C. P. Denton, C. M. Black, R. M. du Bois, and A. U. Wells. 2008. Interstitial lung disease in systemic sclerosis: a simple staging system. Am J Respir Crit Care Med 177:1248-1254.

Gomperts, B. N., and R. M. Strieter. 2007. Fibrocytes in lung disease. J Leukoc Biol 82:449-456.

Hartlapp, I., R. Abe, R. W. Saeed, T. Peng, W. Voelter, R. Bucala, and C. N. Metz. 2001. Fibrocytes induce an angiogenic phenotype in cultured endothelial cells and promote angiogenesis in vivo. Faseb J 15:2215-2224.

Hashimoto, N., H. Jin, T. Liu, S. W. Chensue, and S. H. Phan. 2004. Bone marrow-derived progenitor cells in pulmonary fibrosis. J Clin Invest 113:243-252.

Herzog, E. L., J. Van Arnam, B. Hu, and D. S. Krause. 2006. Threshold of lung injury required for the appearance of marrow-derived lung epithelia. Stem Cells 24:1986-1992.

Kang, H. R., C. G. Lee, R. J. Homer, and J. A. Elias. 2007. Semaphorin 7A plays a critical role in TGF-beta1-induced pulmonary fibrosis. J Exp Med 204:1083-1093.

Kisseleva, T., H. Uchinami, N. Feirt, O. Quintana-Bustamante, J. C. Segovia, R. F. Schwabe, and D. A. Brenner. 2006. Bone marrow-derived fibrocytes participate in pathogenesis of liver fibrosis. J Hepatol 45:429-438.

Lee, C. G., S. J. Cho, M. J. Kang, S. P. Chapoval, P. J. Lee, P. W. Noble, T. Yehualaeshet, B. Lu, R. A. Flavell, J. Milbrandt, R. J. Homer, and J. A. Elias. 2004. Early growth response gene 1-mediated apoptosis is essential for transforming growth factor beta1-induced pulmonary fibrosis. J Exp Med 200:377-389.

Lin, S. L., T. Kisseleva, D. A. Brenner, and J. S. Duffield. 2008. Pericytes and perivascular fibroblasts are the primary source of collagen-producing cells in obstructive fibrosis of the kidney. Am J Pathol 173:1617-1627.

Mathai, S. K., M. Gulati, X. Peng, T. R. Russell, A. C. Shaw, A. N. Rubinowitz, L. A. Murray, J. M. Siner, D. E. Antin-Ozerkis, R. R. Montgomery, R. A. Reilkoff, R. J. Bucala, and E. L. Herzog. 2010. Circulating monocytes from systemic sclerosis patients with interstitial lung disease show an enhanced profibrotic phenotype. Lab Invest 90:812-823.

Mehrad, B., M. D. Burdick, and R. M. Strieter. 2009. Fibrocyte CXCR4 regulation as a therapeutic target in pulmonary fibrosis. Int J Biochem Cell Biol 41:1708-1718.

Mehrad, B., M. D. Burdick, D. A. Zisman, M. P. Keane, J. A. Belperio, and R. M. Strieter. 2007. Circulating peripheral blood fibrocytes in human fibrotic interstitial lung disease. Biochem Biophys Res Commun 353:104-108.

Moeller, A., S. E. Gilpin, K. Ask, G. Cox, D. Cook, J. Gauldie, P. J. Margetts, L. Farkas, J. Dobranowski, C. Boylan, P. M. O'Byrne, R. M. Strieter, and M. Kolb. 2009. Circulating Fibrocytes Are an Indicator for Poor Prognosis in Idiopathic Pulmonary Fibrosis. Am J Respir Crit Care Med.

Moore, B. B., L. Murray, A. Das, C. A. Wilke, A. B. Herrygers, and G. B. Toews. 2006. The role of CCL12 in the recruitment of fibrocytes and lung fibrosis. Am J Respir Cell Mol Biol 35:175-181.

Murray, L. A., Q. Chen, M. S. Kramer, D. P. Hesson, R. L. Argentieri, X. Peng, M. Gulati, R. J. Homer, T. Russell, N. van Rooijen, J. A. Elias, C. M. Hogaboam, and E. L. Herzog. 2011. TGF-beta driven lung fibrosis is macrophage dependent and blocked by Serum Amyloid P. Int J Biochem Cell Biol. 43:154-162.

Niedermeier, M., B. Reich, M. R. Gomez, A. Denzel, K. Schmidbauer, N. Gobel, Y. Talke, F. Schweda, and M. Mack. 2009. CD4+ T cells control the differentiation of Gr1+ monocytes into fibrocytes. Proc Natl Acad Sci U S A 106:17892-17897.

Nihlberg, K., K. Larsen, A. Hultgardh-Nilsson, A. Malmstrom, L. Bjermer, and G. Westergren-Thorsson. 2006. Tissue fibrocytes in patients with mild asthma: a possible link to thickness of reticular basement membrane? Respir Res 7:50.

Nikam, V. S., G. Wecker, R. Schermuly, U. Rapp, K. Szelepusa, W. Seeger, and R. Voswinckel. 2011. Treprostinil Inhibits Adhesion and Differentiation of Fibrocytes via cAMP and Rap Dependent ERK Inactivation. Am J Respir Cell Mol Biol.

Pasterkamp, R. J., and A. L. Kolodkin. 2003. Semaphorin junction: making tracks toward neural connectivity. Curr Opin Neurobiol 13:79-89.

Pasterkamp, R. J., J. J. Peschon, M. K. Spriggs, and A. L. Kolodkin. 2003. Semaphorin 7A promotes axon outgrowth through integrins and MAPKs. Nature 424:398-405.

Peng, X., S. K. Mathai, L. A. Murray, T. Russell, R. Reilkoff, Q. Chen, M. Gulati, J. A. Elias, R. Bucala, Y. Gan, and E. L. Herzog. 2011. Local apoptosis promotes collagen production by monocyte-derived cells in transforming growth factor beta1-induced lung fibrosis. Fibrogenesis Tissue Repair 4:12.

Phillips, R. J., M. D. Burdick, K. Hong, M. A. Lutz, L. A. Murray, Y. Y. Xue, J. A. Belperio, M. P. Keane, and R. M. Strieter. 2004. Circulating fibrocytes traffic to the lungs in response to CXCL12 and mediate fibrosis. J Clin Invest 114:438-446.

Pilling, D., C. D. Buckley, M. Salmon, and R. H. Gomer. 2003. Inhibition of fibrocyte differentiation by serum amyloid P. J Immunol 171:5537-5546.

Pilling, D., T. Fan, D. Huang, B. Kaul, and R. H. Gomer. 2009. Identification of markers that distinguish monocyte-derived fibrocytes from monocytes, macrophages, and fibroblasts. PLoS ONE 4:e7475.

Pilling, D., D. Roife, M. Wang, S. D. Ronkainen, J. R. Crawford, E. L. Travis, and R. H. Gomer. 2007. Reduction of bleomycin-induced pulmonary fibrosis by serum amyloid P. J Immunol 179:4035-4044.

Pilling, D., N. M. Tucker, and R. H. Gomer. 2006. Aggregated IgG inhibits the differentiation of human fibrocytes. J Leukoc Biol 79:1242-1251.

Quan, T. E., S. Cowper, S. P. Wu, L. K. Bockenstedt, and R. Bucala. 2004. Circulating fibrocytes: collagen-secreting cells of the peripheral blood. Int J Biochem Cell Biol 36:598-606.

Reilkoff, R. A., R. Bucala, and E. L. Herzog. 2011. Fibrocytes: emerging effector cells in chronic inflammation. Nature Reviews Immunology in press.

Sakai, N., T. Wada, H. Yokoyama, M. Lipp, S. Ueha, K. Matsushima, and S. Kaneko. 2006. Secondary lymphoid tissue chemokine (SLC/CCL21)/CCR7 signaling regulates fibrocytes in renal fibrosis. Proc Natl Acad Sci U S A 103:14098-14103.

Sargent, J. L., A. Milano, S. Bhattacharyya, J. Varga, M. K. Connolly, H. Y. Chang, and M. L. Whitfield. 2010. A TGFbeta-responsive gene signature is associated with a subset of diffuse scleroderma with increased disease severity. J Invest Dermatol 130:694-705.

Schmidt, M., G. Sun, M. A. Stacey, L. Mori, and S. Mattoli. 2003. Identification of circulating fibrocytes as precursors of bronchial myofibroblasts in asthma. J Immunol 171:380-389.

Shao, D. D., R. Suresh, V. Vakil, R. H. Gomer, and D. Pilling. 2008. Pivotal Advance: Th-1 cytokines inhibit, and Th-2 cytokines promote fibrocyte differentiation. J Leukoc Biol 83:1323-1333.

Steen, V. D., and T. A. Medsger. 2007. Changes in causes of death in systemic sclerosis, 1972-2002. Ann Rheum Dis 66:940-944.

Suzuki, K., T. Okuno, M. Yamamoto, R. J. Pasterkamp, N. Takegahara, H. Takamatsu, T. Kitao, J. Takagi, P. D. Rennert, A. L. Kolodkin, A. Kumanogoh, and H. Kikutani. 2007. Semaphorin 7A initiates T-cell-mediated inflammatory responses through alpha1beta1 integrin. Nature 446:680-684.

Swigris, J. J., A. L. Olson, A. Fischer, D. A. Lynch, G. P. Cosgrove, S. K. Frankel, R. T. Meehan, and K. K. Brown. 2006. Mycophenolate mofetil is safe, well tolerated, and preserves lung function in patients with connective tissue disease-related interstitial lung disease. Chest 130:30-36.

Tashkin, D. P., R. Elashoff, P. J. Clements, J. Goldin, M. D. Roth, D. E. Furst, E. Arriola, R. Silver, C. Strange, M. Bolster, J. R. Seibold, D. J. Riley, V. M. Hsu, J. Varga, D. E. Schraufnagel, A. Theodore, R. Simms, R. Wise, F. Wigley, B. White, V. Steen, C. Read, M. Mayes, E. Parsley, K. Mubarak, M. K. Connolly, J. Golden, M. Olman, B. Fessler, N. Rothfield, and M. Metersky. 2006. Cyclophosphamide versus placebo in scleroderma lung disease. N Engl J Med 354:2655-2666.

Tourkina, E., M. Bonner, J. Oates, A. Hofbauer, M. Richard, S. Znoyko, R. P. Visconti, J. Zhang, C. M. Hatfield, R. M. Silver, and S. Hoffman. 2011. Altered monocyte and fibrocyte phenotype and function in scleroderma interstitial lung disease: reversal by caveolin-1 scaffolding domain peptide. Fibrogenesis Tissue Repair 4:15.

Vakil, V., J. J. Sung, M. Piecychna, J. R. Crawford, P. Kuo, A. K. Abu-Alfa, S. E. Cowper, R. Bucala, and R. H. Gomer. 2009. Gadolinium-containing magnetic resonance image contrast agent promotes fibrocyte differentiation. J Magn Reson Imaging 30:1284-1288.

Wang, C. H., C. D. Huang, H. C. Lin, K. Y. Lee, S. M. Lin, C. Y. Liu, K. H. Huang, Y. S. Ko, K. F. Chung, and H. P. Kuo. 2008. Increased circulating fibrocytes in asthma with chronic airflow obstruction. Am J Respir Crit Care Med 178:583-591.

Yang, L., P. G. Scott, J. Giuffre, H. A. Shankowsky, A. Ghahary, and E. E. Tredget. 2002. Peripheral blood fibrocytes from burn patients: identification and quantification of fibrocytes in adherent cells cultured from peripheral blood mononuclear cells. Lab Invest 82:1183-1192.

8

Inhibition of Thrombin as a Novel Strategy in the Treatment of Scleroderma-Associated Interstitial Lung Disease

Galina S. Bogatkevich[1], Kristin B. Highland[1], Tanjina Akter[1], Paul J. Nietert[1], Ilia Atanelishvili[1], Joanne van Ryn[2] and Richard M. Silver[1]
[1]Medical University of South Carolina, Charleston,
[2]Boehringer Ingelheim GmbH & Co.KG, Biberach,
[1]USA
[2]Germany

1. Introduction

Activation of the coagulation cascade leading to generation of thrombin has been extensively documented in various forms of lung injury including systemic sclerosis-associated interstitial lung disease (SSc-ILD). The molecular mechanisms underlying the pathogenesis and progression of lung fibrosis in SSc-ILD and in idiopathic pulmonary fibrosis (IPF) are not entirely clear. The conceptual process of fibrogenesis involves tissue injury and activation of the coagulation cascade, the release of various fibrogenic factors, and the induction of myofibroblasts culminating in enhanced extracellular matrix deposition. Cells with a myofibroblast phenotype appear in the early stages of fibrosis and are characterized by an increased proliferative capacity and abundant expression of α-SMA, collagens and other extracellular matrix proteins (Hinz et al., 2007). Myofibroblasts can be cultured from bronchoalveolar lavage (BAL) fluid of SSc-ILD patients, and thrombin activity is also significantly greater in BAL fluid from SSc-ILD patients compared with healthy controls (Ludwicka et al., 1992; Ohba et al., 1994). Thrombin differentiates lung fibroblasts to a myofibroblast phenotype, increases lung fibroblast proliferation (Bogatkevich et al., 2001), and enhances the proliferative effect of fibrinogen on fibroblasts (Gray et al., 1993). Thrombin is also a potent inducer of fibrogenic cytokines, such as transforming growth factor-β (TGF-β) (Bachhuber et al., 1997), connective tissue growth factor (CTGF) (Chambers et al., 2000; Bogatkevich et al., 2006), platelet-derived growth factor-AA (PDGF-AA) (Ohba et al., 1994), chemokines (Mercer et al., 2007), and ECM proteins such as collagen, fibronectin, and tenascin in various cells, including lung fibroblasts (Tourkina et al., 2001; Chambers et al., 1998; Armstrong et al., 1996).

Dabigatran is a selective direct thrombin inhibitor that reversibly binds to thrombin and prevents the cleavage of Arg-Gly bonds of fibrinogen needed for the formation of fibrin. Recently, we have demonstrated that binding of dabigatran to thrombin prevents cleavage of the extracellular N-terminal domain of the protease-activated receptor 1 (PAR-1), which is responsible for most profibrotic events induced by thrombin (Bogatkevich et al., 2009). In the absence of dabigatran, thrombin binds to PAR-1, cleaves the peptide bond between residues Arg-41 and Ser-42, thereby unmasking a new amino terminus, SFLLRN, which then can bind to the second extracellular loop of PAR-1 and initiate receptor signaling (Macfarlane et al., 2001). Dabigatran-bound thrombin is unable to cleave and activate PAR-1. The aim of this chapter is to provide a molecular basis for therapeutic interventions in SSc-ILD by inhibition of thrombin.

2. Increased expression of thrombin and PAR-1 in SSc-ILD

Thrombin is a multi-functional serine protease and a key enzyme of blood coagulation, catalyzing the conversion of fibrinogen to fibrin. In addition to its essential role in coagulation, thrombin has several important functions at a cellular level, both in normal health and in multiple disease processes, including pulmonary fibrosis (Chambers, 2008). Our laboratory as well as others has demonstrated dramatically increased levels of thrombin in BALF from scleroderma patients with lung fibrosis and other fibrosing lung diseases (Ohba et al., 1994; Hernadez-Rodriguez et al., 1995). We have reported that BALF from normal subjects contains a low level of thrombin activity ranging from zero to 150 units per mg of BALF protein (48.6 ± 8.7 U/mg, mean ± SEM). BAL fluids of SSc patients express up to 100-fold higher thrombin activity, ranging from 22 to 7,525 units per mg of BALF protein (699.9 ± 201.1 U/mg, mean ± SEM; $P < 0.001$) (Fig. 1A). Elevated levels of thrombin activity have been also observed in bleomycin-induced pulmonary fibrosis in mice (Howell et al., 2005). We found that the level of active thrombin in BAL fluid from bleomycin-treated mice was 35-fold higher (1.3 ± 0.1 ng/ml, mean ± SEM) compared to that in control mice treated with saline (46.1 ± 7.9 ng/ml, mean ± SEM; $P < 0.01$) (Fig. 1B).

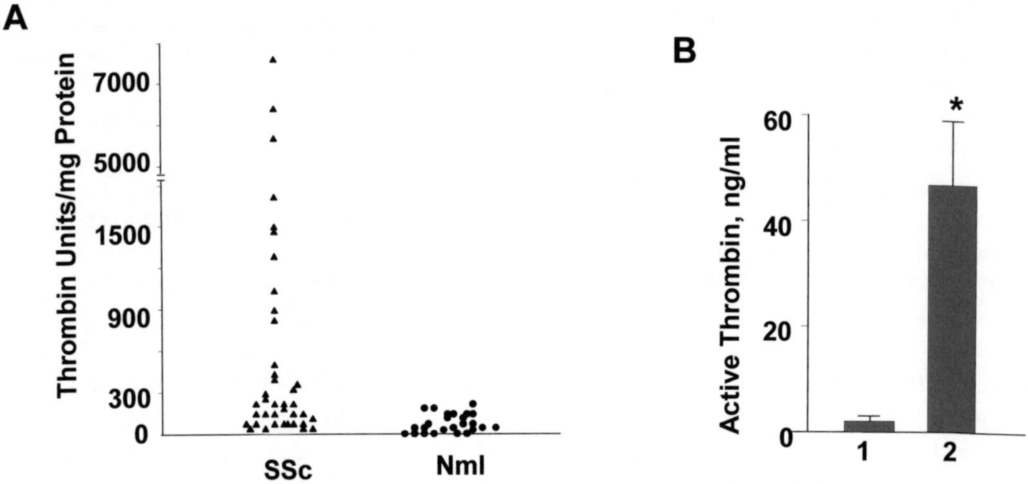

Fig. 1. (A) Thrombin levels in BALF of scleroderma patients (SSc, closed triangles, n = 42) and normal subjects (Nml, closed circles, n = 27). Active thrombin was measured by fluorometric method using a synthetic substrate Boc-Val-Pro-Arg-7-(4-methyl) coumarylamide, and expressed as units per mg of BALF protein. (B) Thrombin levels in BALF of mice treated with saline (1) and with bleomycin-induced pulmonary fibrosis (2).

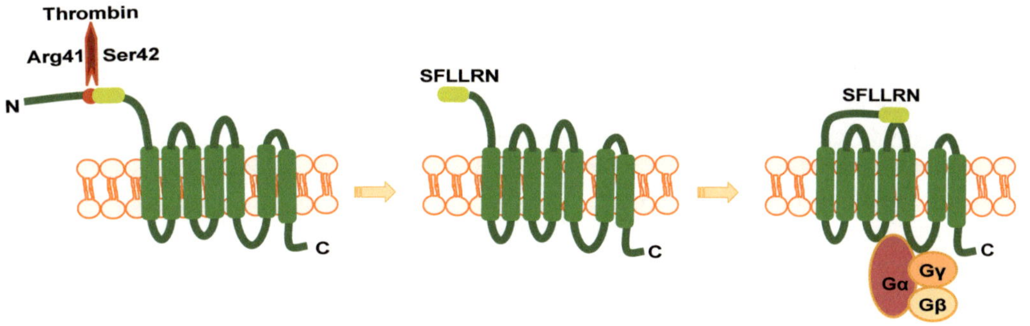

Fig. 2. Mechanism of PAR-1 activation. Proteolytic cleavage of the N-terminus results in the unmasking of a tethered ligand SFLLRN, which in turn interacts with extracellular loop-2 of the receptor and initiates cell signaling via activation of heterotrimeric G-proteins.

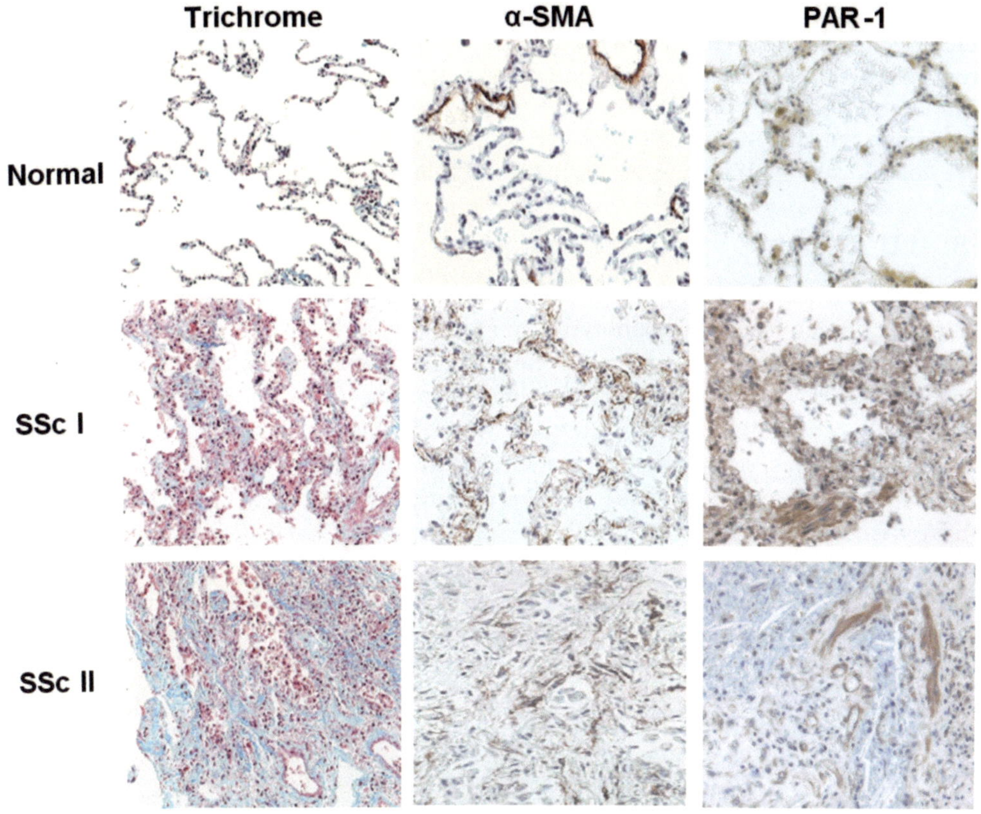

Fig. 3. PAR-1 and α-SMA expression is significantly increased in pulmonary fibrosis associated with scleroderma. Sections of normal and scleroderma (SSc) lung stained by trichrome, α-SMA antibody, and PAR-1 antibody; α-SMA and PAR-1 were visualized as brown color by diaminobenzidine (DAB) and counterstained with hematoxilin. Top panel represents normal lung tissue, middle panel (SSc I) represents lung tissue in early stage of lung involvement and bottom panel (SSc II) represents lung tissue with late stage of fibrosis.

The majority of the cellular responses to thrombin are mediated via the G protein-coupled PAR-1 receptor (Howell et al., 2002; Coughlin 1999). PAR-1 is activated by proteolytic cleavage of N-terminal domains, leading to the exposure of a new amino-terminus, a "tethered ligand" that in turn activates the receptor (Fig. 2). PAR-1 activation has been shown to be an important in the pathophysiology of various lung diseases, including SSc-ILD (Howell et al., 2002; Bogatkevich et al., 2005). PAR-1 is present in a variety of cell types, including leukocytes, platelets, T cells, endothelial cells, vascular smooth muscle cells and fibroblasts (Shrivastava et al., 2007). In the bleomycin model of pulmonary fibrosis, PAR-1 deficient mice show a significant reduction of inflammatory cells in BALF as compared with wild-type mice, and significant protection from lung fibrosis is seen in the PAR-1 deficient mice (Howell et al., 2005). The relative protection from pulmonary fibrosis observed in this model is a reduction in expression of two major fibrogenic growth factors, CTGF and transforming growth factor β- (TGF-β), as well as a reduction of the chemokine (C-C motif) ligand 2 (CCL2)/monocyte chemotactic protein 1 (MCP-1).
Elevated expression of PAR-1 has been shown in patients with IPF and in a murine model of bleomycin-induced lung fibrosis (Chambers, 2008; Howell et al., 2005). In previous studies we demonstrated that PAR-1 expression is also dramatically increased in lung tissue from scleroderma patients, mainly in lung parenchyma in context with myofibroblasts present in inflammatory and fibroproliferative foci (Bogatkevich et al., 2005). PAR-1 expression diminishes in the later stages of pulmonary fibrosis (Fig. 3) suggesting its important role in lung fibroblast activation during the early development of pulmonary fibrosis.

3. SSc-ILD, thrombin, and myofibroblasts

In the pathogenesis of pulmonary fibrosis in general and SSc-ILD in particular, lung fibroblasts undergo specific phenotypic modulation and develop cytoskeletal features similar to those of smooth muscle cells. These phenotypically altered, activated fibroblasts, or "myofibroblasts", express a contractile isoform of actin (α-smooth muscle actin, α-SMA) and promote contractility of lung tissues. Myofibroblasts appear to be the principal mesenchymal cells responsible for tissue remodeling, collagen deposition, and the restrictive nature of the lung parenchyma associated with pulmonary fibrosis (Tomasek et al., 2002).
We have demonstrated that myofibroblasts are present in the BALF of SSc patients and that myofibroblasts cultured from SSc BALF express more collagen I, III, and fibronectin than normal lung fibroblasts (Ludwicka et al., 1992). Myofibroblasts from BALF also show a greater proliferative response upon exposure to TGF-β and PDGF when compared to normal lung fibroblasts. Several groups of investigators have demonstrated a correlation between fibrosis and α-SMA expressing myofibroblasts in a number of different tissues (Tomasek et al., 2002; Zhang et al., 1994; Walker et al., 2001). Myofibroblasts isolated from various fibrotic tissues, including lungs, are thought to be the primary source of collagen and other ECM proteins (Tomasek et al., 2002; Zhang et al., 1994). Studies in animals employing the bleomycin-induced model of pulmonary fibrosis have identified myofibroblasts to be the primary source of increased collagen expression and a major source of cytokines and chemokines as well (Zhang et al., 1996; Vyalow et al., 1993).
The precise source(s) of myofibroblasts is still not well known. Relative contributions from circulating mesenchymal stem cells or from local trans-differentiation of epithelial cells to fibroblasts have been reported (Hinz et al., 2007). It has become generally accepted that lung

fibroblasts may differentiate to a myofibroblast phenotype under the influence of local growth factors and cytokines, such as TGF-β, endothelin-1, and thrombin (Hinz et al., 2007; Bogatkevich et al., 2001; Shi-Wen et al., 2004). Interestingly, thrombin itself has been demonstrated to induce the secretion of TGF-β and endothelin-1 (Shi-Wen et al., 2004; Bachhuber et al., 1997).

4. Thrombin induces differentiation of lung fibroblasts to a myofibroblast phenotype resistant to apoptosis while inducing apoptosis of alveolar epithelial cells

Our previous studies demonstrated that thrombin differentiates normal lung fibroblasts to a myofibroblast phenotype via the PAR-1/PKCε-dependent pathway (Bogatkevich et al., 2001; 2003; 2005). We previously reported that thrombin induces resistance to FasL-induced apoptosis in normal lung fibroblasts and that a similar level of resistance to FasL is observed in SSc lung fibroblasts *de novo* (Bogatkevich et al., 2005). Interestingly, we also found that thrombin-induced resistance to apoptosis is not specific only for FasL. We showed that thrombin also induces resistance to other apoptotic factors such as camptothecin and ceramide, and that SSc lung fibroblasts are also resistant to apoptosis induced by these stimuli. Because of the involvement of Fas-FasL pathway in various pulmonary disorders, we have selected this molecule for further investigations of apoptosis. We demonstrated that FasL induces apoptosis in normal lung fibroblasts in a dose-dependent manner and that this effect is inhibited by thrombin, as well as by overexpression of constitutively-activated PAR-1 or constitutively-activated PKCε (Bogatkevich et al., 2005).

The activation of Akt in different cell lines is necessary for promotion of cell survival and protection from apoptosis. We observed that thrombin induced sustained phosphorylation of Akt at Ser-473 in lung fibroblasts. Phosphorylation of Akt occurred within 10 min of thrombin treatment, reaching a maximum at 30 min and decreasing after 2 hours (Fig. 4 A). Basal levels of total Akt were similar in lung fibroblasts and in A549 alveolar epithelial cells (AEC), and thrombin induced Akt phosphorylation only in lung fibroblasts and not in AEC (Fig.4B) at any time point.

Activation of the thrombin receptor PAR-1 is known to mediate apoptosis of intestinal epithelial and lung epithelial cells (Suzuki et al, 2005; Ando et al., 2007). We incubated human A549 AEC and mouse primary AEC with thrombin to determine if thrombin induces apoptosis in these cells. After 24 hours of incubation with thrombin (1U/ml), A549 cells demonstrated 4.2 times and AT2 cells demonstrated 3.45 times more DNA fragments when compared to control cells, consistent with thrombin induction of apoptosis of these different AEC types (Fig. 4C).

The best recognized hallmark of both early and late stages of apoptosis is the activation of cysteine aspartate-specific proteases, caspases. Upon activation, the caspases cleave specific substrates and thereby mediate many of the typical biochemical and morphological changes in apoptotic cells, such as cell shrinkage, chromatin condensation, DNA fragmentation and plasma membrane blebs (Kohler et al., 2002). Caspase-3 is activated during most apoptotic processes and is believed to be the main executioner caspase. We observed that thrombin activates caspase-3 in AEC, but not in lung fibroblasts (Fig. 4D)

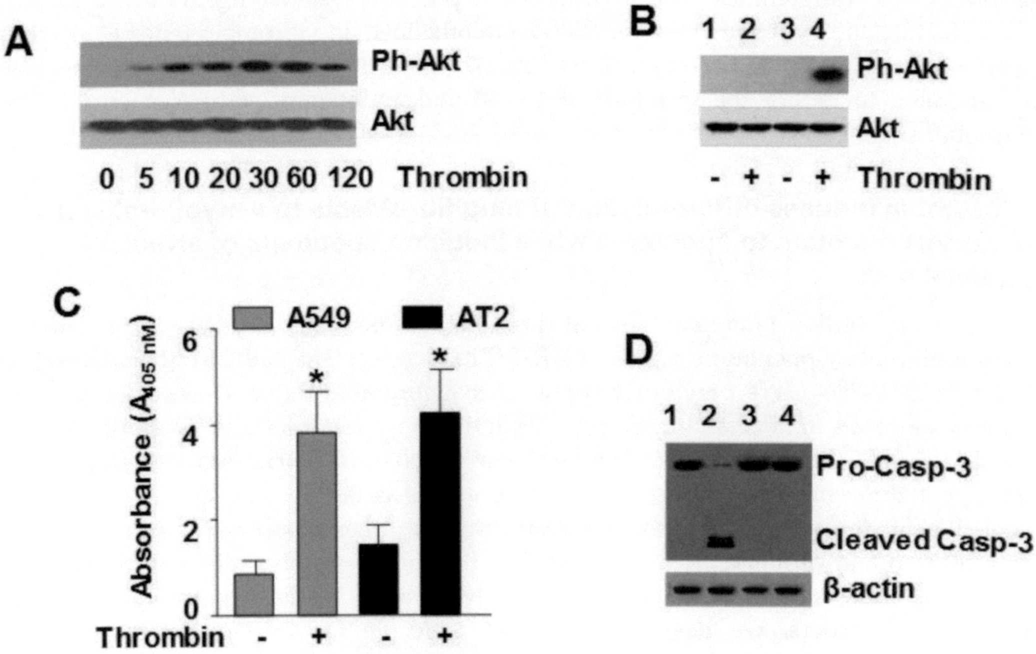

Fig. 4. Distinct effects of thrombin in lung fibroblasts and AEC. (A) Time course of thrombin-induced Akt Phosphorylation was determined in lung fibroblasts treated with 1U/ml thrombin for various time points. (B) AEC (lanes 1 and 2) and lung fibroblasts (lanes 3 and 4) were incubated with or without thrombin for 30 minutes. Cell extracts were immunoblotted with phospho-Akt or total Akt antibody (Cell Signaling Technology). (C) Thrombin-induced apoptosis of human SAEC and mice AT2 cells. Each bar represents the mean ± SD of duplicate determinations in 3 experiments. *Statistically significant differences between cells stimulated with thrombin and dabigatran versus cells stimulated with thrombin ($p<0.05$). (D) Western blot analysis of caspase-3 expression in AEC and lung fibroblasts. Confluent cultures of AEC (lanes 1 and 2) and lung fibroblasts (lanes 3 and 4) were incubated with or without thrombin for 24 hours. Cell were collected with lysis buffer, subjected to SDS-polyacrylamide gels, and analyzed by immunoblotting using anti-caspase-3 antibodies from Cell Signaling Technology. Expression of β-actin is shown to confirm the equal loading of protein. Note that caspase-3 antibody recognizes full length pro-caspase-3 (35kDa) and the fragment (17 kDa) from caspase-3 resulting from cleavage.

5. Effects of direct thrombin inhibitor dabigatran on aec and lung fibroblasts *in vitro*

Thrombin is a well-known mitogen and has been shown to induce human lung fibroblast proliferation. We measured the effect of dabigatran on thrombin-induced lung fibroblast proliferation using a quick cell proliferation assay. This method is based on cleavage of a tetrazolium salt, WST-1, to formazan by cellular mitochondrial dehydrogenases. Expansion of the number of viable cells results in an increase in the activity of the mitochondrial dehydrogenases leading to an increase in the amount of formazan dye detected by spectrometry. Basal levels of viable lung fibroblasts were in a range of between 0.38 and 0.51 OD. Thrombin increased fibroblast proliferation 1.8-fold within 24 hours. The direct thrombin inhibitor, dabigatran, itself had no significant effect on lung fibroblast proliferation, yet dabigatran significantly inhibited thrombin-induced proliferation of lung fibroblasts. Neither thrombin nor dabigatran affected AEC cell proliferation (Fig. 5A). Dabigatran, however, inhibited thrombin-induced apoptosis of AEC A549 (Fig. 5B).

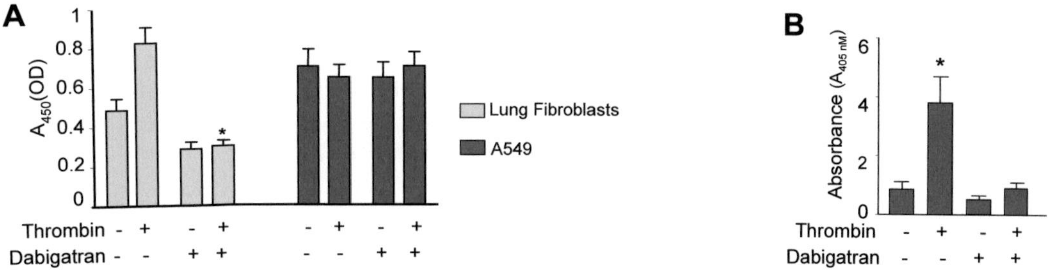

Fig. 5. (A) Dabigatran inhibits thrombin-induced lung fibroblasts proliferation and has no effects on the proliferation of AEC. (B) Dabigatran inhibits thrombin-induced apoptosis of AEC. The *asterisk* represents statistically significant ($p<0.05$) differences between cells stimulated with thrombin *versus* cells stimulated with thrombin and dabigatran.

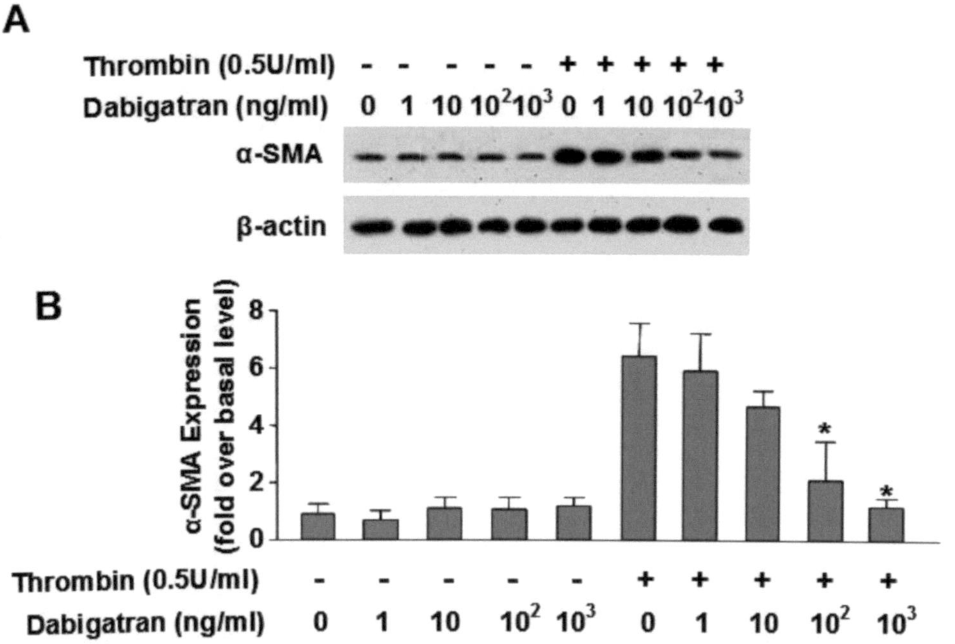

Fig. 6. (A) Dabigatran inhibits α–smooth muscle actin (α–SMA) expression in lung fibroblasts. (B) The images were scanned and analyzed with NIH Imaging software. Densitometric analysis of immunoblots from 3 independent experiments is presented. The *asterisk* represents statistically significant differences ($p<0.05$) between cells stimulated with thrombin and dabigatran *versus* cells treated with thrombin alone.

The appearance of myofibroblasts in areas of active fibrosis strongly suggests that myofibroblasts are key contributors to the pathogenesis of SSc-ILD. Lung fibroblasts from SSc-ILD patients express abundant and highly organized α-SMA (Bogatkevich et al., 2001). Moreover, thrombin receptor PAR-1 and α-SMA co-localize in lung tissue in early stages of lung fibrosis (see Fig. 3). In contrast, normal lung fibroblasts contain relatively small amounts of α-SMA which is not fully organized. Previously we reported that within 24 hours of exposure thrombin increases the amount of highly organized α-SMA in normal lung fibroblasts (Bogatkevich et al., 2001 and 2003). Although dabigatran had no effect on the basal level of α-SMA in normal lung fibroblasts, dabigatran significantly decreased thrombin-induced α-SMA expression in a dose-dependent manner (Fig. 6).

Contractile phenotype is another characteristic feature of myofibroblasts. Contractile forces of the myofibroblast are generated by α-SMA, which is extensively expressed in stress fibers and by large fibronexus adhesion complexes connecting intracellular actin with extracellular fibronectin fibrils (Gabbiani, 2003). Fibroblasts cultured in collagen gel matrices provide an *in vitro* model of fibrocontractility and fibrosing diseases such as scleroderma and IPF (Grinnell, 1999). When cultured within collagen gels fibroblasts recognize collagen fibers leading to contraction of the gels. This is believed to reflect the *in vivo* phenomenon of wound contraction and extracellular remodeling in connective tissue. In lung fibrosis it might also reflect the pathologic stiffness observed in SSc-ILD and other restrictive lung diseases. We previously observed that thrombin induces collagen gel contraction by normal lung fibroblasts in a dose-dependent manner with a maximal effect at 0.5 U/ml (Bogatkevich et al., 2001). To further investigate the effects of dabigatran on collagen gel contraction we used floating and fixed collagen gel assays with normal and SSc lung fibroblasts treated with and without thrombin or dabigatran for 48 hours. Contraction of floating collagen gels is considered to resemble more closely the initial phase of wound contraction and reflects the induction of the myofibroblast phenotype by various growth factors (Grinnell, 1999; Shi-Wen et al., 2004). In contrast, attached or fixed collagen gels serve as a model of the late phase of excessive scarring observed in contractures and reflect the direct ability of proteins to enhance contraction of already formed α-SMA through mechanical stress. SSc lung fibroblasts inherently contain higher levels of α-SMA and readily contracted both floating and fixed collagen gels (Fig. 7). Dabigatran significantly reduced collagen gel contraction by SSc lung fibroblasts and α-SMA in both floating and fixed collagen gels; however, thrombin only slightly induced α-SMA and did not significantly affect collagen gel contraction by SSc lung fibroblasts.

We observed notable differences for floating and fixed collagen gels seeded with normal lung fibroblasts when stimulated with thrombin. Thrombin strikingly contracted floating collagen gels within 48 hours in a similar manner as within 24 hours; in contrast, thrombin only slightly affected fixed collagen gels. Similarly, α-SMA was induced to a much higher extent by thrombin in floating gels as compared to fixed gels. In contrast, dabigatran inhibited collagen gel contraction and α-SMA not only in floating but also in fixed collagen gels, thus blocking differentiation to a myofibroblast phenotype, as well as reversing the already existing myofibroblast phenotype.

Normal lung fibroblasts naturally produce collagen type I and CTGF in very low concentrations. Thrombin and the PAR-1 selective activating peptide PAR1-AP notably increased the production of both of these proteins within 48 hours. Pre-treatment of lung fibroblasts with dabigatran (1μg/ml) prevented the accumulation of collagen type I and CTGF induced by thrombin, but not by PAR1-AP (Fig. 8A).

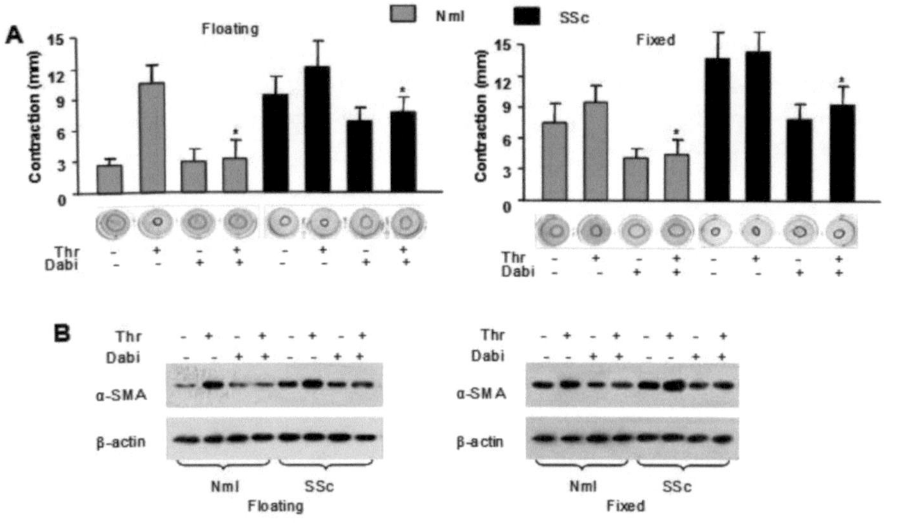

Fig. 7. (A) Inhibition of floating and fixed collagen gel contraction by dabigatran in lung fibroblasts. Data are presented as mean values ± SD of three experiments. The asterisk represents statistically significant differences ($p<0.05$) between cells stimulated with thrombin and dabigatran versus cells treated with thrombin alone. (B) α-SMA expression in floating and fixed collagen gels

Lung fibroblasts from SSc-ILD patients express considerably higher levels of α-SMA, CTGF, and collagen type I when compared with normal lung fibroblasts. To establish whether dabigatran would interfere with the expression of these markers of fibrogenesis, we incubated SSc lung fibroblasts with dabigatran (1μg/ml) for 24, 48, 72, and 96 hours. We observed that the addition of dabigatran for 72 and 96 hours reduced the levels of α-SMA and CTGF; however, treatment of cells with dabigatran for 48 and 24 hours had little or no effect (Fig. 8B). In contrast, the level of collagen type I was not significantly affected by dabigatran even after 72 hours. Yet after 96 hours of incubation with dabigatran SSc lung fibroblasts expressed significantly less collagen type I. To investigate whether, in addition to α-SMA expression, α-SMA organization would also be affected by dabigatran in SSc lung fibroblasts, we performed fluorescence microscopy studies. We observed that prolonged incubation of SSc lung fibroblasts with dabigatran indeed results in decreased α-SMA expression and organization (Fig. 8C). Over-production of collagen with increased expression of CTGF is considered to be a molecular hallmark of fibrosis (Grotendorst et al., 2004). Thrombin increases the expression of collagen type I and CTGF (Chambers et al., 1998 and 2000, Bogatkevich et al., 2006). Importantly, we have demonstrated that dabigatran restrains thrombin-induced accumulation of collagen type I and CTGF in human lung fibroblasts. Although we observed that incubation of SSc-ILD fibroblasts with dabigatran for 24 hours had no effect, upon longer exposure to dabigatran (72 hours) considerable inhibition of CTGF and α-SMA expression/organization was observed. Even longer exposure (96 hours) was required for dabigatran to significantly decrease collagen type I, suggesting that down-regulation of collagen by dabigatran in SSc lung fibroblasts occurs after inhibition of CTGF and α-SMA. It was reported that CTGF induces collagen I by stimulating transcription and promoter activity (Chujo et al., 2005; Gore-Hyer et al., 2002), and diminishing CTGF by small interfering RNA lowers collagens I and IV in rats (Luo et al., 2008). Similarly, the inhibition of α-SMA by the NH2-terminal peptide of α-SMA results in reduction of collagen gene expression (Hinz et al., 2002). Therefore, our data suggest that dabigatran may contribute to collagen type I down-regulation secondarily via reduced expression of CTGF and α-SMA.

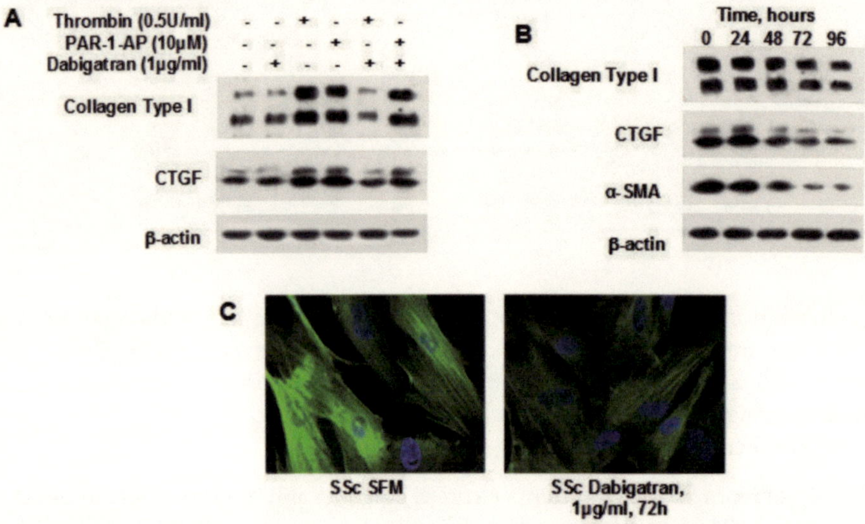

Fig. 8. (A) Dabigatran inhibits thrombin- but not PAR-1-AP-induced collagen type I and CTGF. (B) Dabigatran inhibits collagen type I, CTGF, and α–SMA expression in scleroderma lung fibroblasts. (C) Dabigatran inhibits α–SMA expression and organization in scleroderma lung fibroblasts. The experiments were repeated three times in three different cell lines and representative immunoblots and images are presented.

6. *In vivo* antifibrotic effects of direct thrombin inhibition with dabigatran

Since dabigatran restrained important in vitro profibrotic events in lung fibroblasts, we reasoned that dabigatran would diminish bleomycin-induced pulmonary fibrosis. For in vivo studies we employed dabigatran etexilate, the oral prodrug of dabigatran. The prodrug does not have antithrombin activity; however, after oral administration dabigatran etexilate is rapidly converted by ubiquitous esterases to the active moiety, dabigatran (Sorbera et al., 2005, Wienen et al., 2007). Drugs administrated during the early phase of tissue injury act predominantly as anti-inflammatory agents and should be considered as "preventive treatment", whereas "true" antifibrotic agents might be effective irrespective of timing, particularly if administrated during the "fibrotic" or later phase of the model (Moeller et al., 2008). To distinguish between anti-inflammatory and antifibrotic drug effects, we compared the effect of oral administration of dabigatran etexilate on the day of bleomycin instillation (day 1) and on day 8 after bleomycin instillation in mice.
In control mice that received saline or saline and dabigatran etexilate, lung histology was characterized by alveolar structures composed of septa, vascular components, and connective tissue. Alveolar septa were thin allowing maximum air to occupy the lung. Lung tissue isolated from bleomycin-treated mice demonstrated extensive peribronchial and

interstitial infiltrates of inflammatory cells (H&E staining), thickening of the alveolar walls, and multiple focal fibrotic lesions with excessive amounts of ECM protein shown by trichrome differential staining (Fig. 9A). By contrast, significantly fewer cellular infiltrates, decreased thickness of alveolar septa, and reduced accumulation of ECM proteins were all noted in mice treated with dabigatran etexilate. Importantly, such beneficial effects of dabigatran etexilate on bleomycin-induced pulmonary fibrosis were observed not only in mice receiving dabigatran etexilate beginning on the same day as bleomycin (day 1), but were seen also in mice that received dabigatran etexilate beginning on day 8 after bleomycin administration (Fig. 9A). The overall level of fibrotic changes was quantitatively assessed based on the Ashcroft scoring system (Ashcroft et al., 1988). The score in mice treated with bleomycin + placebo was nearly 9-fold higher compared to control mice (5.76±1.64 and 0.65±0.7 respectively). Fibrosis in mice treated with dabigatran etexilate beginning on day 1 after bleomycin instillation was significantly reduced (2.8-fold, $p < 0.05$) when compared to the bleomycin + placebo group, suggesting an anti-inflammatory effect of dabigatran (Fig. 9B).

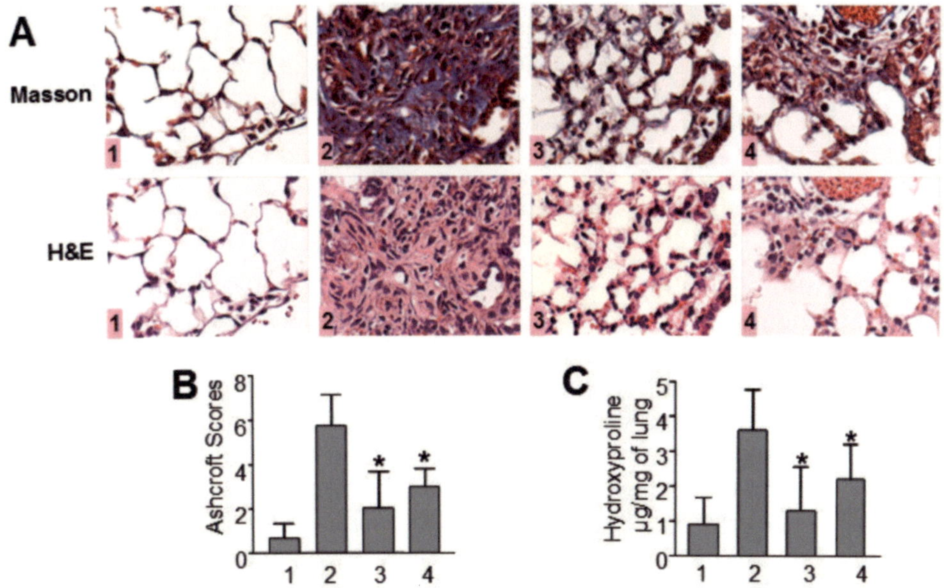

Fig. 9. Effect of dabigatran etexilate on bleomycin-induced pulmonary fibrosis. (A) Representative histological findings of lung inflammation and fibrosis. 1 - control (saline + placebo or saline + dabigatran), 2 - bleomycin + placebo, 3 - bleomycin + dabigatran etexilate (day 1), 4 - bleomycin + dabigatran etexilate (day 8), n = 40 (10 mice per group) (B) Quantitative evaluation of fibrotic changes (Ashcroft scores). (C) Collagen lung content measured by hydroxyproline assay, n = 32 (8 mice per group). Values are the mean ± SD. * = $P < 0.05$ versus bleomycin + placebo-treated mice.

Interestingly, fibrosis in mice that received dabigatran beginning on day 8 after bleomycin instillation was also significantly reduced (1.9-fold, $p < 0.05$) compared to the bleomycin + placebo group, suggesting that in addition to anti-inflammatory properties dabigatran demonstrated a strong anti-fibrotic effect.

The most profound development of fibrosis in the bleomycin model is observed by day 21; therefore, we determined the effect of dabigatran on collagen accumulation in lungs 21 days after bleomycin treatment. To quantify collagen accumulation within the lungs we employed hydroxyproline assay, which is based on colorimetric measurements of hydroxyproline in lung hydrolysates reflecting total collagen in lung tissue. We observed that dabigatran etexilate did not affect the basal level of hydroxyproline (data not shown). However, dabigatran etexilate significantly lowered hydroxyproline in bleomycin-treated mice by 64% and by 39% when administrated beginning on day 1 and day 8, respectively (Fig. 9C). From these studies, we conclude that dabigatran etexilate downregulates lung collagen by exerting an antifibrotic effect via thrombin inhibition.

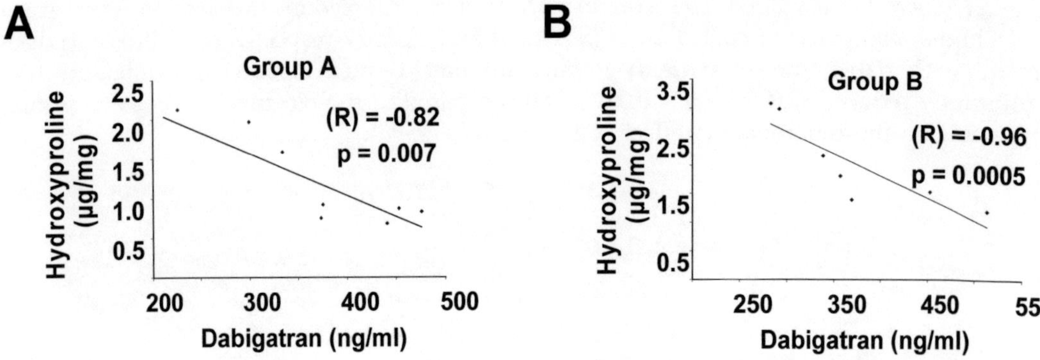

Fig. 10. Negative correlation of collagen content in lung tissue versus dabigatran levels in plasma on day 1 (Group A) and day 8 (Group B), respectively.

The association between hydroxyproline levels in lung tissue and dabigatran concentrations in plasma was tested using the Spearman rank correlation test. The average plasma concentration of dabigatran obtained from mice fed with dabigatran chow was 342.1 ± 90.0 ng/mL (n=21). We observed a strong negative correlation of hydroxyproline versus dabigatran plasma levels (Fig. 10). There was no correlation between hydroxyproline and dabigatran plasma levels in control mice receiving saline and dabigatran chow (data not shown). This suggests that dabigatran affects collagen expression induced by tissue injury (fibrosis) while not interfering with basal levels of collagen in normal lung tissue.

The total nucleated cell count in BALF was markedly higher in the bleomycin-treated group on day 14 as compared to saline control animals (Table 1).

Bronchoalveolar lavage was performed on day 14 after bleomycin administration. Data are presented as mean ± SD (n = 8 mice per treatment group). * = $P < 0.01$ versus bleomycin + placebo-treated mice.

Dabigatran etexilate treatment starting on day 1 and day 8 significantly reduced total nucleated BAL cell counts from bleomycin-treated mice ($p < 0.01$). Dabigatran etexilate alone did not affect BALF cell counts (data not shown). The percentage of BALF neutrophils was significantly decreased in bleomycin/dabigatran etexilate-treated mice when compared to bleomycin/placebo-treated mice ($p < 0.01$). Total BALF protein was increased by 7.9-fold in bleomycin-placebo treated mice when compared to control and was significantly decreased by dabigatran treatment ($p < 0.001$). On day 21 after bleomycin instillation there was notably fewer cells in BALF in mice treated with dabigatran etexilate when compared to placebo-treated mice. However, there were no significant differences in cell numbers among studied groups (data not shown).

Parameters	Control	Bleo/Placebo	Bleo/Dabigatran Day 1	Bleo/Dabigatran Day 8
Total Protein (mg/ml)	0.24±0.09	1.89±0.26	0.87±0.41*	0.89±0.36*
Total Cell ($x10^5$/ml)	8.0±3.5	41.9±17.0	18.2±7.5*	21.0±8.5*
Macrophages (%)	97.8±1.6	71.6±8.3	84.8±9.3*	79.4±9.0
Lymphocytes (%)	2.2±1.4	10.3±4.4	8.7±3.7	9.1±5.8
Neutrophils (%)	0	18.1±5.6	6.5±2.2*	11.5±5.4*

Table 1. Analysis of bronchoalveolar lavage fluid

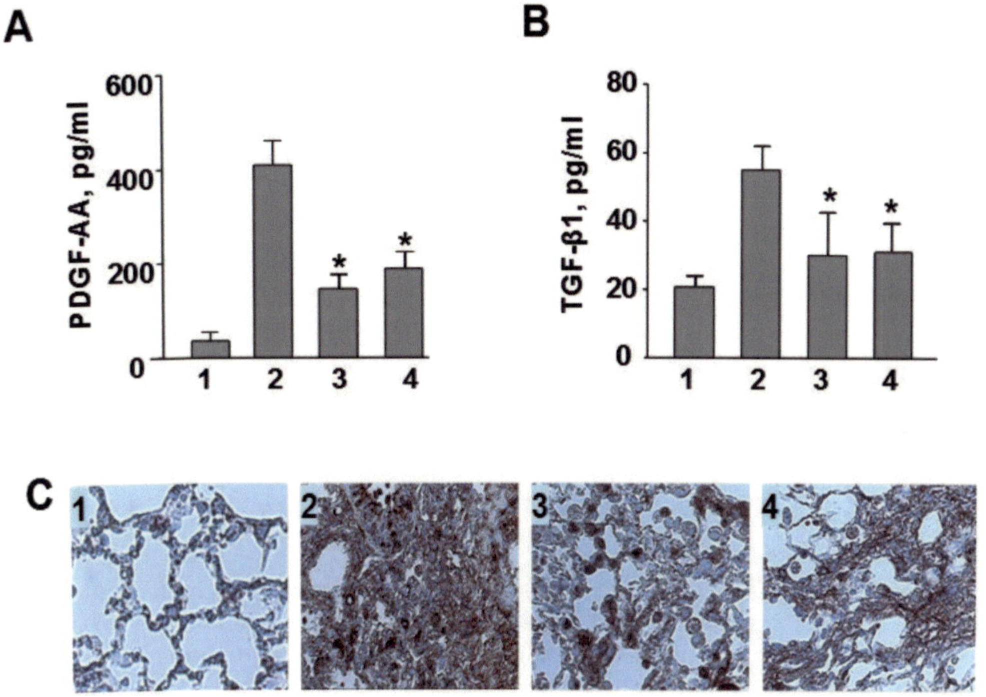

Fig. 11. Effect of dabigatran etexilate on PDGF-AA (A) and TGF-β1 (B) levels in BALF. (C) TGF-β1 expression in lung tissue. 1 – control (saline/placebo), 2 - bleomycin/placebo, 3 – bleomycin/dabigatran etexilate (day 1), 4 – bleomycin/dabigatran etexilate (day 8), n = 24 (6 mice per group). Values are the mean ± SD. * = P < 0.01 versus bleomycin/placebo-treated mice.

We observed that PDGF-AA was up-regulated (11.3-fold) when compared to controls in bleomycin-placebo-treated mice. Dabigatran etexilate significantly reduced PDGF-AA by 65% and 54% when initiated on day 1 and day 8, respectively ($p<0.01$) (Fig. 11A). The level of TGF-β1 in bleomycin-placebo-treated mice was 2.7-fold higher compared to controls (saline/placebo- and saline/dabigatran-treated mice). Dabigatran etexilate significantly reduced TGF-β1 concentrations from 54.9±6.1 pg/ml in bleomycin/placebo-treated mice to 29.9±9.3 and 31.1±8.7 pg/ml when administered beginning on day 1 and day 8, respectively ($p<0.01$, Fig. 11B). TGF-β1 expression was also assessed by immunohistochemistry in lung tissue. In this analysis, TGF-β1 was not detectable in lung from control mice, whereas it was strongly expressed in fibrotic areas of lung tissue from mice treated with bleomycin plus placebo (Fig. 11C). Dabigatran etexilate visibly reduced TGF-β1 expression when used as either early or late treatments. Similar to TGF-β1, CTGF and α-SMA were not detectable in lung tissue from control mice, with the exception of α-SMA expression in smooth muscle cells located in and around blood vessels and airways (Fig. 12). However, CTGF and α-SMA were each strongly upregulated in the lungs of bleomycin-treated mice. Dabigatran etexilate reduced this expression of CTGF and α-SMA in lung tissue, when administered beginning on either day 1 or day 8 of bleomycin treatment.

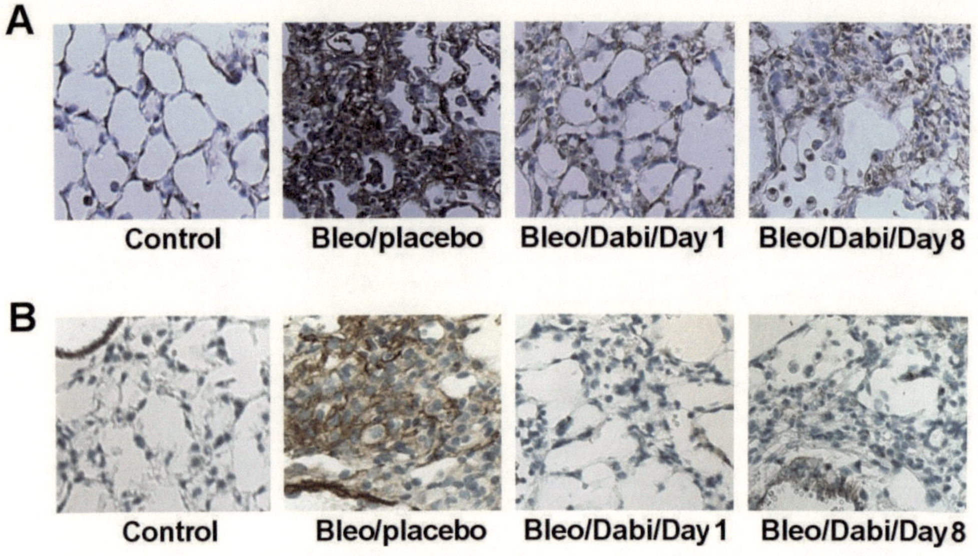

Fig. 12. Immunohistochemical evaluation for CTGF (A) and α-SMA (B) expression in lung tissue.

In this and all other experiments within the study we found that both early and late treatments with dabigatran etexilate were able to inhibit bleomycin-induced pulmonary fibrosis; however, the inhibition of pulmonary fibrosis was more profound with early administration. The efficacy of early treatment with dabigatran etexilate was higher because it targeted the inflammatory stage of fibrosis, while later treatment was introduced at the time of a more developed degree of lung injury. The role of inflammation in the pathogenesis of progressive pulmonary fibrosis remains a controversial issue. Bleomycin causes a severe acute inflammatory response followed by chronic inflammation and fibrosis. It has been shown that the degree of inflammation in bleomycin-induced lung injury is associated with the intensity of fibrosis (Moore & Hogaboam, 2008).

The concentration of dabigatran etexilate used in these experiments yielded plasma levels that are slightly higher than those achieved in patients treated with dabigatran etexilate for various thrombotic diseases (~180 ng/ml peak levels achieved with 150 mg twice daily dose) (Van Ryn et al., 2010). The dose used in this study resulted in a ~2-fold elevation of the aPTT and ~10-fold elevation of the TT (Fig. 13A).

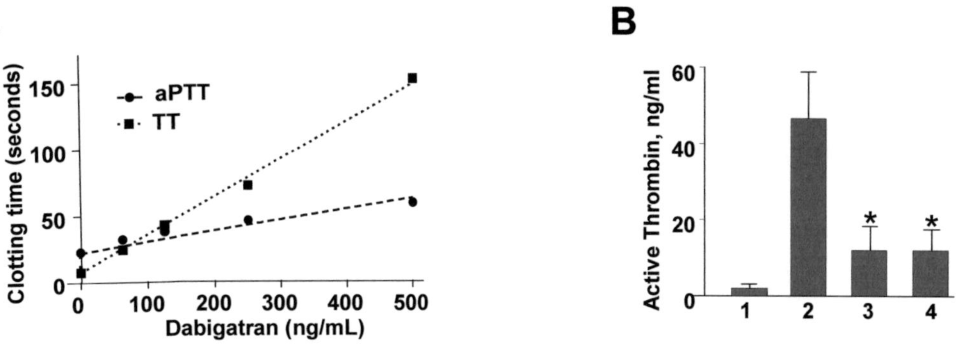

Fig. 13. (A) Effect of increasing concentrations of dabigatran on the thrombin time (TT) and activated partial thromboplastin time (aPTT) clotting times in mouse plasma in vitro. Data expressed as mean of duplicate determinations. (B) Effect of dabigatran etexilate on level of active thrombin in BALF.

Such prolongation in mouse plasma is consistent with findings in human plasma, where it has also been shown that change in the TT is more sensitive to dabigatran than is the aPTT. Though it is not possible to directly relate plasma levels and/or anticoagulation from mice to humans, it is important to note that the antifibrotic effects observed in our studies were achieved at plasma levels and pharmacological effects consistent with human dosing.

It is also important to note that dose of dabigatran etexilate used in this study significantly reduced but did not completely inhibit thrombin activity in BALF (Fig. 13B). We did not observe any bleeding side-effects during the study suggesting that levels of dabigatran in mouse plasma were not sufficient to completely eliminate thrombin from the normal hemostatic process. However, such doses of dabigatran etexilate ameliorated lung fibrosis even after it had been established, indicating that dabigatran etexilate could safely be administered in chronic forms of lung fibrosis, at least in mice.

7. Conclusions

Tissue injury with activation of the coagulation cascade and increased thrombin activity with deposition of fibrin are characteristic features of pulmonary fibrosis – the end result of a heterogeneous group of disorders that includes IPF and SSc-ILD. Characterized by microvascular injury and inflammation, SSc-ILD culminates in excessive deposition of extracellular matrix proteins, often resulting in severe lung dysfunction and death. Although cyclophosphamide treatment may stabilize lung function in some patients, long-term treatment is required and significant toxicity may occur (Berezne et al., 2007; Strange et al., 2008). There is, therefore, a great need for new therapeutic approaches that would be more effective and less toxic than current treatments. Dabigatran etexilate represents the first synthetic oral, reversible, direct inhibitor of thrombin with a very favorable biochemical and pharmacological profile that translates into clinical efficacy and safety in patients with or at risk of thrombotic disorders (Stangier, 2008). The current study provides important preclinical information about the feasibility and efficacy of dabigatran etexilate for the treatment of fibrotic diseases, including IPF and SSc-ILD, in which there is evidence for tissue injury with overexpression of thrombin and downstream fibrogenesis. Any future studies of thrombin inhibition for the treatment of SSc-ILD would need to demonstrate a positive benefit/risk ratio taking into account potential risks such as gastrointestinal tract hemorrhage.

8. Acknowledgment

This work was supported in part by a career award from National Institutes of Health K01AR051052 (to GSB), NIH/NCRR Grant RR029882, the Scleroderma Foundation, and Boehringer Ingelheim International GmbH. Ilia Atanelishvili was sponsored by UICC fellowship ICRETT- 10-087.

9. References

[1] Ando S, Otani H, Yagi Y, Kawai K, Araki H, Nakamura T, Fukuhara S, Inagaki C. Protease-activated receptor 4-mediated Ca2+ signaling in mouse lung alveolar epithelial cells. Life Sci. 2007;81(10):794-802.

[2] Armstrong MT, Fenton JW 2nd, Andersen TT, Armstrong PB. Thrombin stimulation of matrix fibronectin. J Cell Physiol 1996;166:112-20.

[3] Ashcroft T., Simpson J. M., Timbrell V. Simple method of estimating severity of pulmonary fibrosis on a numerical scale. J. Clin. Pathol., 41: 467-470, 1988

[4] Bachhuber BG, Sarembock IJ, Gimple LW, and Owens GK. alpha-Thrombin induces transforming growth factor-beta1 mRNA and protein in cultured vascular smooth muscle cells via a proteolytically activated receptor. J Vasc Res 1997; 34:41-48.

[5] Bérezné A, Valeyre D, Ranque B, Guillevin L, Mouthon L. Interstitial lung disease associated with systemic sclerosis: what is the evidence for efficacy of cyclophosphamide? Ann N Y Acad Sci. 2007;1110:271-84.

[6] Bogatkevich GS, Gustilo E, Oates J, Feghali-Bostwick C, Harley RA, Silver RM, Ludwicka-Bradley A: Distinct PKC isoforms mediate cell survival and DNA synthesis in thrombin-induced myofibroblasts. Am J Physiol: Lung Cell Mol Physiol 2005, 288, L190-L201.

[7] Bogatkevich GS, Ludwicka-Bradley A, Paul J. Nietert, Silver RM: Scleroderma Lung Fibroblasts: Contractility and Connective Tissue Growth Factor. In Myofibroblasts (Gabbiani G, Chaponnier C, Desmouliere A, eds), Landes Bioscience, Georgetown, TX, 2006, 25-31.

[8] Bogatkevich GS, Ludwicka-Bradley A, Silver RM. Dabigatran, a direct thrombin inhibitor, demonstrates antifibrotic effects on lung fibroblasts. Arthritis Rheum. 2009; 60(11):3455-64.

[9] Bogatkevich GS, Tourkina E, Abrams CS, Harley RA, Silver RM, Ludwicka-Bradley A. Contractile activity and smooth muscle alpha-actin organization in thrombin-induced human lung myofibroblasts. Am J Physiol Lung Cell Mol Physiol. 2003;285(2):L334-43.

[10] Bogatkevich GS, Tourkina E, Silver RM and Ludwicka-Bradley A: Thrombin differentiates normal lung fibroblast to a myofibroblast phenotype via proteolytically activated receptor-1 and protein kinase C-dependent pathway. J Biol Chem 2001; 276, 45184-92.

[11] Chambers RC, Dabbagh K, McAnulty RJ, Gray AJ, Blanc-Brude OP, Laurent GJ. Thrombin stimulates fibroblast procollagen production via proteolytic activation of protease-activated receptor 1. Biochem J 1998;333:121-7.

[12] Chambers RC, Leoni P, Blanc-Brude OP, Wembridge DE, Laurent GJ. Thrombin is a potent inducer of connective tissue growth factor production via proteolytic activation of protease-activated receptor-1. J Biol Chem 2000;275:35584-91.

[13]Chambers RC. Procoagulant signalling mechanisms in lung inflammation and fibrosis: novel opportunities for pharmacological intervention? Br J Pharmacol. 2008;153 Suppl 1:S367-78.

[14] Chujo S, Shirasaki F, Kawara S, Inagaki Y, Kinbara T, Inaoki M, Takigawa M, Takehara K. Connective tissue growth factor causes persistent pro α2(I) collagen gene expression

induced by transforming growth factor-β in a mouse fibrosis model. J Cell Physiol 2005;203:447-56.

[15] Coughlin SR. How the protease thrombin talks to cells. Proc Natl Acad Sci USA 1999; 96:11023-11027.

[16] DeMaio L, Tseng W, Balverde Z, Alvarez JR, Kim KJ, Kelley DG, Senior RM, Crandall ED, Borok Z. Characterization of mouse alveolar epithelial cell monolayers. Am J Physiol Lung Cell Mol Physiol. 2009 Jun;296(6):L1051-8.

[17] Gabbiani G. The myofibroblast in wound healing and fibrocontractive diseases. J Pathol 2003; 200:500-03.

[18] Gore-Hyer E, Shegogue D, Markiewicz M, Lo S, Hasen-Martin D, Greene E, Grotendorst G, Trojanowska M. TGF and CTGF have overlapping and distinct fibrogenic effects on human renal cells. Am J Physiol Renal Physiol 2002;283:F707-F716.

[19] Gray AJ, Bishop JE, Reeves JT, Laurent GJ. A alpha and B beta chains of fibrinogen stimulate proliferation of human fibroblasts. J Cell Sci 1993;104:409-13.

[20] Grinnell F. Signal transduction pathways activated during fibroblast contraction of collagen matrices. Curr Top Pathol 1999; 93:61-73.

[21] Grotendorst GR, Rahmanie H, Duncan MR. Combinatorial signaling pathways determine fibroblast proliferation and myofibroblast differentiation. FASEB J. 2004; 18: 469-479.

[22] Hernández-Rodríguez NA, Cambrey AD, Harrison NK, Chambers RC, Gray AJ, Southcott AM, duBois RM, Black CM, Scully MF, McAnulty RJ, et al. Role of thrombin in pulmonary fibrosis. Lancet. 1995;346:1071-3.

[23] Hinz B, Gabbiani G, Chaponnier C. The NH2-terminal peptide of alpha-smooth muscle actin inhibits force generation by the myofibroblast in vitro and in vivo. J Cell Biol 2002;157:657-63.

[24] Hinz B, Phan SH, Thannickal VJ, Galli A, Bochaton-Piallat ML, Gabbiani G. The myofibroblast: one function, multiple origins. Am J Pathol 2007;170:1807-16.

[25] Howell DC, Goldsack NR, Marshall RP, McAnulty RJ, Starke R, Purdy G, Laurent GJ, Chambers RC. Direct thrombin inhibition reduces lung collagen, accumulation, and CTGF mRNA levels in bleomycin-induced pulmonary fibrosis. Am J Pathol 2001;159:1383-95.

[26] Howell DC, Johns RH, Lasky JA, Shan B, Scotton CJ, Laurent GJ, Chambers RC. Absence of proteinase-activated receptor-1 signaling affords protection from bleomycin-induced lung inflammation and fibrosis. Am J Pathol 2005;166:1353-65.

[27]Howell DC, Laurent GJ, Chambers RC. Role of thrombin and its major cellular receptor, protease-activated receptor-1, in pulmonary fibrosis. Biochem Soc Trans. 2002;30:211-6.

[28] Köhler C, Orrenius S, Zhivotovsky B. Evaluation of caspase activity in apoptotic cells. J Immunol Methods. 2002;265(1-2):97-110.

[29] Ludwicka A, Trojanowska M, Smith EA, Baumann M, Strange C, Korn JH, Smith T, Leroy EC, Silver RM. Growth and characterization of fibroblasts obtained from bronchoalveolar lavage of patients with scleroderma. J Rheumatol.1992;19:1716-23.

[30] Luo GH, Lu YP, Song J, Yang L, Shi YJ, Li YP. Inhibition of connective tissue growth factor by small interfering RNA prevents renal fibrosis in rats undergoing chronic allograft nephropathy. Transplant Proc 2008;40:2365-9.

[31] Macfarlane SR, Seatter MJ, Kanke T, Hunter GD, Plevin R. Proteinase-activated receptors. Pharmacol Rev. 2001;53:245-82.

[32] Mercer PF, Deng X, Chambers RC. Signaling pathways involved in proteinase-activated receptor1-induced proinflammatory and profibrotic mediator release following lung injury. Ann N Y Acad Sci 2007;1096:86-8.

[33] Moeller A, Ask K, Warburton D, Gauldie J, Kolb M. The bleomycin animal model: a useful tool to investigate treatment options for idiopathic pulmonary fibrosis? Int J Biochem Cell Biol. 2008;40(3):362-82.
[34] Moore BB, Hogaboam CM. Murine models of pulmonary fibrosis. Am J Physiol Lung Cell Mol Physiol. 2008;294(2):L152-60.
[35] Ohba T, McDonald JK, Silver RM, Strange C, LeRoy EC and Ludwicka A. Scleroderma BAL fluid contains thrombin, a mediator of human lung fibroblast proliferation via induction of the PDGF-alpha receptor. Am J Resp Cell Mol Biol 1994; 10:405-12.
[36] Shi-Wen X, Chen Y, Denton CP, Eastwood M, Renzoni EA, Bou-Gharios G, Pearson JD, Dashwood M, du Bois RM, Black CM, Leask A, Abraham DJ. Endothelin-1 promotes myofibroblast induction through the ETA receptor via a rac/ phosphoinositide 3-kinase/Akt-dependent pathway and is essential for the enhanced contractile phenotype of fibrotic fibroblasts. Mol Biol Cell 2004;15:2707-19.
[37] Shrivastava S, McVey JH, Dorling A. The interface between coagulation and immunity. Am J Transplant. 2007;7:499-506.
[38] Sorbera LA, Bozzo J, Castaner J. Dabigatran/ Dabigatran etexilate. Drugs Fut 2005; 30(9):877.
[39] Stangier J. Clinical pharmacokinetics and pharmacodynamics of the oral direct thrombin inhibitor dabigatran etexilate. Clin Pharmacokinet 2008;47:285-95.
[40] Strange C, Bolster MB, Roth MD, Silver RM, Theodore A, Goldin J, Clements P, Chung J, Elashoff RM, Suh R, Smith EA, Furst DE, Tashkin DP; Scleroderma Lung Study Research Group. Bronchoalveolar lavage and response to cyclophosphamide in scleroderma interstitial lung disease. Am J Respir Crit Care Med. 2008;177(1):91-8.
[41] Suzuki T, Moraes TJ, Vachon E, Ginzberg HH, Huang TT, Matthay MA, Hollenberg MD, Marshall J, McCulloch CA, Abreu MT, Chow CW, Downey GP. Proteinase-activated receptor-1 mediates elastase-induced apoptosis of human lung epithelial cells. Am J Respir Cell Mol Biol. 2005;33(3):231-47.
[42] Tomasek JJ, Gabbiani G, Hinz B et al. Myofibroblasts and mechano-regulation of connective tissue remodeling. Nature Rev Mol Cell Biol 2002; 3:349-363.
[43] Tourkina E, Hoffman S, Fenton JW 2nd, Lipsitz S, Silver RM, Ludwicka-Bradley A. Depletion of protein kinase Cε in normal and scleroderma lung fibroblasts has opposite effects on tenascin expression. Arthritis Rheum 2001;44:1370-81.
[44] van Ryn J, Stangier J, Haertter S, Liesenfeld K-H, Wienen W, Feuring M, Clemens A. Dabigatran etexilate – a novel, reversible, oral direct thrombin inhibitor: Interpretation of coagulation assays and reversal of anticoagulant activity. Thromb Haemost 2010; 103(6):1116-27.
[45] Vyalov SL, Gabbiani G, Kapanci Y: Rat alveolar myofibroblasts acquire -smooth muscle actin expression during bleomycin-induced pulmonary fibrosis. Am J Pathol 1993; 143:1754-1765.
[46] Walker GA, Guerrero IA, Leinwand LA. Myofibroblasts: molecular crossdressers. Curr Top Dev Biol 2001; 51:91-107.
[47] Wienen W, Stassen JM, Priepke H, Ries UJ, Hauel N. In-vitro profile and ex-vivo anticoagulant activity of the direct thrombin inhibitor dabigatran and its orally active prodrug, dabigatran etexilate. Thromb Haemost 2007;98:155-62.
[48] Zhang H, Gharaee-Kermani M, Zhang K, Karmiol S, Phan S: Lung fibroblast α-smooth muscle actin expression and contractile phenotype in bleomycin-induced pulmonary fibrosis. Am J Pathol 1996; 148:527-37.
[49] Zhang K, Rekhter MD, Gordon D et al. Myofibroblasts and their role in lung collagen gene expression during pulmonary fibrosis: A combined immunohistochemical and in situ hybridization. Am J Pathol 1994; 145:114-25.

Part 2

Clinical Features of SSc

9

Emerging Issues in the Immunopathogenesis, Diagnosis and Clinical Management of Primary Biliary Cirrhosis Associated with Systemic Sclerosis

Dimitrios P. Bogdanos[1*], Cristina Rigamonti[2], Daniel Smyk[1], Maria G. Mytilinaiou[1], Eirini I. Rigopoulou[3] and Andrew K. Burroughs[4*]
[1]King's College London School of Medicine/Institute of Liver Studies, London
[2]Università del Piemonte Orientale "A. Avogadro", Department of Clinical and Experimental Medicine, Novara
[3]University of Thessaly Medical School/Department of Medicine, Thessaly, Larissa
[4]The Sheila Sherlock Liver Centre/Royal Free Hospital, London
[1,4]United Kingdom
[2]Italy
[3]Greece

1. Introduction

1.1 Primary biliary cirrhosis

Primary biliary cirrhosis (PBC) is a chronic cholestatic liver disease characterized by immune-mediated, chronic nonsuppurative cholangitis that affects interlobular and septal bile ducts (Kaplan & Gershwin, 2005). PBC is a rare disease, with prevalence ranging from 28 to 402 per million depending on geographical location (Table 1). PBC predominantly affects middle aged women, and is exceedingly rare in males (James et al., 1999). Familial clustering of PBC cases has been observed, which predominantly affects female family members. Several reports indicate that the prevalence and incidence of PBC is increasing globally (James et al., 1999). Concomitant autoimmune diseases are often found in patients with PBC (Kaplan & Gershwin, 2005). The serological hallmark of PBC is the presence of high-titer serum antimitochondrial autoantibodies (AMA), which are present in 90–95% of patients with PBC (Bogdanos et al., 2003; Bogdanos et al., 2008; Bogdanos & Komorowski, 2011; Kaplan & Gershwin, 2005). The presence of AMA in asymptomatic patients is considered predictive of eventual disease development (Metcalf et al., 1996). These autoantibodies are specific to the lipoylated domains within components of the 2-oxoacid dehydrogenase family of enzymes, particularly the E2 component of the pyruvate dehydrogenase complex, located within the inner mitochondrial membrane (Bogdanos et al., 2003; Bogdanos et al., 2008; Bogdanos & Komorowski, 2011, Kaplan & Gershwin, 2005). Indirect immunofluorescence using rodent liver, kidney and stomach sections as substrate are the most widely used screening assays for AMA in the

---

* Equally contributed

routine setting (EASL 2009). Other techniques including immunoblotting and ELISA have a higher sensitivity, and the use of cloned mitochondrial antigens and bead assay testing systems allow for the identification of AMA in the sera of patients previously defined as AMA negative. In addition to AMA, PBC specific anti-nuclear autoantibodies (ANA) are also characteristic of PBC in approximately 30% of patients presenting with multiple nuclear dot (antibodies against Sp100) or nuclear membrane staining patterns (antibodies against gp210) (Bogdanos et al., 2008; Bogdanos & Komorowski 2011; Courvalin & Worman, 1997), which preferentially are identified using HEp-2 cells as substrate . The multiple nuclear dot pattern specific for PBC needs not to be confused with the nuclear dot pattern of anticentromere antibodies (ACA). The autoimmune pathogenesis of PBC is supported by a plethora of experimental and clinical data, such as the presence of autoreactive T cells in PBC patients, and serum autoantibodies characteristic of the disease (Bogdanos et al., 2003; Bogdanos et al., 2010; Bogdanos & Vergani, 2009; Shimoda et al., 1995).

The aetiology of PBC is unknown, however the current view is that both genetic susceptibility, and environmental factors are involved together, although these need further characterization. A number of chemicals and infectious agents have been proposed to induce the disease in genetically predisposed individuals (Bogdanos et al., 2010; Bogdanos & Vergani, 2009; Bogdanos et al., 2004a; Bogdanos et al., 2004b; Gershwin & Mackay, 2008; Smyk et al., 2011; Vergani et al., 2004). The presentation of PBC may include symptoms such as pruritus (the most specific symptom of PBC) and fatigue (the most common non-specific symptom), and/or jaundice (Kaplan & Gershwin, 2005). More severe patients may present with symptoms related to portal hypertension and its complications (Kaplan & Gershwin, 2005). However, a significant proportion of PBC patients are asymptomatic and diagnosed incidentally during treatment for other conditions, which are quite often other concomitant autoimmune conditions (Gershwin et al., 2005; Hudson et al., 2008). Currently, a definite diagnosis of PBC is made on a combination of abnormal serum enzymes indicating cholestasis (i.e. elevated alkaline phosphatase for at least six months), the presence of serum AMA (titre > 1:40), and characteristic liver histology with florid bile duct lesions (EASL 2009, Kaplan & Gershwin, 2005). The presence of two of the three criteria is indicative of a probable PBC diagnosis, but this definition is not globally accepted. Serum AMA may precede disease onset by several years, and many individuals found positive for these autoantibodies in the absence of other criteria eventually develop PBC (Metcalf et al., 1996).

The progression of PBC may extend over many decades, and is highly variable among patients. The final stages of this progression are characterised by cirrhosis, liver failure and death. However, the patterns of clinical disease and natural history have changed significantly in the last two decades after the introduction of medical treatment with ursodeoxycholic acid (UDCA). When UDCA is administered in early PBC at adequate doses (13-15 mg/kg/day), the progression of the disease is often altered, with many patients having a normal life expectancy without additional therapeutic measures.

1.2 Systemic sclerosis (SSc)

Systemic sclerosis (SSc) is a chronic systemic connective tissue disease characterized by vascular and immune dysfunction. The cardinal features are sclerosis of the skin with potential involvement of other organs (kidney, oesophagus, heart and lung are the most frequent targets), but involvement of the liver is relatively rare (Kalabay et al., 2002). The available data indicate a prevalence of scleroderma ranging from 50 to 200 per million (Table 1), with women being at much higher risk for scleroderma than men (Chifflot et al., 2008). The poorly understood pathogenesis of SSc is complex. Familial clustering and the high frequency of other autoimmune disorders in families of patients with scleroderma, is suggestive of a genetic involvement (Kalabay et al., 2002). In addition, infectious agents have been suggested as possible contributing factors to the development and progression of SSc, through mechanisms of molecular mimicry and immunological cross-reactivity involving microbial/self homologues. SSc is extremely heterogeneous in its clinical manifestations, pattern of organ involvement, natural history, and survival. Survival is correlated with internal organ involvement and is inversely related to the severity of restrictive lung disease. In the kidneys, injury to the medium-sized arteries can precipitate scleroderma renal crisis with malignant hypertension, hyper-reninemia, microangiopathic hemolytic anemia, and rapidly progressive renal failure. Pulmonary arterial hypertension develops in 40% of SSc patients, and is a major SSc complication and a leading cause of death (Kalabay et al., 2002). Heart involvement in SSc may include cardiac fibrosis in addition to pulmonary hypertension.

The autoantibody profile in SSc appears specific and is useful for confirming the diagnosis, the disease subset, and for monitoring disease activity (Steen, 2005). Autoantibodies that characterize limited cutaneous SSc (lcSSC) include ACA, anti-Th/To, anti-U1-RNP, and PM/Scl. Diffuse cutaneous SSc (dcSSc) is characterized by anti-Scl 70 antibody (anti-topoisomerase I antibody, TOPO), anti-RNA polymerase III and anti-U3-RNP. Severe lung disease is the hallmark of anti-TOPO positive dcSSC patients. DcSSc patients with anti-RNA polymerase III appear to have the most severe skin disease and the highest frequency of renal crisis. Patients with the nucleolar antibody anti-U3-RNP have dcSSc with multiorgan involvement (Steen, 2005).

2. PBC/SSc

2.1 Epidemiology

The main features of PBC and SSc are shown in Table 1. PBC is the most common liver disorder in SSc patients (Abraham et al., 2004). One case from 1964 reports two patients with SSc and possible (but unconfirmed) PBC. Murray-Lyon et al reports two cases of SSc with PBC (Murray-Lyon et al., 1970). Despite several similar reports over the years, liver disease has not been considered a significant feature of scleroderma, and larger studies have demonstrated that liver disease was more common in the control groups. The association of lcSSc and PBC was first described in 1970 with two cases of PBC and limited scleroderma (Murray-Lyon et al., 1970). A further six cases were also reported, and several other case reports have found an association between lcSSc and PBC. The first case reporting an association of PBC and scleroderma, without features of lcSSc, was described in 1972. The prevalence of clinically evident PBC among patients with SSc was recently reported to be 2.5% in a registry of 1700 SSc patients (Norman et al., 2009), and 2% in a series of 817 patients with SSc (Assassi et al., 2009). On the other hand, the prevalence of SSc in patients with PBC is estimated to be around 8%. However, case reports and some series (Akimoto et al., 1999) reported wider range of prevalence (3-50%) of SSc, mostly lcSSc, in PBC patients.

Large epidemiological studies on PBC note a small number of patients who also have SSc. A large French study found SSc in 1% of a cohort of PBC patients, although 1% of their first degree relatives and 1% of controls also had scleroderma (Corpechot et al., 2010). Gershwin and colleagues found that 2% of PBC patients and 1% of their first degree relatives had scleroderma, which was not found in any of the controls (Gershwin et al., 2005). First degree relatives with scleroderma were more often sisters, followed by daughters of PBC patients, in keeping with the high female predominance (Gershwin et al., 2005; Parikh-Patel et al., 2001). Twin studies in both conditions are scarce. One twin study for SSc found a concordance of 4.2% among monozygotic (MZ) twins, compared to 5.6% in dizygotic (DZ) twins, indicating a small genetic component to the disease (Feghali-Bostwick et al., 2003). However, there was a 90% concordance for ANA among MZ twins, compared to 40% among DZ (Feghali-Bostwick et al., 2003). The only twin study conducted in PBC demonstrated a concordance of 63% among MZ twins (Selmi et al., 2004). Although both twin studies note co-existing autoimmune disease, which was often the same condition in the twin, none have noted SSc in twins with PBC and *vice versa*. If one of the affected twins had SSc, it would be of interest to see whether the other would develop the disease, and within how many years after presentation of the first twin.

2.2 Immunopathogenesis

The immunopathogenesis of PBC has not been fully clarified, but it appears that the interaction between genetic predisposition, antigen-specific autoreactive T and B cells, the innate immune system, and environmental factors are critical in the development of the disease. Although PBC/SSc is relatively uncommon, several common factors found at the genetic and environmental levels may account for the development of the disease in this subgroup of patients.

2.2.1 Genetics

Genetic studies have recently implicated several gene loci in the pathogenesis of PBC (Hirschfield & Invernizzi, 2011). Strong associations between PBC and HLA DQB1, as well as at the IL12A, IL12RB2, STAT4 and CTLA4 loci were found in a large cohort of PBC patients from North America (Hirschfield & Invernizzi, 2011). The role of HLA in PBC is now believed to play a larger role that was previously suspected. Additionally, IRF5-TNPO3, 17q12-21, and MMEL1 loci have also been found to be associated with PBC. A cohort of Japanese PBC patients also showed an association with 17q12-21, however no association was found with IL12A, IL12RB2 or IRF5-TNPO3, and similar findings in an Italian cohort have also been reported. More recently, several new candidate genes have also been identified, including STAT4, DENND1B, CD80, IL7R, CXCR5, TNFRSF1A, CLEC16A and NFKB1. It should be noted that variability in gene associations have been observed between different ethnicities and/or geographical locations.

In regards to SSc, several HLA and non-HLA regions have been identified (Agarwal & Reveille, 2010). Positive HLA associations in whites and Hispanics include HLA-DRB1*1104, DQA1*0501, DQB1*0301 (Assassi et al., 2009). Negative associations in those groups included DRB1*0701, DQA1*0201, DQB1*0202, and DRB1*1501 (Assassi et al., 2009). In African Americans, positive associations have been found with HLA-DRB1*0804, DQA1*0501, DQB1*0301 (Assassi et al., 2009). That study also noted that ACA positivity was closely associated with HLA-DQB1*0501 (Assassi et al., 2009), and another associated TOPO positivity with HLA-DRB1*1104. Similar HLA findings to those noted above were also found in a Spanish cohort. Non-HLA regions have also been identified in SSc, and include STAT4 (Agarwal & Reveille, 2010), IRF5 (Agarwal & Reveille, 2010), BANK1, TNSF4, TBX21, IL-23R , and C8orf13-BLK among others (Agarwal & Reveille, 2010). Overlapping PBC/SSc genes include HLA-DRB1, DQA1, DQB1, IRF5, and STAT4, although it should be noted that DR11, which is positively associated with SSc, is considered protective in PBC (Agarwal & Reveille, 2010; Liu et al., 2010).

	PBC	SSc
Prevalence (highly variable geographically)	28-402/million	50-200/million
Incidence (highly variable geographically)	2.3-27/million	0.6-122/million
Male to Female Ratio	1:8	1 : 1.5-12 (highly variable geographically)
Peak Frequency Age	53 years	45-64 years
Autoantibodies	AMA, ANA	*Limited disease*: ACA, anti-Th/To, anti-U1-RNP *Diffuse disease*: TOPO, anti-RNA polymerase III, anti-U3-RNP
Genes (positive associations)	*HLA*: DRB1, DQA1, DQB1, DQA2 *Non-HLA*: STAT4, IRF5, SPIB, IKZF3-ORMDL3, IL12A, IL12RB, MMEL1, DENND1B, CD80, IL7, CXCR5, TNFRSF1A, CLEC16A, NKFB1	*HLA*: HLA-DRB1*1104, DQA1*0501, DQB1*0301, HLA-DRB1*0804, DQA1*0501, DQB1*0301 *Non-HLA*: STAT4, IRF5, BANK1, TNSF4, TBX21, IL-23R, and C8orf13-BLK

Table 1. Major features of primary biliary cirrhosis (PBC) and systemic sclerosis (SSc)

2.2.2 Cellular immunity

Autoreactive T cells are likely to be involved in the pathogenesis of PBC. Histologically, PBC is characterized by the presence of autoreactive T cells in the periductular spaces. CD4+ and CD8+ lymphocytes purified from biopsy samples of PBC patients recognize PDC-E2 epitopes, and sequence overlap has been demonstrated between PDC-E2 specific T and B cell epitopes (Shimoda et al., 1995). PBC appears to be unique among other classical autoimmune diseases as it seems that there is only one immunodominant CD4+ epitope within the major autoantigen (Shimoda et al., 1995). CD4+ T cell clones have also been shown to recognize other mitochondrial autoantigens, including OGDC-E2, BCOADC-E2, and E3BP (Shimoda et al., 2003). CD8+ T cells have been found to identify amino acids 159-167 and 165-174 of PDC-E2 (Shimoda et al., 1995). As well, a 10 fold increase in these CD8+ cells has been found in liver tissues compared to peripheral blood of PBC patients. In regards to PBC/SSc patients, it has been reported that this patient group has clonally expanded CD8+ T cells expressing one T-cell receptor beta chain variable region, TCRBV3, which may be involved in the disease pathogenesis (Mayo et al., 1999).

2.2.3 Humoral immunity

AMA has been found in approximately one-quarter of patients with scleroderma, and ACA in one-quarter of patients with PBC. Positive ACA is reported in 9–30% of PBC patients (Chan et al., 1994; Marasini et al., 2001; Mayes et al., 2009; Powell et al., 1984) and in 22–25% of all SSc patients, the majority of which have lcSSc. AMA positivity is found in 14-25% of SSc (Gupta et al., 1984). ACA positivity is greater in PBC/SSc than in either disease in isolation, but there is no cross reactivity between mitochondrial and centromere antigens

(Whyte et al., 1994). Because ACA have been detected not only in SSc but also in other autoimmune diseases (Kallenberg et al., 1982; Miyawaki et al., 2005) including PBC (Mayes et al., 2009), the clinical significance of ACA has been investigated. Three major centromere antigens have been recognized: centromere protein A (CENP-A, 18 kD polypeptide), centromere protein B (CENP-B, 80 kD polypeptide), and centromere protein C (CENP-C, 140 kD polypeptide). One study attempted to identify the major centromeric antigen of ACA in sera obtained from patients with PBC, and to classify the clinical characteristics associated with this. Forty one patients with PBC were studied: 10 out of 16 (63%) patients with ACA (all anti-CENP A) had one or more lcSSc feature. The higher incidence of Raynaud's phenomenon seen in ACA positive patients with PBC than in ACA negative patients with PBC suggested a close association of the presence of ACA with clinical features of lcSSc. This led to the proposal that there is a subset of PBC patients with scleroderma who are ACA positive, and differ from both ACA negative PBC/SSc and ACA negative PBC non-SSc patients, based on their clinical features and ACA epitope reactivity. As well, it has been suggested that there may be cross-reactivity between ACA and AMA epitopes, but no such link has been demonstrated (Whyte et al., 1994).

Immunological features of PBC/SSc patients were examined in a study by Akimoto and colleagues (Akimoto et al., 1998), and compared to patients with PBC and SSc alone. ACA positivity was observed in 80% PBC/SSc, 100% PBC/SSc spectrum, 25% PBC alone, and 100% SSc alone patients. AMA positivity was observed in 90% PBC/SSc, 75% PBC/SSc spectrum, 91.7% PBC alone, and 0% SSc alone patients (Akimoto et al., 1998). Interestingly, 100% of PBC/SSc spectrum patients showed reactivity to PDC-E1β, as did 90% PBC/SSc patients, but only 25% of PBC alone patients (Akimoto et al., 1998). Additionally, 70.6% of SSc alone patients showed reactivity to PDC-E2 compared to only 23.8% of controls, and 100% showed PDC-E3 reactivity, although this was also observed in 90.5% of controls (Akimoto et al., 1998). That study has suggested both clinical and immunological similarities in PBC/SSc and PBC/SSc spectrum patients.

2.2.4 Infectious agents and molecular mimicry

Infectious agents have been implicated in the pathogenesis of both SSc and PBC, and pathogens implicated in both are of interest in the pathogenesis of PBC/SSc. *E. coli* has been strongly associated with PBC (Bogdanos et al., 2010; Burroughs et al., 1984), largely due to the high occurrence of recurrent urinary tract infections in women with PBC (Corpechot et al., 2010; Gershwin et al., 2005). Experimental data support the presence of cross-reactive immune responses between human and *E. coli* PDC-E2 at the CD4 and CD8 T-cell level (Shigematsu et al., 2000; Van de Water et al., 2001). Several studies have demonstrated cross reactivity between the human PDC-E2 autoepitope (GDLLAEIETDKATI), and that of *E. coli* (EQSLITVEGDKASM) at the CD4 T cell level (Shimoda et al., 1995). As well, a shared motif, PDC-E2 (ExDK), was found to be critical for T cell epitope recognition (Shimoda et al., 1995). T cells specific for human PDC-E2 have also been shown to be activated by a motif sharing peptide of *E. coli* OGDC-E2 (Shimoda et al., 1995). In another study, 16 T cell clones specific for *E. coli* OGDC-E2 were tested for proliferation when stimulated by human OADC-E2 autoepitopes from PDC-E2, OGDC-E2 and BCOADC-E2. Activation was seen in 13/16 clones when stimulated by human OADC-E2. These studies have demonstrated that cross-reactivity between the highly conserved human and *E. coli* PDC-E2 epitopes may be a factor in the development of PBC, but there is currently no evidence to suggest the association between *E. coli* infection and the development of SSc.

Helicobacter pylori and Chlamydia have been implicated in both PBC and SSc (Grossman et al., 2011; Randone et al., 2008), however some studies indicate the Chlamydia are not involved in the pathogenesis of these diseases (Mayes et al., 2009). DNA of *H. pylori* and *H. hepaticus* have been isolated from livers of patients with PBC, leading to the suggestion that Helicobacter species may be involved in PBC pathogenesis. Anti-helicobacter antibodies have been detected in the serum and the bile of PBC patients. Helicobacter species have induced a PBC-like pathology in experimental models of the disease. In regards to molecular mimicry, it has been reported that a short *H. pylori* urease beta subunit sequence shares significant amino acid similarity with the human PDC-$E2_{212-226}$ autoepitope. The *H. pylori* urease beta subunit mimic has been implicated as a candidate for the initiation of cross-reactive immunity due to a high degree of sequence homology (13/15, 87%), and the fact that the mimic originates from the urease beta subunit, which is a major target antigen of anti-helicobacter immunity during infection. However, experimental studies have not demonstrated evidence of cross-reactive immunity involving *H. pylori* in PBC. *H. pylori* has more recently been implicated in the pathogenesis of SSc. *H. pylori* infection has been found in as many as 78% of SSc patients in one cohort, while another study notes that there is no difference between SSc *and* controls, although 90% of SSc patients had a highly virulent strain compared to only 37% of controls (Danese et al., 2000).
Other pathogens implicated in SSc include herpes-virus, parvovirus B19, retroviruses, and human cytomegalovirus. Sequence homology has been found between retroviral proteins and TOPO, which is the target of anti-Scl 70 antibodies in SSc patients (Jimenez et al., 1995). As well, fibroblast infection with retrovirus' has induced an SSc-like phenotype (Jimenez et al., 1995). It is possible that certain infectious organisms contribute the development of PBC or SSc in isolation, and that other organisms induce the disease in both conditions. Additionally, if common pathogens are implicated in both PBC and SSc, then the possibility of molecular mimicry in one disease may be applicable to the development of the other.

2.3 Screening and diagnosis of PBC in SSc patients and *vice versa*

Given the overlap between PBC with SSc and *vice versa*, including ACA positivity in PBC patients and AMA positivity in SSc patients, the major challenge remains to clarify which screening method would be best for early diagnosis of the associated conditions (Figure 1 and 2).
A recent study investigated the presence of antibodies against PBC disease-specific mitochondrial antigens and antibodies against the sp100 nuclear body antigen in 52 SSc patients using two commercially available ELISAs. In that study, AMA positivity was observed in 13%, ANA in 2% (anti-sp100), and one patient (2%) was diagnosed with symptomatic PBC. These figures were also found by Mytilinaiou et al., who confirmed 13.5% positive results with ELISA testing for antibodies against PBC disease-specific mitochondrial antigens in 37 SSc patients (Mytilinaiou & Bogdanos, 2009). However, this was not confirmed with the conventional indirect immunofluorescence based on unfixed rodent kidney, liver, stomach tissue sections or HEp-2 cells as antigenic substrates, and none of the ELISA positive patients showed features of PBC (Mytilinaiou & Bogdanos, 2009). The specificity of ELISA testing needs clarification in regards to whether it is less specific with false positive results, or that it simply represents a more sensitive method with respect to indirect immunofluorescence, which remains the technique of choice.

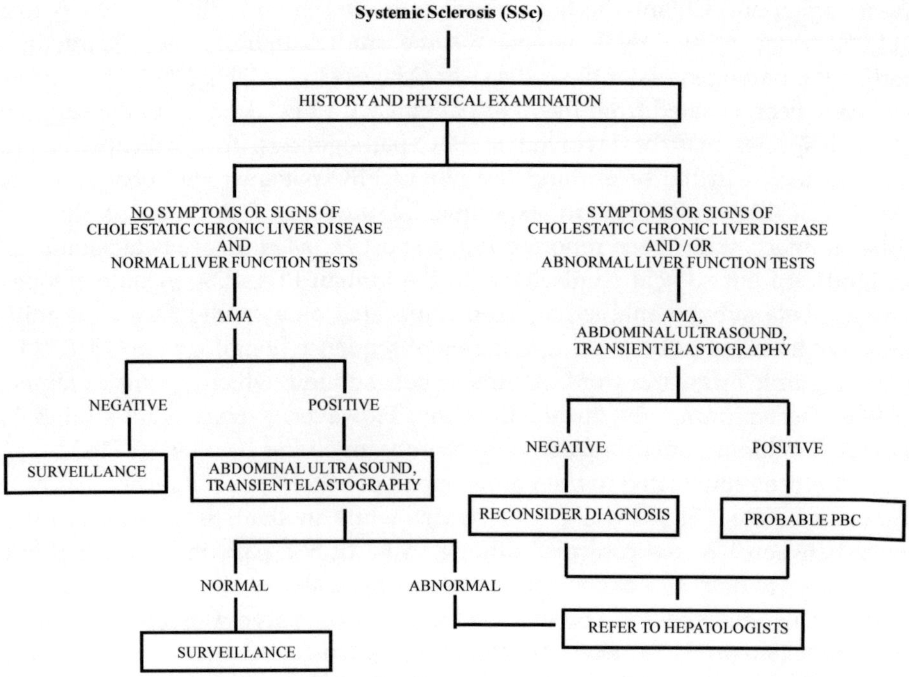

Fig. 1. Diagnostic algorithm for patients with SSc and suspected chronic liver disease

The presence of AMA can precede clinical symptoms of PBC. It has been demonstrated that the vast majority of AMA positive subjects have typical histological features of PBC despite being asymptomatic and having normal liver biochemistry (Metcalf et al., 1996). Furthermore, the study by Prince et al. suggested that 36% of initially asymptomatic PBC patients would become symptomatic within 5 years (Prince et al., 2004). Thus, SSc cases, and in particular those found to be positive for AMA, require urgent attention and long-term monitoring for early detection of symptoms, signs and liver biochemistry suggestive of chronic cholestatic liver disease. Routine follow-up of AMA positive SSc patients should include liver biochemical tests (alaninoaminotransferase, aspartateaminotransferase, gamma-glutamyltranspeptidase, alkaline phosphatase, albumin, bilirubin, international normalized ratio), thyroid function and possibly annual abdominal ultrasound scans. Since transient elastography of the liver has been emerging as a useful screening tool to detect undiagnosed chronic liver disease in apparently healthy subjects, this could be used to detect liver disease by evaluating liver stiffness on a yearly basis, and has the benefit of being non-invasive. In addition, transient elastography is reported to be reliable in the assessment biliary fibrosis. Figure 1 reports a proposed diagnostic and screening algorithm for PBC in SSc patients.

Screening PBC patients for ACA is mandatory. Nakamura et al. reported that in PBC patients, ACA positivity was significantly associated with more severe ductular pathology histologically, and was a significant risk factor for the development of portal hypertension (Nakamura et al., 2007). In another study, ACA positive PBC patients without clinical features of SSc were shown to have similar symptoms and signs at diagnosis. These findings need to be confirmed in large multicenter studies. Although ACA positivity is not pathognomic of SSc, it is associated with an increased risk of developing connective tissue disease. One review reported a sensitivity of 32% (17–56%) for SSc, 57% (32–96%) for lcSSc, and specificity of at least 93%, while ACA positivity was present in 5% of patients with other connective tissue diseases, and less than 1% of disease free controls. Since ACA could be predictive of autoimmune rheumaticological disorders, it has been suggested that an assessment of PBC patients should include careful questioning and evaluation for SSc related symptoms, such as Raynaud's phenomenon and CREST-related symptoms (calcinosis, Raynaud's phenomenon, esophageal dysmotility, sclerodactyly and teleangiectasia). The early diagnosis of SSc was recently defined into three domains containing seven items: skin domain (puffy fingers/puffy swollen digits turning into sclerodactyly), vascular domain (Raynaud's phenomenon, abnormal capillaroscopy with scleroderma pattern) and laboratory domain (ANA, ACA and TOPO antibodies) (Avouac et al., 2011). The use of nailfold video-capillaroscopy in patients suspected of having connective tissue disease may also be a useful indicator. It has been suggested that this assessment would need to be incorporated into the diagnostic and/or clinical management of patients with PBC and suspected SSc. Experimental and clinical observations suggest that endothelial dysfunction is present in PBC patients. One study found nailfold video-capillaroscopy abnormalities in 91% of patients with PBC, and 54% had capillary alterations characteristic of SSc (Fonollosa et al., 2001). Eleven out of the 22 PBC patients (50%) had extrahepatic signs of connective tissue disease with most being related to SSc, while patients with other types of chronic liver disease did not present with rheumatic manifestations (Fonollosa et al., 2001). The high prevalence of nailfold capillary abnormalities characteristic of SSc in patients with PBC, and correlation with sclerodermal manifestations, suggests that this capillaroscopic finding could be a useful indicator to investigate rheumatic manifestations in these patients (Fonollosa et al., 2001). Further clinical assessment of organ involvement (especially lung by spirometry) in association with evaluation of pulmonary artery pressure on echocardiography, should be considered in PBC patients diagnosed with SSc. A proposed diagnostic and screening algorithm for SSc in PBC patients is presented in Figure 2.

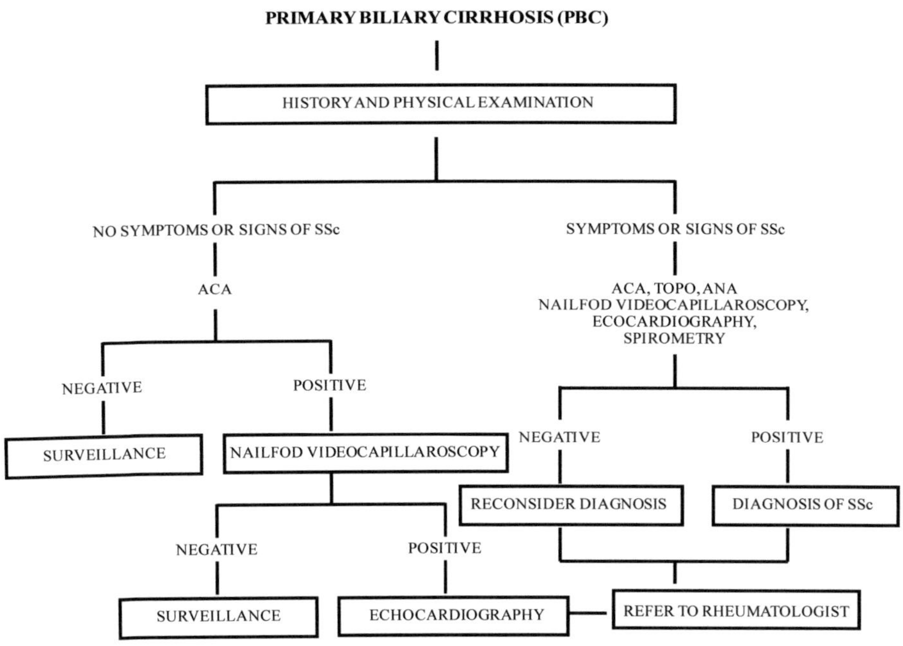

Fig. 2. Diagnostic algorithm for patients with PBC and suspected SSc

2.4 Clinical presentation and prognosis

The clinical presentation of SSc precedes that of PBC in approximately 60% of cases. The demographics of the disease in patients with overlapping features are not well-defined. For example, it is not clear whether in the diagnosis of PBC in the PBC/SSc group occurs at a lower age than in patients with PBC alone. In a study of 43 PBC/SSc patients (Rigamonti et al., 2006), the median age at diagnosis of PBC made after SSc diagnosis was lower (46.1 years) than in PBC diagnosed before SSc (51.1 years). This was lower than the diagnosis in PBC alone, with a median age of 53.2 years at diagnosis. The age difference at diagnosis in the PBC/SSc patients compared to patients with PBC alone, may be attributed to lead time bias (that is, screening for PBC in SSc patients and thus early diagnosis of asymptomatic PBC, since 56% presented with SSc alone).

A higher first incidence of spontaneous bacterial peritonitis is found in PBC/SSc patients, in addition to septicaemia during follow up, when compared to patients with PBC alone. This is likely due to an increased risk of infection due to immune abnormalities and organ system manifestations associated with SSc.

Both SSc and PBC are associated with increased morbidity and mortality (Bryan et al., 1996). Among the disease-related causes of death in SSc patients, pulmonary fibrosis, pulmonary arterial hypertension and cardiac causes (mainly heart failure and arrhythmias) are reported to account for the majority. The most frequent non-SSc-related causes of death are infections, malignancies and cardiovascular causes (Tyndall et al., 2010). In PBC patients, liver-related causes account for roughly 50% of deaths, whereas cardio- and cerebrovascular causes together with malignancies are responsible for the non-liver related deaths. Some case reports suggest that PBC in association with SSc is associated with a more favourable prognosis than PBC alone, whereas increased mortality due to SSc has been reported in others. In the study, which included 43 PBC/SSc patients, liver disease had a slower progression in PBC/SSc compared to matched patients with PBC alone (Rigamonti et al., 2006). A lower rate of liver transplantation and liver related deaths was demonstrated in PBC/SSc patients compared to patients with PBC alone, and these differences were not due to earlier SSc related deaths. However, the improvement in liver related survival in the PBC/SSc cohort was outweighed by an increase in non-liver related deaths due to SSc, and thus overall survival was not different in PBC/SSc patients and those with PBC alone. Prince and colleagues observed an increase in non-hepatic deaths in asymptomatic PBC, even with a reduced liver related mortality, in comparison with symptomatic PBC (Prince et al., 2004). Since the causes of death in PBC/SSc patients are mainly due to SSc and not to liver disease, these patients may need different prognostic models in order to better predict their liver related survival. Prognostic models for PBC alone may not be applicable for PBC associated with SSc, or for other associated autoimmune diseases to assess the risk of liver related mortality and the need for liver transplantation.

2.5 Therapy

All PBC patients with abnormal liver biochemistry should be considered for specific therapy. UDCA at the dose of 13-15 mg/kg/day on a long term basis is currently considered the mainstay of therapy for PBC (EASL 2009). In the early stages of PBC, UDCA protects injured cholangiocytes against the toxic effects of bile acids. In later stages of the disease, UDCA stimulates impaired hepatocellular secretion, mainly by posttranscriptional mechanisms (Beuers, 2006). In addition, stimulation of ductular alkaline choleresis, and inhibition of bile acid-induced hepatocyte and cholangiocyte apoptosis are included among the beneficial effects of UDCA in PBC (Beuers, 2006). UDCA has been demonstrated to

markedly decrease serum bilirubin, alkaline phosphatase, gamma-glutamyltranspeptidase, cholesterol and immunoglobulin M levels, and to ameliorate histological features in patients with PBC in comparison to placebo treatment (Poupon et al., 1991). However, no significant effects on fatigue or pruritus were observed in these large trials, nor were effects on survival. Favorable long-term effects of UDCA are observed in patients with early disease and in those with a good biochemical response, which should be assessed after one year from start of treatment (EASL 2009). A good biochemical response after one year of UDCA treatment is currently defined by a serum bilirubin ≤1 mg / dl (17 micro-mol/l), alkaline phosphatase ≤3 x ULN and aspartate aminotransferase ≤3 x ULN, according to the "Paris criteria". The "Barcelona criteria" indicate a good response with a 40% decrease or normalization of serum alkaline phosphatase.
The appropriate management of SSc is complex and includes early diagnosis of internal organ involvement, identification of patients who are at risk of progressive disease, and treatments tailored for each patient. Raynaud phenomenon and ischaemic digital ulcers are common in patients with SSc and are a cause of disease-related morbidity. The European League against Rheumatism (EULAR) recommended dihydropiridine-type calcium antagonists, such as oral nifedipine, as first-line therapy for Raynaud phenomenon and intravenous prostanoid iloprost for more severe forms (Avouac et al., 2009). The oral treatment with endothelin-1 receptor antagonist bosentan is the treatment of choice for SSc-related pulmonary artery hypertension (Avouac et al., 2009). The reportedly increased incidence of elevated aminotransferases with bosentan (Rubin et al., 2002) gives further support for the continual monitoring of liver function with this treatment, particularly in the special group of patients with associated PBC. Cyclophosphamide given orally should be considered for scleroderma interstitial lung disease (Avouac et al., 2009). Proton-pump inhibitors and prokinetic are used for the management of SSc-related gastrointestinal disease including gastroesophageal reflux, ulcers, strictures and motility disturbances. Scleroderma renal-crisis should be treated with Angiotensin converting-enzyme inhibitors (Avouac et al., 2009).

3. Conclusions

PBC-associated SSc is an intriguing autoimmune syndrome, which provides many challenges to hepatologists and rheumatologists in terms of early diagnosis and management, which should be shared between the two. A major effort should be made for continuing collaborative research in this field aimed at achieving a better understanding of the immunopathogenesis, genetic background, and demographic features of patients at higher risk of developing the associated conditions. Joint outpatient clinics between hepatologists and rheumatologists have been initiated in some large centers, and this may be a good start in the management of these complex patients.

4. References

2009 EASL Clinical Practice Guidelines: management of cholestatic liver diseases. *Journal of Hepatology,* Vol. 51, No. 2, (June 2009), pp. (237-267)

Abraham, S., Begum, S., & Isenberg, D. (2004). Hepatic manifestations of autoimmune rheumatic diseases. *Annals of the Rheumatic Diseases,* Vol. 63, No. 2, (February 2004), pp. (123-129)

Agarwal, S. K., & Reveille, J. D. (2010). The genetics of scleroderma (systemic sclerosis). *Current Opinion in Rheumatology,* Vol. 22, No. 2, (March 2010), pp. (133-138)

Akimoto, S., Ishikawa, O., Muro, Y., Takagi, H., Tamura, T., & Miyachi, Y. (1999). Clinical and immunological characterization of patients with systemic sclerosis overlapping primary biliary cirrhosis: a comparison with patients with systemic sclerosis alone. *J Dermatology,* Vol. 26, No. 1, (January 1999), pp. (18-22)

Akimoto, S., Ishikawa, O., Takagi, H., & Miyachi, Y. (1998). Immunological features of patients with primary biliary cirrhosis (PBC) overlapping systemic sclerosis: a comparison with patients with PBC alone. *Journal of Gastroenterology and Hepatology,* Vol. 13, No. 9, (September 1998), pp. (897-901)

Assassi, S., Fritzler, M. J., Arnett, F. C., Norman, G. L., Shah, K. R., Gourh, P., Manek, N., Perry, M., Ganesh, D., Rahbar, M. H., & Mayes, M. D. (2009). Primary biliary cirrhosis (PBC), PBC autoantibodies, and hepatic parameter abnormalities in a large population of systemic sclerosis patients. *The Journal of Rheumatology,* Vol. 36, No. 10, (October 2009), pp. (2250-2256)

Avouac, J., Fransen, J., Walker, U. A., Riccieri, V., Smith, V., Muller, C., Miniati, I., Tarner, I. H., Randone, S. B., Cutolo, M., Allanore, Y., Distler, O., Valentini, G., Czirjak, L., Muller-Ladner, U., Furst, D. E., Tyndall, A., & Matucci-Cerinic, M. (2011). Preliminary criteria for the very early diagnosis of systemic sclerosis: results of a Delphi Consensus Study from EULAR Scleroderma Trials and Research Group. *Annals of the Rheumatic Diseases,* Vol. 70, No. 3, (March 2011), pp. (476-481)

Avouac, J., Kowal-Bielecka, O., Landewe, R., Chwiesko, S., Miniati, I., Czirjak, L., Clements, P., Denton, C., Farge, D., Fligelstone, K., Foldvari, I., Furst, D. E., Muller-Ladner, U., Seibold, J., Silver, R. M., Takehara, K., Toth, B. G., Tyndall, A., Valentini, G., van den Hoogen, F., Wigley, F., Zulian, F., & Matucci-Cerinic, M. (2009). European League Against Rheumatism (EULAR) Scleroderma Trial and Research group (EUSTAR) recommendations for the treatment of systemic sclerosis: methods of elaboration and results of systematic literature research. *Annals of the Rheumatic Diseases,* Vol. 68, No. 5, (May 2009), pp. (629-634)

Beuers, U. (2006). Drug insight: Mechanisms and sites of action of ursodeoxycholic acid in cholestasis. *Gastroenterology & Hepatology,* Vol. 3, No. 6, (June 2006), pp. (318-328)

Bogdanos, D. P., Baum, H., & Vergani, D. (2003). Antimitochondrial and other autoantibodies. *Clinics in Liver Disease,* Vol. 7, No. 4, (November 2003), pp. (759-777)

Bogdanos, D. P., Baum, H., Vergani, D., & Burroughs, A. K. (2010). The role of E. coli infection in the pathogenesis of primary biliary cirrhosis. *Disease Markers,* Vol. 29, No. 6, (February 2010), pp. (301-311)

Bogdanos, D. P., Invernizzi, P., Mackay, I. R., & Vergani, D. (2008). Autoimmune liver serology: current diagnostic and clinical challenges. *World Journal of Gastroenterology,* Vol. 14, No. 21, (June 2008), pp. (3374-3387)

Bogdanos, D. P., & Komorowski, L. (2011). Disease-specific autoantibodies in primary biliary cirrhosis. *Clinica Chimica Acta,* Vol. 412, No. 7-8, (March 2011), pp. (502-512)

Bogdanos, D. P., Pares, A., Baum, H., Caballeria, L., Rigopoulou, E. I., Ma, Y., Burroughs, A. K., Rodes, J., & Vergani, D. (2004). Disease-specific cross-reactivity between mimicking peptides of heat shock protein of Mycobacterium gordonae and dominant epitope of E2 subunit of pyruvate dehydrogenase is common in Spanish but not British patients with primary biliary cirrhosis. *Journal of Autoimmunity,* Vol. 22, No. 4, (June 2004), pp. (353-362)

Bogdanos, D. P., Pares, A., Rodes, J., & Vergani, D. (2004). Primary biliary cirrhosis specific antinuclear antibodies in patients from Spain. *The American Journal of Gastroenterology,* Vol. 99, No. 4, (April 2004), pp. (763-764) author reply 765.

Bogdanos, D. P., & Vergani, D. (2009). Bacteria and primary biliary cirrhosis. *Clinical Reviews in Allergy & Immunology,* Vol. 36, No. 1, (February 2009), pp. (30-39)

Bryan, C., Howard, Y., Brennan, P., Black, C., & Silman, A. (1996). Survival following the onset of scleroderma: results from a retrospective inception cohort study of the UK patient population. *British Journal of Rheumatology,* Vol. 35, No. 11, (November 1996), pp. 1122-1126

Burroughs, A. K., Rosenstein, I. J., Epstein, O., Hamilton-Miller, J. M., Brumfitt, W., & Sherlock, S. (1984). Bacteriuria and primary biliary cirrhosis. *Gut,* Vol. 25, No. 2, (February 1984), pp. 133-137

Chan, H. L., Lee, Y. S., Hong, H. S., & Kuo, T. T. (1994). Anticentromere antibodies (ACA): clinical distribution and disease specificity. *Clinical and Experimental Dermatology,* Vol. 19, No. 4, (July 1994), pp. (298-302)

Chifflot, H., Fautrel, B., Sordet, C., Chatelus, E., & Sibilia, J. (2008). Incidence and prevalence of systemic sclerosis: a systematic literature review. *Seminars in Arthritis and Rheumatism,* Vol. 37, No. 4, (February 2008), pp. (223-235)

Corpechot, C., Chretien, Y., Chazouilleres, O., & Poupon, R. (2010). Demographic, lifestyle, medical and familial factors associated with primary biliary cirrhosis. *Journal of Hepatology,* Vol. 53, No. 1, (July 2010), pp. (162-169)

Courvalin, J. C., & Worman, H. J. (1997). Nuclear envelope protein autoantibodies in primary biliary cirrhosis. *Seminars in Liver Disease,* Vol. 17, No. 1, (February 1997), pp. (79-90)

Danese, S., Zoli, A., Cremonini, F., & Gasbarrini, A. (2000). High prevalence of Helicobacter pylori type I virulent strains in patients with systemic sclerosis. *The Journal of Rheumatology,* Vol. 27, No. 6, (June 2000), pp. (1568-1569)

Feghali-Bostwick, C., Medsger, T. A., Jr., & Wright, T. M. (2003). Analysis of systemic sclerosis in twins reveals low concordance for disease and high concordance for the presence of antinuclear antibodies. *Arthritis and Rheumatism,* Vol. 48, No. 7, (July 2003), pp. (1956-1963)

Fonollosa, V., Simeon, C. P., Castells, L., Garcia, F., Castro, A., Solans, R., Lima, J., Vargas, V., Guardia, J., & Vilardell, M. (2001). Morphologic capillary changes and manifestations of connective tissue diseases in patients with primary biliary cirrhosis. *Lupus,* Vol. 10, No. 9, (September 2001), pp. (628-631)

Gershwin, M. E., & Mackay, I. R. (2008). The causes of primary biliary cirrhosis: Convenient and inconvenient truths. *Hepatology,* Vol. 47, No. 2, (February 2008), pp. (737-745)

Gershwin, M. E., Selmi, C., Worman, H. J., Gold, E. B., Watnik, M., Utts, J., Lindor, K. D., Kaplan, M. M., & Vierling, J. M. (2005). Risk factors and comorbidities in primary biliary cirrhosis: a controlled interview-based study of 1032 patients. *Hepatology,* Vol. 42, No. 5, (November 2005), pp. (1194-1202)

Grossman, C., Dovrish, Z., Shoenfeld, Y., & Amital, H. (2011). Do infections facilitate the emergence of systemic sclerosis? *Autoimmunity reviews,* Vol. 10, No. 5, (March 2011), pp. (244-247)

Gupta, R. C., Seibold, J. R., Krishnan, M. R., & Steigerwald, J. C. (1984). Precipitating autoantibodies to mitochondrial proteins in progressive systemic sclerosis. *Clinical and Experimental Immunology,* Vol. 58, No. 1, (October 1984), pp. (68-76)

Hirschfield, G. M., & Invernizzi, P. (2011). Progress in the genetics of primary biliary cirrhosis. *Seminars in Liver Disease,* Vol. 31, No. 2, (May 2011), pp. (147-156)

Hudson, M., Rojas-Villarraga, A., Coral-Alvarado, P., Lopez-Guzman, S., Mantilla, R. D., Chalem, P., Baron, M., & Anaya, J. M. (2008). Polyautoimmunity and familial autoimmunity in systemic sclerosis. *Journal of Autoimmunity,* Vol. 31, No. 2, (Spetember 2008), pp. (156-159)

James, O. F., Bhopal, R., Howel, D., Gray, J., Burt, A. D., & Metcalf, J. V. (1999). Primary biliary cirrhosis once rare, now common in the United Kingdom? *Hepatology,* Vol. 30, No. 2, (August 1999), pp. (390-394)

Jimenez, S. A., Diaz, A., & Khalili, K. (1995). Retroviruses and the pathogenesis of systemic sclerosis. *International Reviews of Immunology,* Vol. 12, No. 2-4, (1995), pp. (159-175)

Kalabay, L., Fekete, B., Czirjak, L., Horvath, L., Daha, M. R., Veres, A., Fonyad, G., Horvath, A., Viczian, A., Singh, M., Hoffer, I., Fust, G., Romics, L., & Prohaszka, Z. (2002). Helicobacter pylori infection in connective tissue disorders is associated with high levels of antibodies to mycobacterial hsp65 but not to human hsp60. *Helicobacter,* Vol. 7, No. 4, (August 2002), pp. (250-256)

Kallenberg, C. G., Pastoor, G. W., Wouda, A. A., & The, T. H. (1982). Antinuclear antibodies in patients with Raynaud's phenomenon: clinical significance of anticentromere antibodies. *Annals of the Rheumatic Diseases,* Vol. 41, No. 4, (August 1982), pp. (382-387)

Kaplan, M. M., & Gershwin, M. E. (2005). Primary biliary cirrhosis. *The New England Journal of Medicine,* Vol. 353, No. 12, (September 2005), pp. (1261-1273)

Liu, X., Invernizzi, P., Lu, Y., Kosoy, R., Lu, Y., Bianchi, I., Podda, M., Xu, C., Xie, G., Macciardi, F., Selmi, C., Lupoli, S., Shigeta, R., Ransom, M., Lleo, A., Lee, A. T., Mason, A. L., Myers, R. P., Peltekian, K. M., Ghent, C. N., Bernuzzi, F., Zuin, M., Rosina, F., Borghesio, E., Floreani, A., Lazzari, R., Niro, G., Andriulli, A., Muratori, L., Muratori, P., Almasio, P. L., Andreone, P., Margotti, M., Brunetto, M., Coco, B., Alvaro, D., Bragazzi, M. C., Marra, F., Pisano, A., Rigamonti, C., Colombo, M., Marzioni, M., Benedetti, A., Fabris, L., Strazzabosco, M., Portincasa, P., Palmieri, V. O., Tiribelli, C., Croce, L., Bruno, S., Rossi, S., Vinci, M., Prisco, C., Mattalia, A., Toniutto, P., Picciotto, A., Galli, A., Ferrari, C., Colombo, S., Casella, G., Morini, L., Caporaso, N., Colli, A., Spinzi, G., Montanari, R., Gregersen, P. K., Heathcote, E. J., Hirschfield, G. M., Siminovitch, K. A., Amos, C. I., Gershwin, M. E., & Seldin, M. F. (2010). Genome-wide meta-analyses identify three loci associated with primary biliary cirrhosis. *Nature Genetics,* Vol. 42, No. 8, (August 2010), pp. (658-660)

Marasini, B., Gagetta, M., Rossi, V., & Ferrari, P. (2001). Rheumatic disorders and primary biliary cirrhosis: an appraisal of 170 Italian patients. *Annals of the Rheumatic Diseases,* Vol. 60, No. 11, (November 2001), pp. (1046-1049)

Mayes, M. D., Whittum-Hudson, J. A., Oszust, C., Gerard, H. C., & Hudson, A. P. (2009). Lack of evidence for bacterial infections in skin in patients with systemic sclerosis. *The American Journal of the Medical Sciences,* Vol. 337, No. 4, (April 2009), pp (233-235)

Mayo, M. J., Jenkins, R. N., Combes, B., & Lipsky, P. E. (1999). Association of clonally expanded T cells with the syndrome of primary biliary cirrhosis and limited scleroderma. *Hepatology,* Vol. 29, No. 6, (June 1999), pp. (1635-1642)

Metcalf, J. V., Mitchison, H. C., Palmer, J. M., Jones, D. E., Bassendine, M. F., & James, O. F. (1996). Natural history of early primary biliary cirrhosis. *Lancet,* Vol. 348, No. 9039), pp. (1399-1402)

Miyawaki, S., Asanuma, H., Nishiyama, S., & Yoshinaga, Y. (2005). Clinical and serological heterogeneity in patients with anticentromere antibodies. *The Journal of Rheumatology,* Vol. 32, No. 8, (August 2005). pp. (1488-1494)

Murray-Lyon, I. M., Thompson, R. P., Ansell, I. D., & Williams, R. (1970). Scleroderma and primary biliary cirrhosis. *British Medical Journal,* Vol. 3, No. 5717, (August 1970), pp. (258-259)

Mytilinaiou, M. G., & Bogdanos, D. P. (2009). Primary biliary cirrhosis-specific autoantibodies in patients with systemic sclerosis. *Digestive and Liver Disease,* Vol. 41, No. 12: 916, (December 2009), pp. (916-917)

Nakamura, M., Kondo, H., Mori, T., Komori, A., Matsuyama, M., Ito, M., Takii, Y., Koyabu, M., Yokoyama, T., Migita, K., Daikoku, M., Abiru, S., Yatsuhashi, H., Takezaki, E., Masaki, N., Sugi, K., Honda, K., Adachi, H., Nishi, H., Watanabe, Y., Nakamura, Y., Shimada, M., Komatsu, T., Saito, A., Saoshiro, T., Harada, H., Sodeyama, T., Hayashi, S., Masumoto, A., Sando, T., Yamamoto, T., Sakai, H., Kobayashi, M., Muro, T., Koga, M., Shums, Z., Norman, G. L., & Ishibashi, H. (2007). Anti-gp210 and anti-centromere antibodies are different risk factors for the progression of primary biliary cirrhosis. *Hepatology,* Vol. 45, No. 1, (January 2007), pp. (118-127)

Norman, G. L., Bialek, A., Encabo, S., Butkiewicz, B., Wiechowska-Kozlowska, A., Brzosko, M., Shums, Z., & Milkiewicz, P. (2009). Is prevalence of PBC underestimated in patients with systemic sclerosis? *Digestive and Liver Disease,* Vol. 41, No. 10, (October 2009), pp. (762-764)

Parikh-Patel, A., Gold, E. B., Worman, H., Krivy, K. E., & Gershwin, M. E. (2001). Risk factors for primary biliary cirrhosis in a cohort of patients from the united states. *Hepatology,* Vol. 33, No. 1, (January 2001), pp (16-21)

Poupon, R. E., Balkau, B., Eschwege, E., & Poupon, R. (1991). A multicenter, controlled trial of ursodiol for the treatment of primary biliary cirrhosis. UDCA-PBC Study Group. *The New England Journal of Medicine,* Vol. 324, No. 22, (May 1991), pp. (1548-1554)

Powell, F. C., Winkelmann, R. K., Venencie-Lemarchand, F., Spurbeck, J. L., & Schroeter, A. L. (1984). The anticentromere antibody: disease specificity and clinical significance. *Mayo Clinic Proceedings,* Vol. 59, No. 10, (October 1984), pp (700-706)

Prince, M. I., Chetwynd, A., Craig, W. L., Metcalf, J. V., & James, O. F. (2004). Asymptomatic primary biliary cirrhosis: clinical features, prognosis, and symptom progression in a large population based cohort. *Gut,* Vol. 53, No. 6, (June 2004), pp. (865-870)

Randone, S. B., Guiducci, S., & Cerinic, M. M. (2008). Systemic sclerosis and infections. *Autoimmunity Reviews,* Vol. 8, No. 1, (October 2008), pp. (36-40)

Rigamonti, C., Shand, L. M., Feudjo, M., Bunn, C. C., Black, C. M., Denton, C. P., & Burroughs, A. K. (2006). Clinical features and prognosis of primary biliary cirrhosis associated with systemic sclerosis. *Gut,* Vol. 55, No. 3, (March 2006), pp. (388-394)

Rubin, L. J., Badesch, D. B., Barst, R. J., Galie, N., Black, C. M., Keogh, A., Pulido, T., Frost, A., Roux, S., Leconte, I., Landzberg, M., & Simonneau, G. (2002). Bosentan therapy for pulmonary arterial hypertension. *The New England Journal of Medicine,* Vol. 346, No. 12, (March 2002), pp. (896-903)

Selmi, C., Mayo, M. J., Bach, N., Ishibashi, H., Invernizzi, P., Gish, R. G., Gordon, S. C., Wright, H. I., Zweiban, B., Podda, M., & Gershwin, M. E. (2004). Primary biliary cirrhosis in monozygotic and dizygotic twins: genetics, epigenetics, and environment. *Gastroenterology,* Vol. 127, No. 2, (August 2004), pp. (485-492)

Shigematsu, H., Shimoda, S., Nakamura, M., Matsushita, S., Nishimura, Y., Sakamoto, N., Ichiki, Y., Niho, Y., Gershwin, M. E., & Ishibashi, H. (2000). Fine specificity of T cells reactive to human PDC-E2 163-176 peptide, the immunodominant autoantigen in primary biliary cirrhosis: implications for molecular mimicry and cross-recognition among mitochondrial autoantigens. *Hepatology,* Vol. 32, No. 5, (November 2000), pp. (901-909)

Shimoda, S., Nakamura, M., Ishibashi, H., Hayashida, K., & Niho, Y. (1995). HLA DRB4 0101-restricted immunodominant T cell autoepitope of pyruvate dehydrogenase complex in primary biliary cirrhosis: evidence of molecular mimicry in human autoimmune diseases. *The Journal of Experimental Medicine,* Vol. 181, No. 5, (May 1995), pp. (1835-1845)

Shimoda, S., Nakamura, M., Ishibashi, H., Kawano, A., Kamihira, T., Sakamoto, N., Matsushita, S., Tanaka, A., Worman, H. J., Gershwin, M. E., & Harada, M. (2003). Molecular mimicry of mitochondrial and nuclear autoantigens in primary biliary cirrhosis. *Gastroenterology,* Vol. 124, No. 7, (June 2003), pp. (1915-1925)

Smyk, D., Rigopoulou, E. I., Baum, H., Burroughs, A. K., Vergani, D., & Bogdanos, D. P. (2011). Autoimmunity and Environment: Am I at risk? *Clinical Reviews in Allergy & Immunology,* Epub ahead of print, (February 2011)

Steen, V. D. (2005). Autoantibodies in systemic sclerosis. *Seminars in Arthritis and Rheumatism,* Vol. 35, No. 1, (August 2005), pp. (35-42)

Tyndall, A. J., Bannert, B., Vonk, M., Airo, P., Cozzi, F., Carreira, P. E., Bancel, D. F., Allanore, Y., Muller-Ladner, U., Distler, O., Iannone, F., Pellerito, R., Pileckyte, M., Miniati, I., Ananieva, L., Gurman, A. B., Damjanov, N., Mueller, A., Valentini, G., Riemekasten, G., Tikly, M., Hummers, L., Henriques, M. J., Caramaschi, P., Scheja, A., Rozman, B., Ton, E., Kumanovics, G., Coleiro, B., Feierl, E., Szucs, G., Von Muhlen, C. A., Riccieri, V., Novak, S., Chizzolini, C., Kotulska, A., Denton, C., Coelho, P. C., Kotter, I., Simsek, I., de la Pena Lefebvre, P. G., Hachulla, E., Seibold, J. R., Rednic, S., Stork, J., Morovic-Vergles, J., & Walker, U. A. (2010). Causes and risk factors for death in systemic sclerosis: a study from the EULAR Scleroderma Trials and Research (EUSTAR) database. *Annals of the Rheumatic Diseases,* Vol. 69, No. 10, (October 2010), pp. (1809-1815)

Van de Water, J., Ishibashi, H., Coppel, R. L., & Gershwin, M. E. (2001). Molecular mimicry and primary biliary cirrhosis: premises not promises. *Hepatology,* Vol. 33, No. 4, (April 2001), pp. (771-775)

Vergani, D., Bogdanos, D. P., & Baum, H. (2004). Unusual suspects in primary biliary cirrhosis. *Hepatology,* Vol. 39, No. 1, (January 2004), pp. (38-41)

Whyte, J., Hough, D., Maddison, P. J., & McHugh, N. J. (1994). The association of primary biliary cirrhosis and systemic sclerosis is not accounted for by cross reactivity between mitochondrial and centromere antigens. *Journal of Autoimmunity,* Vol. 7, No. 3, (June 1994), pp. (413-424).

10

Capillary Dimension Measured by Computer Based Digitalized Image in Patients with Systemic Sclerosis

Hyun-Sook Kim
Division of Rheumatology, Department of Internal Medicine, College of Medicine, The Chosun University of Korea, Gwangju Republic of Korea

1. Introduction

Systemic sclerosis (SSc) is an autoimmune disease characterized by fibrotic vasculopathy and excessive organ fibrosis. Endothelial and vascular damage are main leading disability in SSc. The goal of treatment lies in the prevention of excessive fibrosis affecting major organs such as lung, esophagus or skin, and in minimizing microvascular injury to lessen the deterioration in quality of life. Raynaud's phenomenon is the clue of early diagnosis that present vascular damage developing in the preclinical stage of SSc in 80-90% of patients. Nailfold capillaroscopy (NFC) is a easily accessible diagnostic tool in secondary Raynaud's phenomenon. Examination of the nailfold capillaries can reveal the nature and extent of microvascular pathology in patients with SSc. Several prominent nailfold capillary changes, for example, megacapillary, capillary hemorrhage, loss in capillary distribution, is distinctively apparent in SSc.

The main cytokines that induce fibrosis from fibroblasts and endothelial cells are transforming growth factor-β (TGF-β), interleukin-1 (IL-1), endothelin-1 (ET-1), tumor necrosis factor-α (TNF-α). Especially, ET-1 was reported to play an important role in vasoconstriction, stimulation of fibroblasts growth incurring serious complications of SSc, such as, pulmonary fibrosis or pulmonary hypertension. These aberrant biochemical processes may involve systemic microcirculation and, thus, cause diffuse vascular abnormalities.

2. Optimal NFC parameter in SSc

Nailfold capillary is represent microcirculation (Figure 1). NFC is a well-established imaging technique widely used for diagnostic purposes in rheumatology as well as in other diseases, to assess features of microcirculation in vivo. Nailfold videocapillaroscopy enables the study of several aspects of capillary vessels, including morphology, distribution, density and blood flow. For Significant correlation between the results of NFC and microvascular injury and lung involvement was reported. Therefore, severity of the disease or response to the treatment could be estimated. Recently, researches on new factors in NFC, that would enable earlier detection of change in clinical conditions and microvascular injury with computer-based digitalied analysis, are underway. Despite these advantages, there is some debate regarding the optimal parameter in assessing microvascular injury reflecting clinical status.

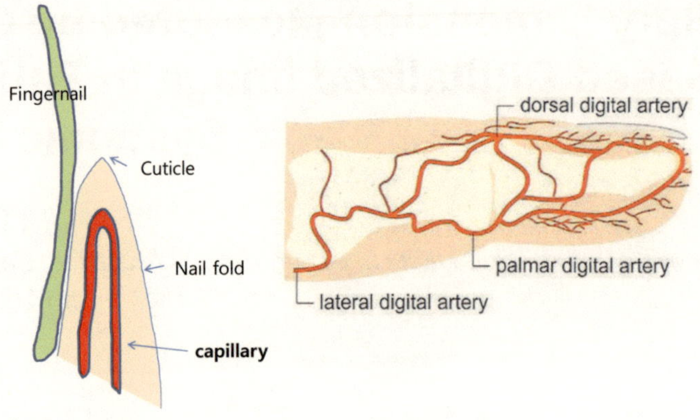

Fig. 1. Scheme of nailfold capillary

2.1 Study design

We carried out this study to define the value of optimal NFC parameter in patients diagnosed as SSc, by investigating correlation between clinical manifestations and plasma ET-1 which are known to reflect disease activity.

2.1.1 Patients and investigations of clinical manifestations

Sixty patients were randomly selected from those fulfilling American College of Rheumatology criteria for SSc and whom visited outpatient clinic. 30 healthy controls were chosen from adults with no known medical history, and 23 disease controls were chosen from the patients with connective tissue disorders other than SSc. The disease control group consisted of 14 systemic lupus erythematosus (SLE), 4 primary Sjogren's syndrome (pSS), 2 dermatomyositis (DM), 2 mixed connective tissue disease (MCTD) and 1 rheumatoid arthritis (RA) patient.

All patients and controls underwent NFC and blood sampling. After removing plasma from blood, the sample was stored at -70°C freezer (ULT-1386-5D-40) in order to measure ET-1. Evaluation of patient group's clinical manifestations was done with following exams; manometry and gastrofiberscopy to discover gastric involvement, pulmonary function test (PFT) and chest HRCT to discover pulmonary fibrosis, echocardiography to discover pulmonary hypertension, urinalysis and kidney sonography to discover renal involvement. Symptomatically, the presence of arthralgia, arthritis and digital ulceration was investigated. Assessment of skin sclerosis was done by an experienced rheumatologist, converting the severity into score using Modified Rodnan Score (MRS) (range : 0-51). Antinuclear antibody (ANA), Anti scl-70 antibody, Anti centromere antibody, extracellular nuclear antigen (ENA) was measured by immunoblot method.

2.1.2 Nailfold capillaroscopy

Patients were kept inside the procedure room for a minimum of 15 minutes before the nailfold analysis can be performed, to adapt to the room temperature of 20–25 ℃. Each subject seated with dorsum of hand facing upwards, and with halogen lightings illuminating upon the nails coated with immersion oil, under nailfold microscopy. The NFC examination was performed by an experienced examiner without the patient's clinical information and nailfolds of second, third and fourth digits of both hands were observed with light microscope (Olympus SZ-PT, Japan) under 100 times and 400 times magnification (Figure 2). All microphotographs were transmitted to computer by digital camera (Polaroid, USA) and after saving the images, enhancement was done by color filtering using Adobe Photoshop® ver. 7.0 for analysis. Quantitative analysis was done by counting total number of capillaries and number of capillaries with deletion, which were observed within 3mm width of the central part of digits. The results were recorded in average value of 6 digits. Also, an experienced rheumatologist measured the apical limb width and capillary width of 3 capillary rings located at the center, where resolution is the finest, directly from computer screen, from all 6 digits (Figure 3). Previous reports have suggested that activity of SSc is in strong correlation with capillary width and apical limb width, but not capillary length. Therefore, we presumed that measuring capillary dimension at fixed capillary length (25um) could be a new parameter. We defined capillary dimension as the sum of pixel numbers of the area set by measuring capillary boundary at capillary length of 25 um. (1cm on x 400) Adobe Photoshop® ver. 7.0 was used in this process (Figure 4).

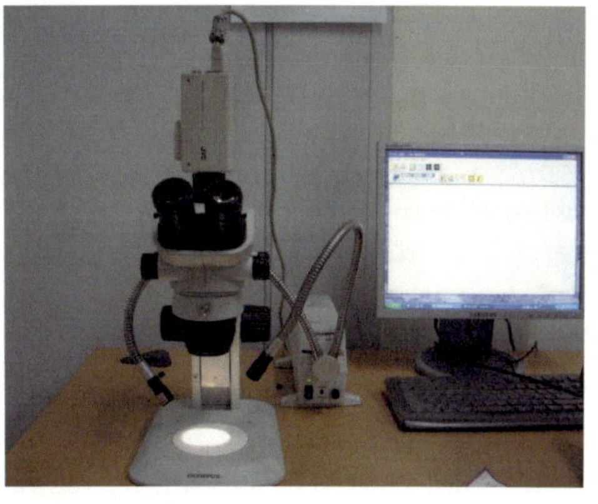

Fig. 2. Nailfold capillaroscopy is a safe and noninvasive tool that possible to detect the progression of the morphological changes.

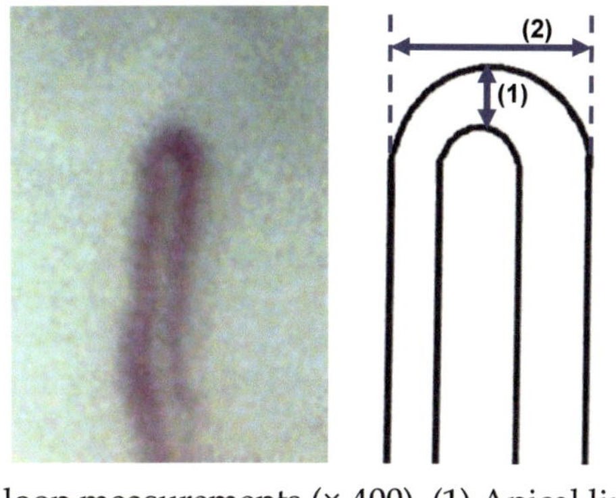

Fig. 3. Scheme of capillary loop measurements (× 400). (1) Apical limb width, (2) Capillary width.

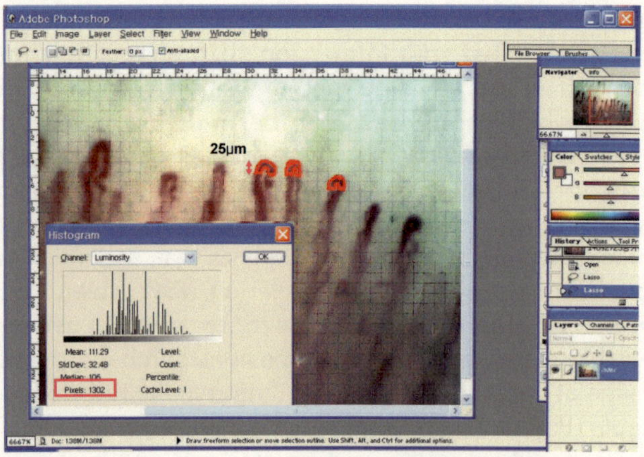

Fig. 4. The method of calculating "the sum of pixel number" with Adobe Photoshop® version 7.0 as reflect of capillary dimension: A perpendicular length of 25um tangent to internal limit of a capillary loop transverse segment defined the transverse segment area.

2.1.3 Measurement of plasma endothelin-1 and Statistical analysis

Plasma concentration of ET-1 was measured with ELISA (enzyme-linked immunosorbent assay) method. 500 uL of plasma ET-1 in EDTA tube was evenly mixed with 750ul of extraction solvent (acetone : 1N HCl :Water (40 : 1 : 5)) and then microcentrifuged. The supernant was dried down for 7 hours using speedVac concentrator and ET-1 ELISA kit (R&D, Minneapolis, MN, USA) was used for measurement. The results were interpreted using a microplate reader set to 450 nm as reference wavelength. The results were expressed in median values and inter-quartile range. SPSS ver. 17.0 program for Windows (SPSS, Chicago, IL) was used for statistical analysis. Mann-Whitney test was used for the comparison of NFC parameters and continual variables of ET-1, and Chi-square test and Fisher's exact test was used for the comparison of clinical manifestations, between the SSc patient group and the control groups. Spearman's correlation coefficient was used to express the relationship between MRS, measurement parameters of NFC, and plasma levels of ET-1 in SSc. All results were interpreted to be statistically significant when p value < 0.05.

2.1.4 Results

There were 30 people of diffuse type of systemic sclerosis (dSSc), and 30 people of limited type (lSSc). The mean age of 60 patients is 47 years old (12 - 66 years); 52 people are women (84%), the mean prevalence period is 4 years (0.1-18 years), which is similar in the sexual ratio and the age compared to the control groups. 57 people (95%) of SSc have Raynaud phenomena and it was more frequent than the disease control group. Raynaud phenomenon period is 12 months (1-120 months), statistically longer than the disease control group, which is 6 months (3-24months). Among the clinical manifestations, dysfunction due to gastrointestinal sclerosis, pulmonary fibrosis, arthralgia, arthritis, and digital ulcer were significantly frequent in SSc (Table 1). The difference in clinical patterns due to the subtypes of SSc was significantly elevated in the outbreak frequency of MRS high scores, gastrointestinal dysfunction, pulmonary fibrosis, and digital ulcer in the dSSc than the lSSc. On the contrary, there was no difference in Raynaud phenomenon, pulmonary hypertension, renal diseases, arthralgia, and arthritis. Statistically, autoantibody such as ANA, anti scl-70 antibody, ENA showed more positive incidence in the dSSc (Table 2).

	Healthy Controls (N =30) (%)	Disease control* (N =23) (%)	SSc (dSSc=30, lSSc=30) (%)
Female sex , n (%)	30 (100)	23 (100)	52 (83.87)
Age, yrs, median (IQR)	30 (24-53)	41 (18-57)	47 (12-66)
Disease duration, yrs, median (IQR)		5 (0.5-10)	4 (0.1-18)
Raynaud's phenomenon	0 (0)	10 (43.48)	57 (95.0)
Duration of Raunaud's ph, months, median (IQR)		6 (3-24)	12 (1-120)
GI manifestation	0 (0)	0 (0)	29 (48.33) #
Pulmonary fibrosis	0 (0)	2 (8.70)	33 (55.0) #
Pulmonary Hypertension	0 (0)	2 (8.70)	3 (5.0)
Renal disease	0 (0)	1 (4.35)	3 (5.0)
Arthralgia	0 (0)	11 (47.83)	45 (75.0) #
Arthritis	0 (0)	2 (8.70)	14 (23.33) #
Digital ulceration	0 (0)	5 (21.74)	27 (45.0) #

Table 1. Clinical characteristics of control and patients with SSc.

	Diffuse type of SSc (N =30) (%)	Limited type of SSc (N=30) (%)	*p*- value
Clinical			
Raynaud's phenomenon	28 (93.33)	29 (96.67)	NS
Modified Rodnan score, IQR	10.5 (4-33)	4 (2-18)	$p<0.05$*
GI manifestation	19 (63.33)	10 (33.33)	$p<0.05$*
Pulmonary fibrosis	19 (63.33)	14 (46.67)	$p<0.05$*
Pulmonary Hypertension	1 (3.33)	2 (6.67)	NS
Renal disease	1 (3.33)	2 (6.67)	NS
Arthralgia	23 (76.67)	22 (73.33)	NS
Arthritis	7 (23.33)	7 (23.33)	NS
Digital ulceration	17 (56.67)	10 (33.33)	$p<0.05$*
Serological positivity			
ANA (>1:160)	30 (100)	24 (80.0)	$p<0.05$*
Anti scl-70 Ab	18 (60.0)	12 (40.0)	$p<0.05$*
Anticentromere Ab	3 (10.0)	4 (13.33)	NS
ENA	15 (50.0)	6 (20.0)	$p<0.05$*

Table 2. Clinical and serological finding according to type of SSc

2.1.5 Results of NFC parameter

In healthy control, nailfold capillary looks like comb-like patten with minor disorganization and tortousity (Figure 5). Not like uniformly ordered capillary shape in the healthy control group, there was statistical significance in the smaller number of capillaries within 3mm, increased deletion numbers, apical limb with, capillary width, capillary hemorrhage and dimension of capillary loop in SSc patient group.

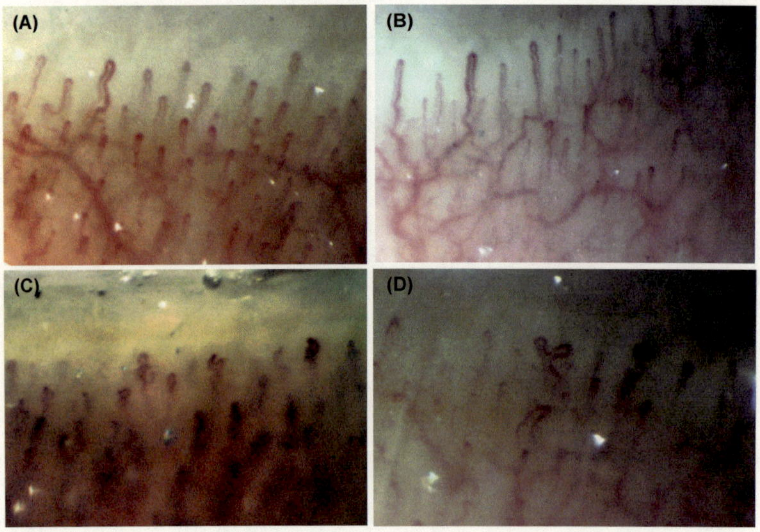

Fig. 5. The example of NFC finding (x400): (A)(B) In healthy control, the field of observation is rather uniform as comb-like appearance. (C)(D) Minimal change of capillary dilatation and increased tortousity are also seen even in healthy control.

The nailfold capillaroscopic pattern of early SSc is characterized by the massive dilatation and presence of giant capillaries (homogeneous and symmetrical capillary enlargement over 10 times compared with normal pattern) and microhemorrages (Figure 6-A,B) (early to active pattern). At the late phase of SSc progresses into fibrosis, the capillaroscopic pattern most likely reflects the effects of capillary destruction, loss of capillaries, and avascular areas are observed along with ramifications and bushy capillaries (Figure 6-C,D) (late pattern).

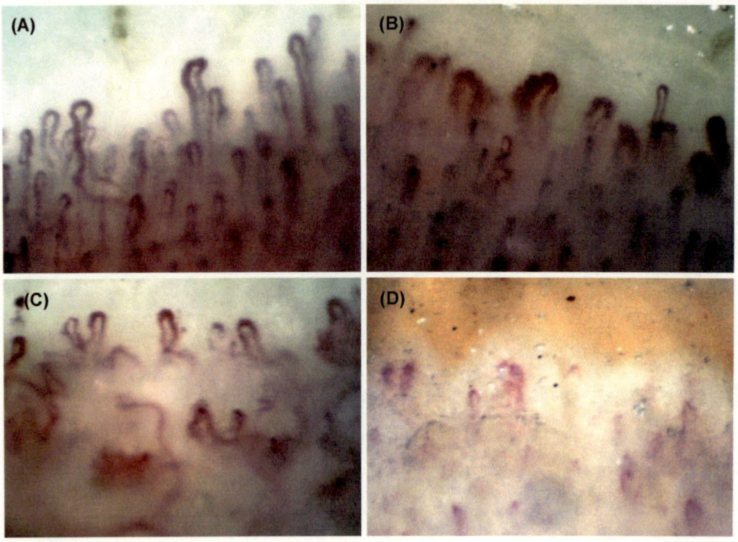

Fig. 6. The example of NFC finding (x400): (A)(B) In early to active phase of SSc, typically many giant capillary and microhemorrage is noted. (C)(D) At the late phase, ramified capillaries and avascular areas are observed along with bushy capillaries.

Above all, the capillary dimension presented as the sum of pixel numbers per 25 um capillary length was 1097, which showed the biggest difference; 516 from the healthy control group, 561 from disease control group (p <0.001) (Table3-1). Median and range of plasma ET-1 of the SSc patient group, normal control group and disease control group are on Table 3-1. The SSc patient group and disease control group had higher plasma ET-1 level than normal control group.

	Healthy Controls	Disease control	SSc
	(N =30)	(N =23)	(N =30)
NFC feature, median (IQR)			
No. of loop (in 3mm)	21.8 (16-28)	20 (13.5-25)	11.8 (1-19.5)*
Deletion No. of loop	0.5 (0-2)	1 (0.5-5.5)	3 (0-13)*
Apical width (um)	9.2 (6.7-13.3)	9.5 (6.7-11.8)	14.23 (7.9-30)*
Capillary width (um)	19.6 (12.5-26.7)	25 (15-49.7)	37.5 (15-100.9)*
Capillary dimension#	515.9 (357-566)	561.0(420-920)	1096.7(312.6-2134)*
Endothelin-1(pg/ml), median (IQR)	1.7 (0.5-2.5)	2.1 (1.2-4.1)#a	2.4 (0.9-6.3)#b

#Capillary dimension is presented by the sum of pixel number
IQR: Inter-quartile range, median(range: minimum-maximum)
* : p <0.05 is significant value
#a : p <0.05 between disease control and heatrhy control group
#b : p <0.05 between SSc and heatrhy control group

Table 3-1. Nailfold capillary microscopic feature and plasma endothelin-1 level

Other than that the capillary dimension of the dSSc was significantly wider than that of the lSSc, there was no difference between the two subtypes. There was no difference in the levels of plasma ET-1 among the subtypes of SSc patient group (Table 3-2).

	dSSc	lSSc	
	(N =30)	(N =30)	p- value
NFC feature, median (IQR)			
No. of loop (in 3mm)	10.1 (3-30)	13.5(3.5-23)	NS
Deletion No. of loop	3 (0.5-13)	3 (0-8)	NS
Apical width (um)	14.75(7.5-35)	12.75(8-30)	NS
Capillary width (um)	40.25(8-100.75)	35.13(21.68-88.35)	NS
Capillary dimension#	1312.7(313-2097)	965.1(527-2156)	p<0.05*
Endothelin-1 (pg/ml), median (IQR)	2.63(0.86-4.54)	2.21(1.09-6.31)	NS

Table 3-2. Nailfold capillary microscopic feature and plasma endothelin-1 between diffuse and limited type in patients with Systemic sclerosis.

The NFC parameters did not differ in the presence of pulmonary fibrosis, renal diseases, arthralgia and arthritis in SSc. However, the number of capillaries in 3mm and capillary deletion had statistically significant smaller in gastrointestinal dysfunction and pulmonary hypertension. When there is a digital ulcer, all parameters of NFC showed significant

disparity, especially in number of capillary deletions ($p < 0.01$) and capillary dimension ($p < 0.001$) (Table 4).
Comparison of plasma ET-1 of SSc patient group divided according to clinical characteristics showed notably high in the group with digital ulcer and pulmonary hypertension ($p < 0.01$, $p < 0.05$) (Table 4). It should be noted that plasma ET-1 is statistically proportional to MRS. Moreover, there was a statistic correlation between the level of plasma ET-1 and the capillary dimension in NFC (Table 5).

	Clinical manifestation						
	G-I	Pul. fibrosis	Pul. HTN	Renal dis.	Arthralgia	Arthritis	Digital ulcer
NFC feature							
No. of loop (in 3mm)	$p < 0.01$*	NS	$p < 0.01$*	NS	NS	NS	$p < 0.05$*
Deletion No. of loop	$p < 0.05$*	NS	$p < 0.01$*	NS	NS	NS	$p < 0.01$*
Apical width	NS	NS	NS	NS	NS	NS	$p < 0.05$*
Capillary width	NS	NS	NS	NS	NS	NS	$p < 0.01$*
Capillary dimension#	NS	NS	NS	NS	NS	NS	$p < 0.001$*
Endothelin-1	NS	NS	$p < 0.05$*	NS	NS	NS	$p < 0.01$*

#Capillary dimension is presented by the sum of pixel number
G-I:abnormal finding in manometry including of GERD (gastro-esophageal reflux disease)
Pul. fibrosis: Pulmonary fibrosis
Pul. HTN: Pulmonary Hypertension
Renal dis.: Renal disease
NS: not significant
$p < 0.05$* is significant value

Table 4. Correlation of clinical manifestations with NFC parameters and cytokines in patients with SSc.

	Endothelin-1
Skin hardness (MRS)	$p < 0.05$*
NFC feature	
No. of loop	NS
Deletion No. of loop	NS
Apical width	NS
Capillary width	NS
Capillary dimension#	$p < 0.05$*

MRS: modified rodnan score
SSc: Systemic sclerosis
#Capillary dimension is presented by the sum of pixel number
NS: not significant
$p < 0.05$* is significant value by Spearmam's correlation.

Table 5. Correlation of plasma endothelin-1 with skin hardness and NFC parameters in patients with SSc

The level of plasma ET-1 and the capillary dimension were notably correlated in all of healthy, disease control group and SSc patient group (Rs = 0.82 / p<0.001, Rs = 0.83 / p<0.001, Rs = 0.31 / p<0.05) (Figure 7). The results suggest that computer-based microscopic analysis of NFC is a useful method that potentially provides information on organ involvement and plasma ET-1.

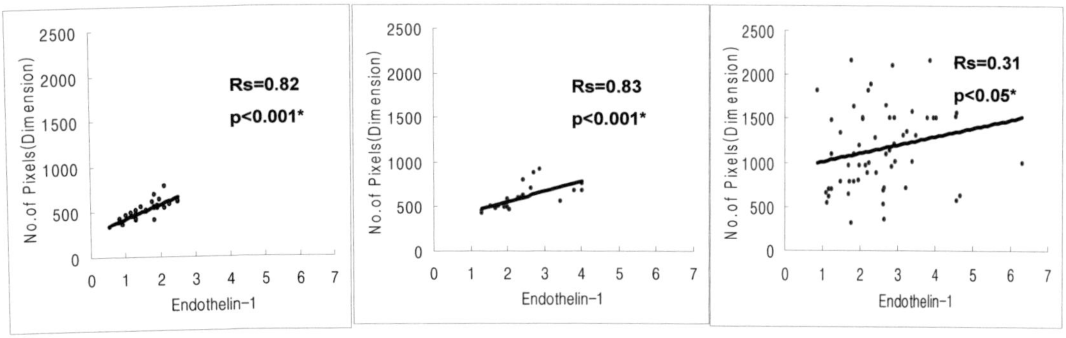

Fig. 7. Relationship between plasma Endothelin-1 and capillary dimension; Capillary dimension showed strong correlation with the level of endothelin-1 in (A) healthy control, (B) disease control, (C) SSc (p <0.05* is significant value by Spearmam's correlation).

3. Conclusion

NFC is a non-invasive, relatively inexpensive modality in diagnosing secondary Raynaud's phenomenon and it detects characteristic changes of SSc. NFC is able to indirectly evaluate vascular function of the connective tissue disorder. Recent researches reported the correlation between the NFC change and the occurrence of gastrointestinal invasion, pulmonary fibrosis, portal hypertension; thereby there is increasing the possibilities of the early detection of internal organ invasion or the marker for the follow-up after treatment based with digitalized computer-based analysis. Many clinical findings and plasma cytokines was compared with traditionally used NFC parameter, which to observe the number of capillaries and deletions in 3mm, apical limb width and the capillary width itself; however, we suggest that a computer can generate a more powerful relation which predicts the capillary dimension presented as the sum of pixel number in 25um of length.

Previously anderson et al. asserted that capillary dimension could be a new parameter for Raynaud phenomenon; there were differences in capillary dimension according with diabetic's vasospastic symptoms. Also in our study, the capillary dimension positively correlates with the apical limb width and capillary width in healthy control group. In disease control and SSc group, the capillary dimension negatively correlates with the number of capillary and showed positive correlations to the rest parameters, which advocates as a new optimal parameter. The capillary dimension also is illustrated statistic correlation to MRS which is the distinctive symptom in SSc. Additionally, the capillary dimension increases the most with the incidence of digital ulcer, which best reflects the activity of the disease in general. Not only in SSc, capillary dimension represented an authentic correlation to plasma ET-1 level in both the healthy control and the disease control group. For those reasons, the capillary dimension can be a factor that speaks for plasma ET-1, regardless of the disease types.

The endothelial cell or the smooth muscle cell secretes ET-1, which is a strong vasoconstrictor related to the onset of numerous diseases. ET-1 is known to the main cytokine which causes capillary deletion and directly to the development of fatal diseases such as pulmonary fibrosis and portal hypertension in SSc. As like in other studies, in SSc, plasma ET-1 level was increased than the healthy control group, but there was no statistic difference with the disease control group. The reason is that ET-1 is also increased in other connective tissue disorders that involve microvessel disruption due to vasoconstriction. Scala et al. emphasized the research and control of essential cytokines that overproduces or causes unbalance in extracellular materials in connective tissue cells, among many causes of fibrosis, is adequate for pathophysiologic approach to the disease and to prevent the progress of the disease. On the other hand, it is troublesome to measure the changes of cytokines all the time and the relationship to internal organ invasion is uncertain.
From this study, plasma ET-1 is elevated in SSc than the healthy control group proportionately to MRS, and meaningfully high in digital ulcer and pulmonary hypertension. For that reason, ET-1 could be considered to be closely related to the disease progression and severity of SSc. In our study, the capillary dimension is the best reflects of plasma ET-1 in the NFC parameters. Consequently, capillary dimension using computer pixel number is able to assume according to increasing in the plasma ET-1 and disease activity. Capillary dimension maybe a powerful parameter, could be advantageous for early diagnosis of complications as a result of organ involvement, and for the regular follow-ups to assessments of the treatment in the patients with SSc.

4. Acknowledgment

This is supported by Chosun University.

5. References

LeRoy EC, Black C, Fleischmajer R et al (1988) Scleroderma (systemic sclerosis): classification, subsets and pathogenesis. J Rheumatol 15:202–205

Bukhari M, Hollis S, Moore T et al (2000) Quantitation of microcirculatory abnormalities in patients with primary Raynaud's phenomenon and systemic sclerosis by video capillaroscopy. Rheumatology (Oxford) 39: 506-512

Markus B, Ricardo MX, Karina GC et al (2004) Nailfold Capillary Microscopy Can Suggest Pulmonary Disease Activity in Systemic Sclerosis. J Rheumatol 31:286-294

Czirjak L, Kiss CG, Lovei C et al (2005) Survey of Raynaud's phenomenon and systemic sclerosis based on a representative study of 10,000 south-Transdanubian Hungarian inhabitants. Clin Exp Rheumatol 23:801-808

JH Do, HY Kim (2004) Increased plasma endothelin-1 and abnormal nailfold capillaroscopic findings in patients with connective tissue diseases. The Korean J of Med 66: 275-283

Pucinelli ML, Atra E, Sato EI et al (1995) Nailfold capillaroscopy in systemic sclerosis: correlations with involvement of lung and esophagus. Rev Bras Rheumatol 35:136-142

11

Scleroderma Renal Crisis

Lola Chabtini[1,*], Marwan Mounayar[1,*], Jamil Azzi[1], Vanesa Bijol[1],
Sheldon Bastacky[2], Helmut G. Rennke[1] and Ibrahim Batal[1]
[1]*Brigham and Women's Hospital and Harvard University*
[2]*University of Pittsburgh Medical Center*
USA

1. Introduction

Scleroderma renal crisis (SRC) is an infrequent complication of a rare disease. To date, many aspects of the pathophysiology of SRC are still mysterious. Since SRC biopsies are not frequently encountered in practice, our understanding of the spectrum of histologic changes is derived from a combination of a limited personal experience and data obtained from several relatively small pathologic studies.

This book chapter will be devoted to discuss the pathophysiology and the histologic manifestations of SRC and will cover the most important aspects of clinical and laboratory findings as well as treatment of SRC.

Systemic sclerosis (SSc) is a chronic systemic autoimmune disease characterized by excess collagen production. According to the extent of cutaneous sclerosis, SSc can be classified as either diffuse cutaneous (dc) or limited cutaneous (lc) variant (Sakkas, 2005). Many studies have been conducted to explore the pathogenesis of SSc. Activation of T-cells, B-cells and macrophages have been described and linked to the development and progression of fibrosis (Sakkas, Chikanza, & Platsoucas, 2006). Activated T-cells, mainly T helper lymphocyte type-2 (TH-2), are associated with increased IL-4 and IL-13 production and collagen accumulation. Activated B-cells produce autoantibodies that can facilitate transformation of fibroblasts into more fibrotic phenotypes while activated macrophages can accumulate in the perivascular spaces to produce transforming growth factor-B and platelet derived growth factor, which can also promote fibrosis. In addition to collagen accumulation, endothelial cell injury appears to play a central role in the pathogenesis of SSc. Increased permeability of the nail fold capillaries (Bollinger, Jager, & Siegenthaler, 1986) and increased endothelial apoptosis (Sgonc et al., 1996)have been described in SSc patients. Endothelial cell injury in SSc may be triggered by anti-endothelial antibody (Worda et al., 2003), cytokines (Kahaleh, 2004), complement abnormalities (Venneker, van den Hoogen, Boerbooms, Bos, & Asghar, 1994) and/or cellular cytotoxicity (Sgonc et al., 2000). Scleroderma renal crisis (SRC) can complicate the course of up to 10-20% of patients with SSc. SRC is most commonly encountered in patients with dcSSc; however, it can still occur in patients with lcSSc(Sugimoto, Sanada, & Kashiwagi, 2008; Sugimoto et al., 2006) and even in patients with no significant dermal sclerosis, termed systemic sclerosis sine scleroderma (ssSSc) (Gonzalez, Schmulbach, & Bastani, 1994). Compared to SSc, much less is known

* Contributed equally

about the pathophysiology of SRC. This is largely attributed to the rarity of the disease and the absence of acceptable animal models for SRC. However, accumulating data suggest an important role of antibody-mediated injury in the pathogenesis of SRC. The histologic picture of SRC is not entirely specific for this disease. A similar histologic picture may be encountered in a number of primary vascular diseases and clinical conditions that may present as thrombotic microangiopathy. In addition to confirming the clinical diagnosis, renal biopsy can help predict the clinical outcome and optimize therapy in SRC patients. The mortality associated with SRC has decreased because of early diagnosis and angiotensin-converting enzyme inhibitor therapy (Collins, Patel, Eastwood, & Bourke, 1996; Steen, Costantino, Shapiro, & Medsger, 1990). Kidney transplantation remains as a treatment option for a subset of SRC patients who develop end-stage renal failure despite aggressive therapy. Unfortunately, the post-transplantation outcome for these patients continues to be worse than that of the general renal transplant population.

2. Clinical and laboratory features

SRC occurs more frequently in females than males and in Caucasians compared to African American (Sakkas, 2005). It is also much more common in patients with dcSSc than patients with lcSSc. However, only 10-20% of patients with dcSSc develop SRC (Ferri et al., 2002; Steen & Medsger, 2000b). SRC usually occurs early in the course of SSc. Up to 75% of SRC develop within the first four years from the diagnosis of SSc (Steen, 1994, 2003). SRC is classically associated with a sudden increase in blood pressure (>150/90 mm Hg) (Mouthon et al.; Steen, 2003). This is usually accompanied by an acute deterioration in renal function. In addition, such patients often complain of headache, blurred vision and dyspnea as a result of hypertensive encephalopathy, congestive heart failure and pulmonary edema. Nevertheless, up to 10% of SRC patients present with blood pressures below malignant hypertension levels ("normotensive SRC")(Helfrich, Banner, Steen, & Medsger, 1989; Kagan, Nissim, Green, & Bar-Khayim, 1989). In these subjects, although blood pressure is within the normal range, it is commonly increased from its baseline value (Helfrich, et al., 1989; Steen, 2003).
Thrombotic microangiopathy, characterized by thrombocytopenia, normocytic hemolytic anemia, elevated levels of LDH and low serum haptoglobin can be encountered in approximately 50% of SRC patients at clinical presentation (Penn et al., 2007; Steen, 2003; Walker et al., 2003). In SRC patients, serum creatinine and blood urea nitrogen (BUN) are consistently elevated and are usually proportional to the severity of renal involvement (Steen, 2003). Renin blood levels are significantly elevated, especially in patients with malignant hypertension (Traub et al., 1983). Urinalysis may reveal microscopic hematuria and mild to moderate proteinuria (usually 0.5 to 2.5 grams per 24 hours) (Mouthon, et al.; Steen, 2003).
With regard to autoantibodies, ANA is detected in up to 90% of SRC patients. The pattern of ANA immunofluorescence is usually speckled (Penn, et al., 2007). Anti-centromere antibody, which is typically observed in lcSSc, has been infrequently reported in SRC patients (Mouthon, et al.; Steen, 2005; Teixeira et al., 2008). Some investigators even consider the detection of anti-centromere antibody to be protective against renal crises (Penn, et al., 2007). Anti-topoisomerase antibody, formerly known as Scl-70 antibody, is typically described in dSSc patients. This antibody has been shown to have some association with renal involvement as well as pulmonary fibrosis and cardiac disease (Steen, Powell, & Medsger, 1988). Anti-RNA polymerase III antibody is seen at a high frequency in patients

with SSc who develop SRC (B. Nguyen, Assassi, Arnett, & Mayes; Okano, Steen, & Medsger, 1993). Anti Th/To antibodies have been reported in some cases of SRC without pulmonary involvement (Gunduz, Fertig, Lucas, & Medsger, 2001) while anti-RNP3 or fibrillarin antibodies have a stronger association with pulmonary hypertension and skeletal muscle involvement than SRC (Aggarwal, Lucas, Fertig, Oddis, & Medsger, 2009). Compared to other autoimmune connective tissue diseases, SRC has the worst prognosis (Ferri, et al., 2002; LeRoy et al., 1988). Predictors of poor outcome in SRC include male gender, age above fifty years, cardiac disease and dcSSc with extensive skin sclerosis (higher skin score) (Denton, Lapadula, Mouthon, & Muller-Ladner, 2009; Teixeira, et al., 2008). Normal blood pressure at presentation has also been associated with a poor prognosis (Medsger, Masi, Rodnan, Benedek, & Robinson, 1971; Penn, et al., 2007; Teixeira, et al., 2008). Patients with normotensive SRC could possibly have lower activation of their renin-angiotensin system and therefore a lower blood pressure at presentation(Penn, et al., 2007). The poor prognosis observed in the latter group might be attributed to a possible delay in diagnosis and treatment (Haviv & Safadi, 1998; Helfrich, et al., 1989).

3. Pathophysiology

Despite efforts to investigate the underlying immune mechanisms, the pathophysiology of SRC remains incompletely understood. Injury to the vascular endothelium appears to play a key role in activating the pathological cascade of SRC. Endothelial injury leads to increased endothelial permeability, vascular edema, accumulation of mucopolysaccharide material, and proliferation of intimal cells. If the injury is sufficiently severe, endothelial damage can initiate arteriolar and arterial fibrinoid necrosis and vascular thrombosis through platelet activation and adhesion to the sub-endothelium (Batal, Domsic, Medsger, & Bastacky, 2010; Fisher & Rodnan, 1958; Steen, 2003). With time, these changes can organize leading to fibrointimal thickening and narrowing of the small arteries (Cannon et al., 1974; Fisher & Rodnan, 1958). Intimal arteritis, manifested as lymphocytic and mononuclear cell infiltration, is typically absent in SRC (Steen, 2003). Even though collagen overproduction and accumulation is well established in the skin and lung lesions of SSc patients, collagen's role in early kidney lesions appears less important. Increased collagen appears later in the form of vascular fibrointimal and adventitial thickening or as interstitial fibrosis. The latter is often attributed to decreased perfusion due to chronic ischemic vasculopathy.

Intermittent vasospasm of renal arteries, also known as renal Raynaud's phenomenon, has also been proposed as a potential contributor to SRC-induced kidney injury (Cannon, et al., 1974); Traub et al. reported an increase in the frequency of SRC in the winter suggesting cold-induced vasoconstriction of renal arteries (Traub, et al., 1983). Vasospasm can also participate in renal injury in SSc patients even in the absence of SRC. Following cold pressor testing, Cannon et al. demonstrated a significant reduction in renal cortical blood flow in SSc patients when compared to control subjects (Cannon, et al., 1974). In addition, Doppler studies showed increased vascular resistance in SSc patients without concurrent renal damage (Rivolta et al., 1996). Nevertheless, Raynaud's phenomenon does not appear to be the only explanation of renal injury in SSc patients without SRC. In an autopsy-based study, Trostle et al. were able to show well established anatomic vascular changes in the form of fibrointimal thickening in SSc patients without SRC (Trostle, Helfrich, & Medsger, 1986).

Regardless of the cause, reduction in kidney perfusion causes subsequent hyperplasia of the juxtaglomerular apparatus (JGA) and increased renin secretion (Stone, Tisher, Hawkins, &

Robinson, 1974). Kovalchik et al. (Kovalchik, Guggenheim, Silverman, Robertson, & Steigerwald, 1978) proposed that renin production in SSc patients may be proportional to the severity of vascular lesions. These authors also suggested that a substantial increment in plasma renin activity in response to cold pressor testing could identify SSc subjects with a preclinical renal involvement. However, more recent studies revealed that plasma renin levels are neither sensitive nor predictive for SRC. Hyperreninemia has been described in asymptomatic SSc patients who did not develop SRC (Mouthon, et al.). The potential mechanisms of kidney injury in SRC are summarized in (Figure 1).

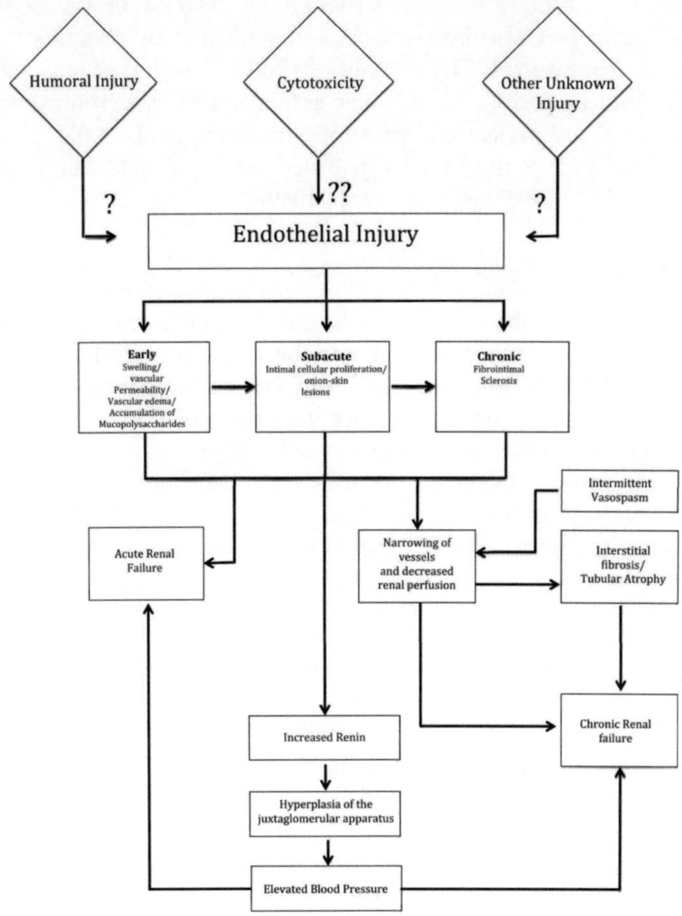

Abbreviation: ?, Potential strong association; ??, potential weaker association; MPS, mucopolysaccharide

Fig. 1. Potential mechanisms of injury in scleroderma renal crisis.

Endothelin-1 is a peptide produced mainly by endothelial cells. It has three isoforms ET-1, ET-2 and ET-3. ET-1 binds to ET type A and ET type B receptors on muscular and endothelial cells (Tirapelli et al., 2005). It modulates vascular constriction and smooth muscle cell proliferation (Hirata, 1989; Takuwa, Takuwa, Yanagisawa, Yamashita, & Masaki, 1989). Accumulating data suggest that the latter might play an important role in the pathogenesis of scleroderma. Higher serum ET-1 levels were detected in SSc compared to healthy controls (Vancheeswaran et al., 1994). In kidney specimens, overexpression of ET-1 and ET type B receptors were described in two patients who died following SRC (Kobayashi et al., 1999). Mouthon et al. extended the aforementioned observations by studying the pattern of ET-1 expression in kidney biopsies utilizing the immunoperoxidase technique (Mouthon et al.). These investigators found glomerular and vascular overexpression of ET-1 in SRC specimens. In comparison, normal kidney biopsies revealed negative ET-1 glomerular staining and only weak vascular staining. In contrast, biopsies from patients with hemolytic uremic syndrome (HUS) showed increased ET-1 expression on the glomerular but not the vascular endothelium. ET-1 expression was largely detected in areas of glomerular capillary wall thickening, glomerular and vascular thrombosis, and vessels with either mucoid changes, onion-skin lesions, or fibrointimal thickening. Of note, ET-1 was recently identified as one of the most up regulated endothelial transcripts in allografts following antibody-mediated rejection [48, 49].

C4d is an early complement split product of the classical pathway of activation. When detected in the peritubular capillary of an allograft biopsy, it is very suggestive of the diagnosis of antibody-mediated rejection (Racusen et al., 2003). Using immunoperoxidase techniques, we could detect similar pattern of C4d staining in a subset of SRC patients who had poor renal outcome (Batal et al., 2009). Nevertheless, the presence and/or significance of C4d deposits in SRC should be confirmed in larger studies using the more specific immunofluorescence techniques.

In summary, accumulating data suggest the contribution of antibody-mediated injury in the pathogenesis of SRC; First, specific autoantibodies have been associated with the development of SRC. Second, the detection of peritubular capillary C4d staining has been demonstrated in occasional patients with SRC. Third, ET-1 is overly expressed in SRC biopsies.

In contrast, while the role of cytotoxicity is well accepted in SSc, cytotoxicity was not systematically studied in SRC. The presence of peritubular capillary and tubulointerstitial inflammation in some SRC biopsies suggests a possible contribution of cytotoxicity to kidney injury. An immunohistochemical study to look at granzyme-B+ cells in such biopsy in association with apoptosis of endothelial cells might be an initial step to investigate such possibility.

Several factors such as pericardial effusion, arrhythmia(McWhorter & LeRoy, 1974; Satoh et al., 1995; Steen et al., 1984), pregnancy (Karlen & Cook, 1974), sepsis (Steen, 2003) , non steroidal anti-inflammatory drugs (NSAID) and cocaine(Lam & Ballou, 1992) can decrease renal perfusion and precipitate or aggravate SRC in SSc patients. Corticosteroids are also believed to trigger SRC; high dose prednisone might inhibit prostacyclin levels, increase in angiotensin converting enzyme (ACE) activity and subsequent vasoconstriction (Sharnoff, Carideo, & Stein, 1951).

Animal models are important tools to expand our knowledge of a particular disease process. They offer the advantage of developing targeted therapies to diseases without placing patients at risk of a direct intervention. Several experimental animal models of scleroderma have been developed (Yamamoto). One of the better-known models is bleomycin-induced scleroderma. A repeated intradermal or subcutaneous injection of bleomycin into rats and mice leads to the development of dermal sclerosis (Mountz et al., 1983; Yamamoto; Yamamoto & Nishioka, 2001, 2002, 2004; Yamamoto et al., 1999; Yamamoto, Takahashi, Takagawa, Katayama, & Nishioka, 1999). The latter is microscopically characterized by the deposition of thick collagen bundles, homogeneous acellular material, and cellular infiltrates of T-cells, macrophages, and mast cells. Ishikawa et al. has recently shown that the adoptive transfer of CD4+ T-cells from bleomycin-treated mice into untreated BALB/c nude mice induced a similar pathological picture with autoantibody production (Ishikawa, Takeda, Okamoto, Matsuo, & Isobe, 2009). Dermal sclerosis in this animal model is generally limited to the areas of bleomycin-injection and sclerotic changes are not observed in fingers or abdominal skin. In addition to rodent animal models, UCD-200 chicken is another extensively studied SSc animal model. In addition to clinical manifestations, UCD-200 is one of the very few SSc models that display renal abnormalities. Endothelial cell apoptosis has been described in the kidneys of such animals. However, the histologic picture is different from what is typically observed in humans with SRC. In contrast to the typical thrombotic microangiopathic pattern of injury, the kidneys of UCD-200 chicken are characterized by the presence of glomerulonephritis associated with IgG deposition and thickening of the muscular vascular layer (Gershwin et al., 1981; V. A. Nguyen, Sgonc, Dietrich, & Wick, 2000). From this model, one can conclude that SRC falls behind cutaneous sclerosis with regard to *in vivo* models. To date, SRC still lack a well-accepted animal model.

Finally, one should remember that despite its importance in facilitating our understanding of the pathophysiology and treatment options, differences do exist between human and murine immune systems. The use of "humanized mouse model"(Pearson, Greiner, & Shultz, 2008; Zhang, Meissner, Chen, & Su, 2010), a small immune compromised murine model possessing a functional reconstituted human immune system, might offer a potential way to overcome some existing frustrations in improving scleroderma treatment.

4. Gross pathology

Macroscopic changes observed in SRC are relatively nonspecific, since similar changes can be encountered in other thrombotic microangiopathic disorders. Petechial hemorrhages are frequently observed on the surface of the affected kidneys while cut sections commonly reveal small wedge shaped infarcts or, less often, larger foci of cortical necrosis (Fisher & Rodnan, 1958).

5. Microscopic pathology

5.1 Light microscopy

In the absence of acceptable animal models, our current knowledge of the renal pathologic changes in SRC is largely derived from histologic assessment of kidney biopsy specimens performed during such crises. Autopsy materials provide another source to study the morphologic alterations of this disease, although the histologic changes in autopsy specimens often reflect a clinically severe and prolonged form of the disease typically associated with end stage renal failure. A complete understanding of the spectrum of pathologic changes in SRC is also limited by the low incidence of the disease and the fact that renal biopsies are not routinely performed during the crisis. Such biopsies are basically recommended when doubt exists about the etiology of renal dysfunction or, alternatively, to exclude the coexistence of other diseases.

The histologic manifestations may vary during the course of the disease and the pathologic changes predominate in small vessels and arterioles rather than larger arteries. Early vascular changes can manifest as intimal edema and accumulation of acid mucopolysaccharide material (Figure 2), which is positively stained with Alcian blue or toluidine blue. Other early vascular changes include thrombosis (Figure 3) and/or fibrinoid necrosis. Onion-skin lesions develop later as a result of cellular proliferation (Figure 4).

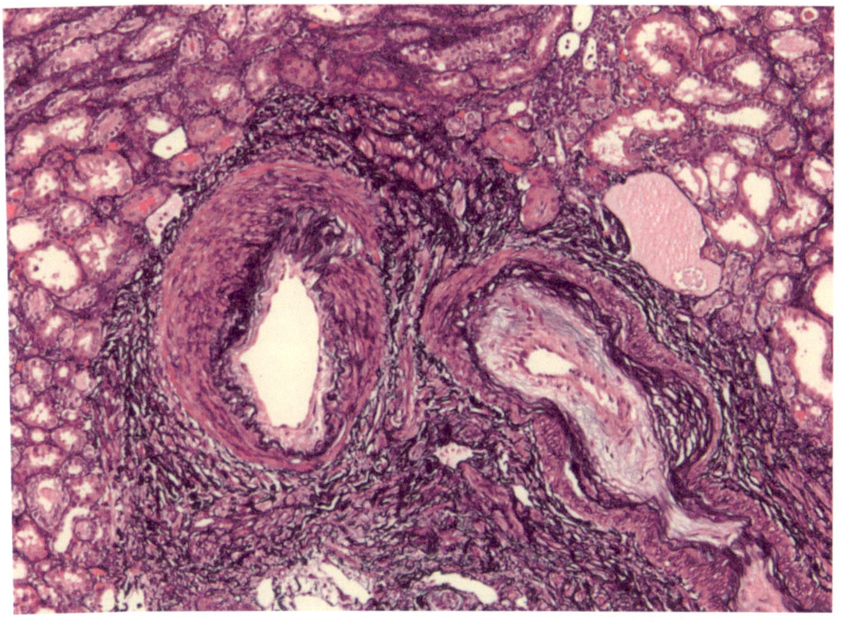

Fig. 2. Intimal accumulation of mucoid material (artery on the right) with associated adventitial fibrosis (artery of the left) in a patient with scleroderma renal crisis. (Methenamine silver stain; original magnification x100) (Batal, et al., 2010).

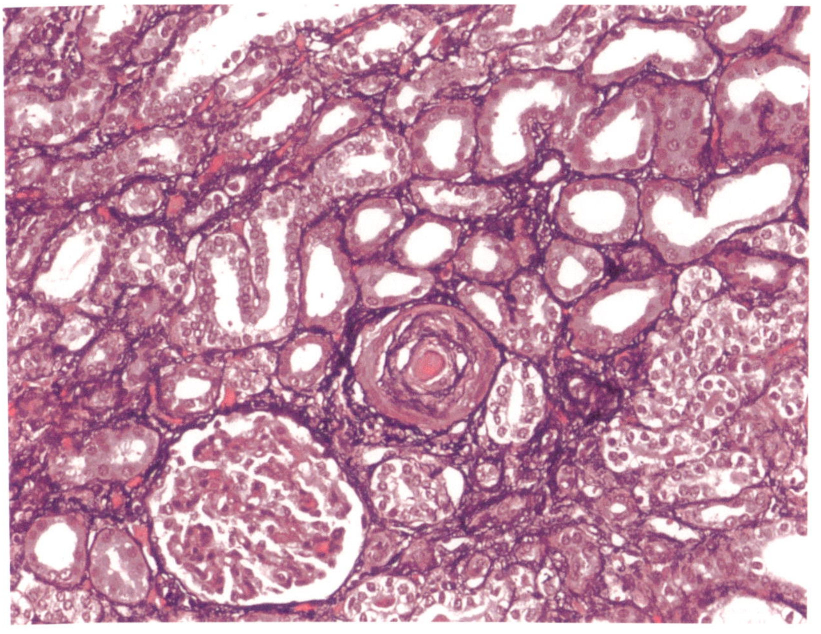

Fig. 3. Arterial thrombosis (middle) and glomerular ischemic collapse (lower left) in a patient with scleroderma renal crisis (Methenamine silver stain; original magnification x100) (Batal, et al., 2010)

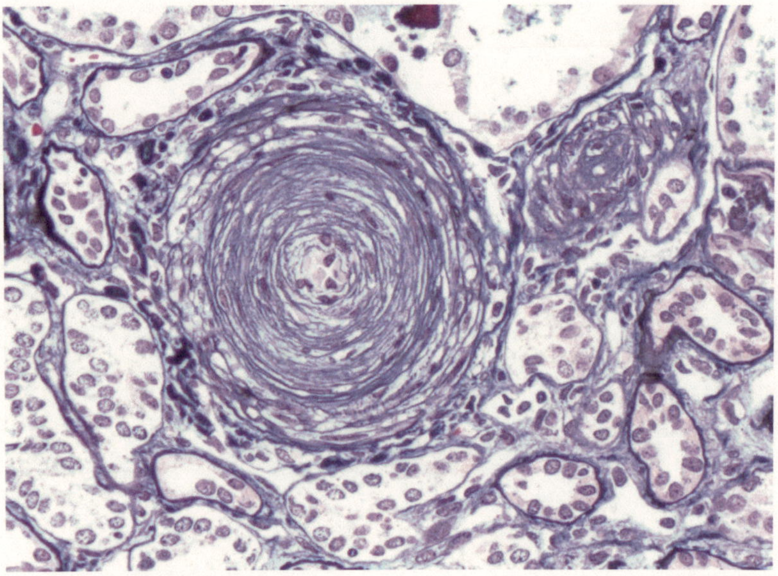

Fig. 4. Onion skin lesion causing severe vascular narrowing in a patient with scleroderma renal crisis (Methenamine silver stain; original magnification x400) (Batal, et al., 2010).

Fibrointimal sclerosis with or without adventitial fibrosis may be the result of chronic ongoing damage or, alternatively, can represent a manifestation of burned-out injury from a previous attack. Glomerular changes can be classified as acute or chronic. Acute glomerular changes manifests usually as endothelial swelling and glomerular capillary thrombosis (Figure 5).

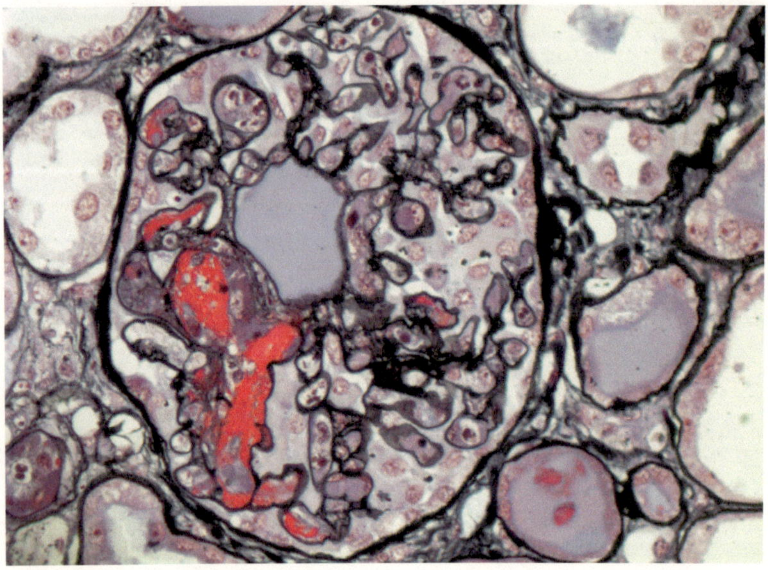

Fig. 5. Glomerular thrombosis in a patient with scleroderma renal crisis. Note the associated mild podocytic proliferation (Methenamine silver stain; original magnification x600) (Batal, et al., 2010).

Severe glomerular injury can lead to segmental glomerular fibrinoid necrosis or mesangiolysis. Fragmentation of red blood cells and fibrin deposits can be observed within the glomerular capillaries. These findings might sometime reflect a concurrent peripheral micro-hemolytic anemia (Salyer, Salyer, & Heptinstall, 1973). A common form of secondary glomerular injury is glomerular ischemic collapse due to decreased arterial perfusion. Glomerular ischemic collapse is characterized by wrinkling and thickening of the capillary walls and shrinkage of the glomerular tuft. Repetitive glomerular endothelial cell damage results in significant remodeling of the glomerular capillary walls, with glomerular basement membrane double contours (tram tracking) and a membranoproliferative pattern of injury. In more subtle cases, these changes can be focal and segmental, but over time and with more extensive injury, the remodeling becomes more complex and involves the majority of the glomerular capillary loops. The membranoproliferative pattern in thrombotic microangiopathies is usually associated with less mesangial proliferation, when compared to immune complex-mediated diseases with a similar pattern of injury by light microscopy. Endothelial cell injury, however, may result in mesangiolysis and resultant mesangial expansion that leads to nodular glomerulosclerosis as the process heals.

Tubulointerstitial changes, usually occurring secondary to vasculopathy, are frequently manifested acutely as ischemic acute tubular injury/necrosis or, chronically, as tubular atrophy and interstitial fibrosis. A lymphohistiocytic interstitial inflammatory infiltrate can infrequently be observed. Mild leukocytic margination in the peritubular capillaries can occasionally be encountered. Small renal infarcts might be observed secondary to vascular injury. Early in the course of infarction, neutrophils accumulate at the junction between affected and non-affected areas while mononuclear cells predominate later.

The overall histologic picture is that of a thrombotic microangiopathic process (Fisher & Rodnan, 1958; Mouthon et al., 2011). No histologic feature is absolutely pathognomonic for SRC. However, in contrast to hemolytic uremic syndrome/thrombotic thrombocytopenic purpura, small vessel changes predominate over glomerular changes in SRC. In hemolytic uremic syndrome, Tostivint et al. showed that thrombotic microangiopathic alterations were more frequently encountered in the glomeruli compared to small vessels [11/12 (92%) versus 4/12 (33%), p = .009] (Tostivint et al., 2002). In SRC, thrombi were more commonly detected in small vessels [11/17 (65%) small vessels thrombi versus 3/17 (18%) glomerular thrombi, P = .01] (Batal, et al., 2009).

Small vessels in SRC may display thinning of the media and/or adventitial expansion.

A few investigators suggest that the latter (Figure 2) is specific for SRC, but more data are needed to support this concept (Cannon, et al., 1974). Juxtaglomerular (JGA) hyperplasia can be observed in SRC and is believed to be associated with increased renin production (Stone, et al., 1974)(Figure 6). However, this feature is not entirely specific for SRC (Okada, Lertprasertsuke, & Tsutsumi, 2000), and is not a consistent finding. We detected a prominent JGA hyperplasia only in 12% of our SRC cases (Batal, et al., 2009).

Finally, it should be noted that vascular pathologic changes in scleroderma patients are not restricted to SRC. Trostle et al. used morphometric techniques to study vascular changes in autopsy specimens (Trostle, et al., 1986). In the absence of SRC, Trostle et al. were able to demonstrate a significant increase in arterial fibrointimal thickness in dcSSc patients, and to a lesser extent in lcSSc patients, compared to age and sex matched controls. These observations might be explained by a possible existence of mild ongoing renal vascular injury below the threshold needed to trigger SRC.

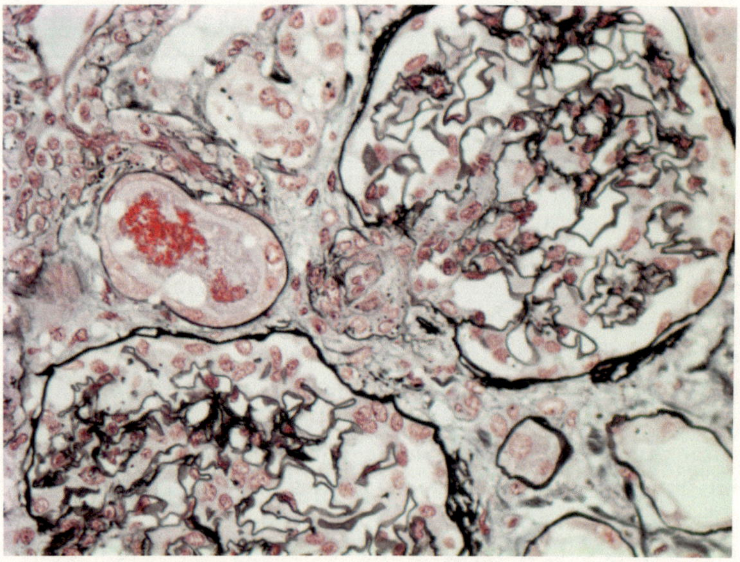

Fig. 6. Prominent juxtaglomerular apparatus (middle) in a patient with scleroderma renal crisis (Methenamine silver stain; original magnification x400) (Batal, et al., 2010).

5.2 Immunofluorescence microscopy studies

Immunofluorescence microscopy studies typically reveal no evidence of an immune complex-mediated renal disease, unless the patient suffers from overlap syndrome. IgM deposition, which is frequently attributed to nonspecific entrapment, is the most frequently detected immunoglobulin in the glomeruli and/or blood vessels (Lapenas, Rodnan, & Cavallo, 1978; McCoy, Tisher, Pepe, & Cleveland, 1976; McGiven, De Boer, & Barnett, 1971). Similarly, complement deposits are frequently detected. Fibrin or fibrinogen deposition might also be observed in severely affected vessels or along the glomerular capillaries, usually with dull continuous reactivity. Identical findings are seen also in thrombotic angiopathies within other clinical settings.

5.3 Electron microscopy

Ultrastructural evaluation typically reveals severe endothelial cell injury. Well-formed electron dense deposits are not detected in SRC. However, hyaline material, which can sometime be difficult to distinguish from definite immune deposits, might accumulate in the sub-endothelium of the glomeruli and/or blood vessels (Silva & Pirani, 1988). Endothelial cell swelling and accumulation of sub-endothelial flocculent material and cell debris is a common finding in SRC (Figure 7). Injured endothelial cells detach from the underlying basement membrane and in most severe cases, the endothelial cells may be completely sloughed off and missing. As the endothelium recovers from the injury, it will re-grow the remodeled endocapillary surface and form a new basement membrane layer, resulting in double contour formation. The repair is usually irregular, resulting in complex asymmetrical glomerular basement membrane with projections and deposits of cellular debris in the expanded subendothelial space. The resultant pattern of glomerular wall injury is membranoproliferative in the absence of electron dense deposits. Within the expanded fibrointima of the small vessels, myointimal cells can also be demonstrated (Salomon, Lamovec, & Tchertkoff, 1978).

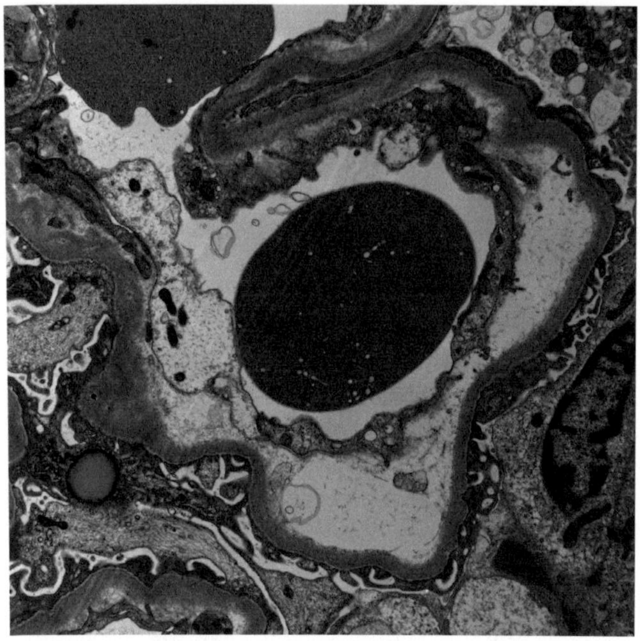

Fig. 7. Electron microscopic picture from a patient with scleroderma renal crisis. Note the prominent sub-endothelial electron lucent fluffy material (Electron microscopy; original magnification x5600)(Batal, et al., 2010).

6. Differential diagnosis (native kidneys)

As alluded to in paragraph four (Microscopic Pathology), acute SRC is very difficult if not impossible to be differentiated from other thrombotic microangiopathies based on histologic examination alone. Thrombotic microangiopathy is a pathologic term that encompasses a number of clinical conditions that appear to be triggered by endothelial injury. In addition to the rare SRC, this pattern of injury includes, although it is not limited to, thrombotic thrombocytopenic purpura (TTP), typical and atypical HUS, preeclampsia, antiphospholipid antibody syndrome, drug-induced thrombotic angiopathy(chemotherapy, cocaine, calcineurin inhibitors), and what is known as "idiopathic malignant hypertension". Disseminated intravascular coagulation (DIC) also enters the differential diagnosis. The latter is usually characterized by diffuse cortical necrosis and widespread glomerular, vascular and intratubular microthrombi(Kawasaki, Hayashi, & Awai, 1987). However, arterial mucoid changes and fibrinoid necrosis are usually absent. DIC is very rarely encountered in surgical pathology samples compared to autopsy specimens.

The differential diagnosis of chronic/burned-out SRC is broad. These cases often show signs of organization such as glomerular capillary double contours and glomerular scarring, and vascular sclerosis and fibrointimal thickening. In some cases, the aforementioned glomerular double contour can be associated with mesangial sclerosis and mild hypercellularity reminiscent to membranoproliferative glomerulonephritis pattern of glomerular injury. Membranoproliferative pattern of glomerular injury is typically seen in three types of disorders, including immune complex-mediated disorders (such as autoimmune diseases and chronic infections), paraprotein and other deposition diseases (such as monoclonal immunoglobulin deposition disease, fibrillary glomerulonephritis, and immunotactoid glomerulopathy), and thrombotic microangiopathies. Immunofluorescence and ultrastructural studies are essential in distinguishing these three groups of disorders. The presence of polyclonal or monoclonal immunoglobulin deposition that show dense deposits with or without organized substructures, favors immune complex and other deposition diseases. In contrast, the absence of immunoglobulin deposition and the dull continuous reactivity for fibrin along the glomerular capillary loops by immunofluorescence studies, together with the absence of dense deposits by electron microscopy, characterize various forms of thrombotic microangiopathies.

From a clinical perspective, one should remember that not all acute renal failure in SSc patients is due to SRC. Distinguishing SRC from crescentic GN is important since immunosuppressive therapy can exacerbate the former, but is used to treat the latter. The hallmark of crescentic GN is the presence of glomerular extracapillary proliferative lesions (crescents). As in non SSc patients, the most common form of crescentic GN in SSc patients is pauci-immune ANCA-associated GN, followed by immune complex GN (Ramaswami et al., 2008) and anti-glomerular basement membrane GN (Namba et al., 2008). In these cases, immunofluorescence studies are necessary for a correct sub classification. They are negative in the first; reveal granular immune complex deposits in the second, and linear glomerular basement membrane IgG staining in the third group of diseases. In contrast, crescents are typically absent in typical SRC, and if present, they are rare and very small (Kamen, Wigley, & Brown, 2006; Ramaswami, et al., 2008). Ischemic glomerulopathy lesions in SRC can sometime be accompanied by extracapillary epithelial cell proliferation, which can occasionally mimic a crescentic proliferative process. However, these ischemic "pseudocrescents" are characterized by the absence of necrotizing lesions, extracapillary fibrin, or glomerular basement membrane destruction. Furthermore, although each of crescentic glomerulonephritis and thrombotic microangiopathies can show vascular thrombosis and/or fibrinoid necrosis, one should remember that small vessel vasculitis/ inflammatory changes are frequently observed in the former but are typically absent in the latter.

Lastly, in addition to confirming the diagnosis, renal biopsy may help in predicting the clinical outcome in SRC patients. A few studies have investigated the prognostic values of different histologic parameters in SRC. When expressed as binary variables (presence/absence), Penn et al. found that the presence of mucoid edema or vascular thrombosis was associated with a suboptimal renal outcome (Penn, et al., 2007). We extended Penn et al. observations by demonstrating that the severity and extent of acute vascular damage and its consequences, namely arterial thrombosis/fibrinoid changes and glomerular ischemic collapse, were indeed predictors of poor prognosis (Batal, et al., 2009). In contrast to the study by Penn et al., we could not associate mucoid changes with poor renal outcome.

7. Treatment

Before the advent of angiotensin converting enzymes (ACE) inhibitors, nephrectomy or dialysis were the only available treatment options for SRC (Mitnick & Feig, 1978; Traub, et al., 1983). At that time, less than 10% of patients with SRC survived more than five months(Steen, 2003). ACE inhibitors were first introduced as a potential treatment of SRC in the late 1970s (Lopez-Ovejero et al., 1979). Since then, they have altered the management and outcome of this disease (Thurm & Alexander, 1984; Zawada et al., 1981), considerably increased patients' five year survival (up to 65%) (Steen, 2003) and rapidly became the first line of treatment of both hypertensive and normotensive SRC (Steen, 2003). Bosentan is an endothelin receptor blocker which is also considered a first line therapy (Dhaun, MacIntyre, Bellamy, & Kluth, 2009). However, Bosentan did not show any significant advantage over ACE inhibitors in regards to mortality and outcome (Patel et al., 2009). While angiotensin receptor blockers (ARBs) had promising results in animals with hypertension, clinical experience with these agents has not been very convincing (Siragy, de Gasparo, El-Kersh, & Carey, 2001). Currently, these medications are only considered in patients who cannot tolerate ACE inhibitors (Caskey, Thacker, Johnston, & Barnes, 1997; Mouthon, et al.; Steen, 2003).

In patients with SRC started on ACE inhibitors, one should aim for a blood pressure of 120/70 mm Hg (Steen, 2003). If this is not achieved within 12 hours of initiation of therapy, then intravenous calcium channel blocker therapy should be considered. Conservative medical treatment alone can successfully control blood pressure in approximately 30-40% of SRC patients. These patients usually have a good prognosis. However, despite this aggressive therapy, a proportion of patients (~20%) die within three months of the onset of SRC due to multiorgan failure. Subjects in this group are often older males, presenting with highly elevated serum creatinine and have pre-existing cardiac conditions (Steen & Medsger, 2000a). In the remaining patients, the aforementioned medications fail to normalize blood pressure and dialysis should be initiated. Of note, patients requiring temporary dialysis (up to 18 months) had a five-year survival comparable to SSc patients who never had SRC (90%). In contrast, patients who required permanent dialysis had a considerably lower five-year survival (40%). A large subset of these patients fails to recover renal function and require renal transplantation (Penn, et al., 2007; Steen & Medsger, 2000a).

8. Transplantation

Transplantation should be considered when renal failure persists beyond 18 months from initiation of dialysis (Steen, 2003). In SRC, graft and patient survival post-transplantation is inferior to general renal transplant patient (Pham et al., 2005). Recurrence of scleroderma may participate in this poor outcome (Cheung, Gibson, Rush, Jeffery, & Karpinski, 2005). Post-transplant recurrence of SRC has been reported even after transplantation from a twin sister (Caplin, Dikman, Winston, Spiera, & Uribarri, 1999; Woodhall, McCoy, Gunnells, & Seigler, 1976). Pham et al. (Pham, et al., 2005) suggested that SRC recurrence occurs early in the post-transplantation course. However, Cheung et al. (Cheung, et al., 2005) challenged this view when describing a late SRC recurrence observed seven years post-transplantation.

From a histologic perspective, establishing a diagnosis of recurrent SRC in a renal allograft is more difficult than in a native kidney biopsy. The differential diagnosis in this case is broader and includes acute antibody-mediated rejection, acute calcineurin inhibitor toxicity, and occasionally infections such as CMV. Any other thrombotic microangiopathic disease described in native kidneys can also manifest in the allograft as *de novo* thrombotic microangiopathic process (Liptak & Ivanyi, 2006). Chronic SRC changes are even more challenging. Glomerular double contour resulting from SRC can be indistinguishable from chronic transplant glomerulopathy, which has been recognized as a histologic manifestation of chronic antibody-mediated rejection. Therefore, a careful clinicopathological and immunological correlation with serum creatinine changes, blood pressure, circulating donor-specific antibody, calcineurin inhibitor levels, and opportunistic infections are highly important to achieve a correct diagnosis. A careful assessment of C4d in allograft biopsies could also suggest the diagnosis of antibody-mediated rejection (Racusen, et al., 2003). However, one should keep in mind that a few patients with SRC might show some levels of peritubular capillary C4d staining while in contrast, C4d staining may be absent in some cases of antibody-mediated rejection. C4d negative antibody-mediated rejection cases have also been recently described (Haas, 2011; Sis & Halloran, 2010).

9. References

Aggarwal, R., Lucas, M., Fertig, N., Oddis, C. V., & Medsger, T. A., Jr. (2009). Anti-U3 RNP autoantibodies in systemic sclerosis. *Arthritis Rheum, 60*(4), 1112-1118.

Batal, I., Domsic, R. T., Medsger, T. A., & Bastacky, S. (2010). Scleroderma renal crisis: a pathology perspective. *Int J Rheumatol, 2010*, 543704.

Batal, I., Domsic, R. T., Shafer, A., Medsger, T. A., Jr., Kiss, L. P., Randhawa, P., et al. (2009). Renal biopsy findings predicting outcome in scleroderma renal crisis. *Hum Pathol, 40*(3), 332-340.

Bollinger, A., Jager, K., & Siegenthaler, W. (1986). Microangiopathy of progressive systemic sclerosis. Evaluation by dynamic fluorescence videomicroscopy. *Arch Intern Med, 146*(8), 1541-1545.

Cannon, P. J., Hassar, M., Case, D. B., Casarella, W. J., Sommers, S. C., & LeRoy, E. C. (1974). The relationship of hypertension and renal failure in scleroderma (progressive systemic sclerosis) to structural and functional abnormalities of the renal cortical circulation. *Medicine (Baltimore), 53*(1), 1-46.

Caplin, N. J., Dikman, S., Winston, J., Spiera, H., & Uribarri, J. (1999). Recurrence of scleroderma in a renal allograft from an identical twin sister. *Am J Kidney Dis, 33*(4), e7.

Caskey, F. J., Thacker, E. J., Johnston, P. A., & Barnes, J. N. (1997). Failure of losartan to control blood pressure in scleroderma renal crisis. *Lancet, 349*(9052), 620.

Cheung, W. Y., Gibson, I. W., Rush, D., Jeffery, J., & Karpinski, M. (2005). Late recurrence of scleroderma renal crisis in a renal transplant recipient despite angiotensin II blockade. *Am J Kidney Dis, 45*(5), 930-934.

Collins, D. A., Patel, S., Eastwood, J. B., & Bourke, B. E. (1996). Favourable outcome of scleroderma renal crisis. *J R Soc Med, 89*(1), 49P-50P.

Denton, C. P., Lapadula, G., Mouthon, L., & Muller-Ladner, U. (2009). Renal complications and scleroderma renal crisis. *Rheumatology (Oxford), 48 Suppl 3*, iii32-35.

Dhaun, N., MacIntyre, I. M., Bellamy, C. O., & Kluth, D. C. (2009). Endothelin receptor antagonism and renin inhibition as treatment options for scleroderma kidney. *Am J Kidney Dis, 54*(4), 726-731.

Ferri, C., Valentini, G., Cozzi, F., Sebastiani, M., Michelassi, C., La Montagna, G., et al. (2002). Systemic sclerosis: demographic, clinical, and serologic features and survival in 1,012 Italian patients. *Medicine (Baltimore), 81*(2), 139-153.

Fisher, E. R., & Rodnan, G. P. (1958). Pathologic observations concerning the kidney in progressive systemic sclerosis. *AMA Arch Pathol, 65*(1), 29-39.

Gershwin, M. E., Abplanalp, H., Castles, J. J., Ikeda, R. M., van der Water, J., Eklund, J., et al. (1981). Characterization of a spontaneous disease of white leghorn chickens resembling progressive systemic sclerosis (scleroderma). *J Exp Med, 153*(6), 1640-1659.

Gonzalez, E. A., Schmulbach, E., & Bastani, B. (1994). Scleroderma renal crisis with minimal skin involvement and no serologic evidence of systemic sclerosis. *Am J Kidney Dis, 23*(2), 317-319.

Gunduz, O. H., Fertig, N., Lucas, M., & Medsger, T. A., Jr. (2001). Systemic sclerosis with renal crisis and pulmonary hypertension: a report of eleven cases. *Arthritis Rheum, 44*(7), 1663-1666.

Haas, M. (2011). C4d-negative antibody-mediated rejection in renal allografts: evidence for its existence and effect on graft survival. *Clin Nephrol, 75*(4), 271-278.

Haviv, Y. S., & Safadi, R. (1998). Normotensive scleroderma renal crisis: case report and review of the literature. *Ren Fail, 20*(5), 733-736.

Helfrich, D. J., Banner, B., Steen, V. D., & Medsger, T. A., Jr. (1989). Normotensive renal failure in systemic sclerosis. *Arthritis Rheum, 32*(9), 1128-1134.

Hirata, Y. (1989). Endothelin-1 receptors in cultured vascular smooth muscle cells and cardiocytes of rats. *J Cardiovasc Pharmacol, 13 Suppl 5*, S157-158.

Ishikawa, H., Takeda, K., Okamoto, A., Matsuo, S., & Isobe, K. (2009). Induction of autoimmunity in a bleomycin-induced murine model of experimental systemic sclerosis: an important role for CD4+ T cells. *J Invest Dermatol, 129*(7), 1688-1695.

Kagan, A., Nissim, F., Green, L., & Bar-Khayim, Y. (1989). Scleroderma renal crisis without hypertension. *J Rheumatol, 16*(5), 707-708.

Kahaleh, M. B. (2004). Vascular involvement in systemic sclerosis (SSc). *Clin Exp Rheumatol, 22*(3 Suppl 33), S19-23.

Kamen, D. L., Wigley, F. M., & Brown, A. N. (2006). Antineutrophil cytoplasmic antibody-positive crescentic glomerulonephritis in scleroderma--a different kind of renal crisis. *J Rheumatol, 33*(9), 1886-1888.

Karlen, J. R., & Cook, W. A. (1974). Renal scleroderma and pregnancy. *Obstet Gynecol, 44*(3), 349-354.

Kawasaki, H., Hayashi, K., & Awai, M. (1987). Disseminated intravascular coagulation (DIC). Immunohistochemical study of fibrin-related materials (FRMs) in renal tissues. *Acta Pathol Jpn, 37*(1), 77-84.

Kobayashi, H., Nishimaki, T., Kaise, S., Suzuki, T., Watanabe, K., & Kasukawa, R. (1999). Immunohistological study endothelin-1 and endothelin-A and B receptors in two patients with scleroderma renal crisis. *Clin Rheumatol, 18*(5), 425-427.

Kovalchik, M. T., Guggenheim, S. J., Silverman, M. H., Robertson, J. S., & Steigerwald, J. C. (1978). The kidney in progressive systemic sclerosis: a prospective study. *Ann Intern Med, 89*(6), 881-887.

Lam, M., & Ballou, S. P. (1992). Reversible scleroderma renal crisis after cocaine use. *N Engl J Med, 326*(21), 1435.

Lapenas, D., Rodnan, G. P., & Cavallo, T. (1978). Immunopathology of the renal vascular lesion of progressive systemic sclerosis (scleroderma). *Am J Pathol, 91*(2), 243-258.

LeRoy, E. C., Black, C., Fleischmajer, R., Jablonska, S., Krieg, T., Medsger, T. A., Jr., et al. (1988). Scleroderma (systemic sclerosis): classification, subsets and pathogenesis. *J Rheumatol, 15*(2), 202-205.

Liptak, P., & Ivanyi, B. (2006). Primer: Histopathology of calcineurin-inhibitor toxicity in renal allografts. *Nat Clin Pract Nephrol, 2*(7), 398-404; quiz following 404.

Lopez-Ovejero, J. A., Saal, S. D., D'Angelo, W. A., Cheigh, J. S., Stenzel, K. H., & Laragh, J. H. (1979). Reversal of vascular and renal crises of scleroderma by oral angiotensin-converting-enzyme blockade. *N Engl J Med, 300*(25), 1417-1419.

McCoy, R. C., Tisher, C. C., Pepe, P. F., & Cleveland, L. A. (1976). The kidney in progressive systemic sclerosis: immunohistochemical and antibody elution studies. *Lab Invest, 35*(2), 124-131.

McGiven, A. R., De Boer, W. G., & Barnett, A. J. (1971). Renal immune deposits in scleroderma. *Pathology, 3*(2), 145-150.

McWhorter, J. E. t., & LeRoy, E. C. (1974). Pericardial disease in scleroderma (systemic sclerosis). *Am J Med, 57*(4), 566-575.

Medsger, T. A., Jr., Masi, A. T., Rodnan, G. P., Benedek, T. G., & Robinson, H. (1971). Survival with systemic sclerosis (scleroderma). A life-table analysis of clinical and demographic factors in 309 patients. *Ann Intern Med, 75*(3), 369-376.

Mitnick, P. D., & Feig, P. U. (1978). Control of hypertension and reversal of renal failure in scleroderma. *N Engl J Med, 299*(16), 871-872.

Mountz, J. D., Downs Minor, M. B., Turner, R., Thomas, M. B., Richards, F., & Pisko, E. (1983). Bleomycin-induced cutaneous toxicity in the rat: analysis of histopathology and ultrastructure compared with progressive systemic sclerosis (scleroderma). *Br J Dermatol, 108*(6), 679-686.

Mouthon, L., Berezne, A., Bussone, G., Noel, L. H., Villiger, P. M., & Guillevin, L. Scleroderma renal crisis: a rare but severe complication of systemic sclerosis. *Clin Rev Allergy Immunol, 40*(2), 84-91.

Mouthon, L., Berezne, A., Bussone, G., Noel, L. H., Villiger, P. M., & Guillevin, L. (2009). Scleroderma Renal Crisis: A Rare but Severe Complication of Systemic Sclerosis. *Clin Rev Allergy Immunol.*

Mouthon, L., Berezne, A., Bussone, G., Noel, L. H., Villiger, P. M., & Guillevin, L. (2011). Scleroderma renal crisis: a rare but severe complication of systemic sclerosis. *Clin Rev Allergy Immunol, 40*(2), 84-91.

Namba, T., Hatanaka, M., Takahashi, A., Takeji, M., Takahara, K., Uzu, T., et al. (2008). [Case of scleroderma with rapid progressive glomerulonephritis associated with both MPO-ANCA and anti-GBM antibodies]. *Nippon Jinzo Gakkai Shi, 50*(1), 64-68.

Nguyen, B., Assassi, S., Arnett, F. C., & Mayes, M. D. Association of RNA polymerase III antibodies with scleroderma renal crisis. *J Rheumatol, 37*(5), 1068; author reply 1069.

Nguyen, V. A., Sgonc, R., Dietrich, H., & Wick, G. (2000). Endothelial injury in internal organs of University of California at Davis line 200 (UCD 200) chickens, an animal model for systemic sclerosis (Scleroderma). *J Autoimmun, 14*(2), 143-149.

Okada, M., Lertprasertsuke, N., & Tsutsumi, Y. (2000). Quantitative estimation of renin-containing cells in the juxtaglomerular apparatus in Bartter's and pseudo-Bartter's syndromes. *Pathol Int, 50*(2), 166-168.

Okano, Y., Steen, V. D., & Medsger, T. A., Jr. (1993). Autoantibody reactive with RNA polymerase III in systemic sclerosis. *Ann Intern Med, 119*(10), 1005-1013.

Patel, J. D., Bonomi, P., Socinski, M. A., Govindan, R., Hong, S., Obasaju, C., et al. (2009). Treatment rationale and study design for the pointbreak study: a randomized, open-label phase III study of pemetrexed/carboplatin/bevacizumab followed by maintenance pemetrexed/bevacizumab versus paclitaxel/carboplatin/bevacizumab followed by maintenance bevacizumab in patients with stage IIIB or IV nonsquamous non-small-cell lung cancer. *Clin Lung Cancer, 10*(4), 252-256.

Pearson, T., Greiner, D. L., & Shultz, L. D. (2008). Humanized SCID mouse models for biomedical research. *Curr Top Microbiol Immunol, 324*, 25-51.

Penn, H., Howie, A. J., Kingdon, E. J., Bunn, C. C., Stratton, R. J., Black, C. M., et al. (2007). Scleroderma renal crisis: patient characteristics and long-term outcomes. *QJM, 100*(8), 485-494.

Pham, P. T., Pham, P. C., Danovitch, G. M., Gritsch, H. A., Singer, J., Wallace, W. D., et al. (2005). Predictors and risk factors for recurrent scleroderma renal crisis in the kidney allograft: case report and review of the literature. *Am J Transplant, 5*(10), 2565-2569.

Racusen, L. C., Colvin, R. B., Solez, K., Mihatsch, M. J., Halloran, P. F., Campbell, P. M., et al. (2003). Antibody-mediated rejection criteria - an addition to the Banff 97 classification of renal allograft rejection. *Am J Transplant, 3*(6), 708-714.

Ramaswami, A., Kandaswamy, T., Rajendran, T., Jeyakrishnan, K. P., Aung, H., Iqbal, M., et al. (2008). Scleroderma with crescentic glomerulonephritis: a case report. *J Med Case Reports, 2*, 151.

Rivolta, R., Mascagni, B., Berruti, V., Quarto Di Palo, F., Elli, A., Scorza, R., et al. (1996). Renal vascular damage in systemic sclerosis patients without clinical evidence of nephropathy. *Arthritis Rheum, 39*(6), 1030-1034.

Sakkas, L. I. (2005). New developments in the pathogenesis of systemic sclerosis. *Autoimmunity, 38*(2), 113-116.

Sakkas, L. I., Chikanza, I. C., & Platsoucas, C. D. (2006). Mechanisms of Disease: the role of immune cells in the pathogenesis of systemic sclerosis. *Nat Clin Pract Rheumatol, 2*(12), 679-685.

Salomon, M. I., Lamovec, J., & Tchertkoff, V. (1978). Renal lesions in scleroderma. *Angiology, 29*(8), 569-578.

Salyer, W. R., Salyer, D. C., & Heptinstall, R. H. (1973). Scleroderma and microangiopathic hemolytic anemia. *Ann Intern Med, 78*(6), 895-897.

Satoh, M., Tokuhira, M., Hama, N., Hirakata, M., Kuwana, M., Akizuki, M., et al. (1995). Massive pericardial effusion in scleroderma: a review of five cases. *Br J Rheumatol, 34*(6), 564-567.

Sgonc, R., Gruschwitz, M. S., Boeck, G., Sepp, N., Gruber, J., & Wick, G. (2000). Endothelial cell apoptosis in systemic sclerosis is induced by antibody-dependent cell-mediated cytotoxicity via CD95. *Arthritis Rheum, 43*(11), 2550-2562.

Sgonc, R., Gruschwitz, M. S., Dietrich, H., Recheis, H., Gershwin, M. E., & Wick, G. (1996). Endothelial cell apoptosis is a primary pathogenetic event underlying skin lesions in avian and human scleroderma. *J Clin Invest, 98*(3), 785-792.

Sharnoff, J. G., Carideo, H. L., & Stein, I. D. (1951). Cortisone-treated scleroderma; report of a case with autopsy findings. *J Am Med Assoc, 145*(16), 1230-1232.

Silva, F. G., & Pirani, C. L. (1988). Electron microscopic study of medical diseases of the kidney: update--1988. *Mod Pathol, 1*(4), 292-315.

Siragy, H. M., de Gasparo, M., El-Kersh, M., & Carey, R. M. (2001). Angiotensin-converting enzyme inhibition potentiates angiotensin II type 1 receptor effects on renal bradykinin and cGMP. *Hypertension, 38*(2), 183-186.

Sis, B., & Halloran, P. F. (2010). Endothelial transcripts uncover a previously unknown phenotype: C4d-negative antibody-mediated rejection. *Curr Opin Organ Transplant, 15*(1), 42-48.

Steen, V. D. (1994). Renal involvement in systemic sclerosis. *Clin Dermatol, 12*(2), 253-258.

Steen, V. D. (2003). Scleroderma renal crisis. *Rheum Dis Clin North Am, 29*(2), 315-333.

Steen, V. D. (2005). Autoantibodies in systemic sclerosis. *Semin Arthritis Rheum, 35*(1), 35-42.

Steen, V. D., Costantino, J. P., Shapiro, A. P., & Medsger, T. A., Jr. (1990). Outcome of renal crisis in systemic sclerosis: relation to availability of angiotensin converting enzyme (ACE) inhibitors. *Ann Intern Med, 113*(5), 352-357.

Steen, V. D., & Medsger, T. A., Jr. (2000a). Long-term outcomes of scleroderma renal crisis. *Ann Intern Med, 133*(8), 600-603.

Steen, V. D., & Medsger, T. A., Jr. (2000b). Severe organ involvement in systemic sclerosis with diffuse scleroderma. *Arthritis Rheum, 43*(11), 2437-2444.

Steen, V. D., Medsger, T. A., Jr., Osial, T. A., Jr., Ziegler, G. L., Shapiro, A. P., & Rodnan, G. P. (1984). Factors predicting development of renal involvement in progressive systemic sclerosis. *Am J Med, 76*(5), 779-786.

Steen, V. D., Powell, D. L., & Medsger, T. A., Jr. (1988). Clinical correlations and prognosis based on serum autoantibodies in patients with systemic sclerosis. *Arthritis Rheum, 31*(2), 196-203.

Stone, R. A., Tisher, C. C., Hawkins, H. K., & Robinson, R. R. (1974). Juxtaglomerular hyperplasia and hyperreninemia in progressive systemic sclerosis complicated acute renal failure. *Am J Med, 56*(1), 119-123.

Sugimoto, T., Sanada, M., & Kashiwagi, A. (2008). Is scleroderma renal crisis with anti-centromere antibody-positive limited cutaneous systemic sclerosis overlooked in patients with hypertension and/or renal dysfunction? *Nephrology (Carlton), 13*(2), 179-180.

Sugimoto, T., Soumura, M., Danno, K., Kaji, K., Kondo, M., Hirata, K., et al. (2006). Scleroderma renal crisis in a patient with anticentromere antibody-positive limited cutaneous systemic sclerosis. *Mod Rheumatol, 16*(5), 309-311.

Takuwa, N., Takuwa, Y., Yanagisawa, M., Yamashita, K., & Masaki, T. (1989). A novel vasoactive peptide endothelin stimulates mitogenesis through inositol lipid turnover in Swiss 3T3 fibroblasts. *J Biol Chem, 264*(14), 7856-7861.

Teixeira, L., Mouthon, L., Mahr, A., Berezne, A., Agard, C., Mehrenberger, M., et al. (2008). Mortality and risk factors of scleroderma renal crisis: a French retrospective study of 50 patients. *Ann Rheum Dis, 67*(1), 110-116.

Thurm, R. H., & Alexander, J. C. (1984). Captopril in the treatment of scleroderma renal crisis. *Arch Intern Med, 144*(4), 733-735.

Tirapelli, C. R., Casolari, D. A., Yogi, A., Montezano, A. C., Tostes, R. C., Legros, E., et al. (2005). Functional characterization and expression of endothelin receptors in rat carotid artery: involvement of nitric oxide, a vasodilator prostanoid and the opening of K+ channels in ETB-induced relaxation. *Br J Pharmacol, 146*(6), 903-912.

Tostivint, I., Mougenot, B., Flahault, A., Vigneau, C., Costa, M. A., Haymann, J. P., et al. (2002). Adult haemolytic and uraemic syndrome: causes and prognostic factors in the last decade. *Nephrol Dial Transplant, 17*(7), 1228-1234.

Traub, Y. M., Shapiro, A. P., Rodnan, G. P., Medsger, T. A., McDonald, R. H., Jr., Steen, V. D., et al. (1983). Hypertension and renal failure (scleroderma renal crisis) in progressive systemic sclerosis. Review of a 25-year experience with 68 cases. *Medicine (Baltimore), 62*(6), 335-352.

Trostle, D. C., Helfrich, D., & Medsger, T. A., Jr. (1986). Systemic sclerosis (scleroderma) and multiple sclerosis. *Arthritis Rheum, 29*(1), 124-127.

Vancheeswaran, R., Magoulas, T., Efrat, G., Wheeler-Jones, C., Olsen, I., Penny, R., et al. (1994). Circulating endothelin-1 levels in systemic sclerosis subsets--a marker of fibrosis or vascular dysfunction? *J Rheumatol, 21*(10), 1838-1844.

Venneker, G. T., van den Hoogen, F. H., Boerbooms, A. M., Bos, J. D., & Asghar, S. S. (1994). Aberrant expression of membrane cofactor protein and decay-accelerating factor in the endothelium of patients with systemic sclerosis. A possible mechanism of vascular damage. *Lab Invest, 70*(6), 830-835.

Walker, J. G., Ahern, M. J., Smith, M. D., Coleman, M., Pile, K., Rischmueller, M., et al. (2003). Scleroderma renal crisis: poor outcome despite aggressive antihypertensive treatment. *Intern Med J, 33*(5-6), 216-220.

Woodhall, P. B., McCoy, R. C., Gunnells, J. C., & Seigler, H. F. (1976). Apparent recurrence of progressive systemic sclerosis in a renal allograft. *JAMA, 236*(9), 1032-1034.

Worda, M., Sgonc, R., Dietrich, H., Niederegger, H., Sundick, R. S., Gershwin, M. E., et al. (2003). In vivo analysis of the apoptosis-inducing effect of anti-endothelial cell antibodies in systemic sclerosis by the chorionallantoic membrane assay. *Arthritis Rheum, 48*(9), 2605-2614.

Yamamoto, T. Animal model of systemic sclerosis. *J Dermatol, 37*(1), 26-41.

Yamamoto, T., & Nishioka, K. (2001). Animal model of sclerotic skin. IV: induction of dermal sclerosis by bleomycin is T cell independent. *J Invest Dermatol, 117*(4), 999-1001.

Yamamoto, T., & Nishioka, K. (2002). Animal model of sclerotic skin. V: Increased expression of alpha-smooth muscle actin in fibroblastic cells in bleomycin-induced scleroderma. *Clin Immunol, 102*(1), 77-83.

Yamamoto, T., & Nishioka, K. (2004). Animal model of sclerotic skin. VI: Evaluation of bleomycin-induced skin sclerosis in nude mice. *Arch Dermatol Res, 295*(10), 453-456.

Yamamoto, T., Takagawa, S., Katayama, I., Yamazaki, K., Hamazaki, Y., Shinkai, H., et al. (1999). Animal model of sclerotic skin. I: Local injections of bleomycin induce sclerotic skin mimicking scleroderma. *J Invest Dermatol, 112*(4), 456-462.

Yamamoto, T., Takahashi, Y., Takagawa, S., Katayama, I., & Nishioka, K. (1999). Animal model of sclerotic skin. II. Bleomycin induced scleroderma in genetically mast cell deficient WBB6F1-W/W(V) mice. *J Rheumatol, 26*(12), 2628-2634.

Zawada, E. T., Jr., Clements, P. J., Furst, D. A., Bloomer, H. A., Paulus, H. E., & Maxwell, M. H. (1981). Clinical course of patients with scleroderma renal crisis treated with captopril. *Nephron, 27*(2), 74-78.

Zhang, L., Meissner, E., Chen, J., & Su, L. (2010). Current humanized mouse models for studying human immunology and HIV-1 immuno-pathogenesis. *Sci China Life Sci, 53*(2), 195-203.

12

Pregnancy and Scleroderma

Charlotte Gorgiard, Alice Bérezné and Luc Mouthon
Université Paris Descartes, Faculté de Médecine, Pôle de Médecine Interne, Centre de Référence pour les vascularites nécrosantes et la sclérodermie systémique, Hôpital Cochin, Assistance Publique-Hôpitaux de Paris (AP-HP), Paris, France

1. Introduction

More than 30 years ago, pregnancy was not recommended for patients with systemic sclerosis (SSc) because of the overrepresentation in the literature of pregnancies with poor outcome. Thus, women with SSc had been strongly advised against pregnancy and often counseled to terminate ongoing pregnancies.
Retrospective studies found an increased frequency of pre-term births and small full-term infants in cohorts of patients with SSc. However, it turned out that finally the frequency of miscarriage and neonatal survival rate did not differ from that observed in the general population. Thus, in recent retrospective studies, maternal prognosis has improved as compared to historical series, possibly as a consequence of a better knowledge of the natural history of SSc and complications that may occur during pregnancy and a better multidisciplinary management of pregnancies occurring in patients with SSc.

2. Epidemiology

SSc is a rare disease with a prevalence of 50 to 250 cases per million inhabitants [1]. SSc predominantly affects women (3-8 for women one man) with a peak incidence between 45 and 64 years. However, women tend to develop SSc earlier than men and 1 out of 2 women have early symptoms of the disease while of childbearing age. As a consequence, pregnancies in patients with SSc are infrequent. In the past, this connective-tissue disease ordinarily affected patients in the late reproductive and post-reproductive age [2]. In the more recent decades, many women have postponed childbearing into their 30s and 40s year. For this reason, the number of women who develop SSc and may become pregnant is likely to increase. Interestingly, Johnson et al reported in 1988 that in 17% of women with SSc, the onset of disease occur during pregnancy [3].
The number of gestations before the onset of SSc might influence the age at which the disease starts [4], since nulliparous women are younger at SSc onset and present with a more aggressive clinical course. Thus, the average age at SSc onset in women with a past history of pregnancy is 44 years, whereas, in women in whom SSc started before or occurred at the time of pregnancy, the average age at disease onset is 26 years [5]. This result, in favor of a bimodal distribution, suggests that there may be differences in the pathogenesis of SSc in these two groups of women.

The type of SSc is associated with marked differences in term of number of pregnancies. Thus, patients with limited SSc experience more pregnancies and get more children than those with diffuse SSc, most probably because of the severity of the disease. In addition, an association between the sex of the offspring and SSc has been suggested, women with SSc being more likely to give birth to male children [6]. However, the underlying explanation for this observation is not known and these data remain to be confirmed.

3. Pathogenesis

SSc is characterized by vascular hyperreactivity and collagen deposition. Endothelial cells, fibroblasts and lymphocytes abnormalities have been reported in SSc. Endothelial cells produce an excess of endothelin 1 and inducible NO synthase and undergo increased apoptosis. Oxydative stress seems to play a major role in disease progression.

Fibroblasts dysfunction is characterized by an uncontrolled activation of the transforming growth factor-β (TGF-β) pathway, an excess in synthesis of connective tissue growth factor (CTGF) and free radicals, favoring the accumulation of extra-cellular matrix. Increased levels of interleukine 4, a pro-fibrosing cytokine, have been detected in plasma and skin of SSc patients. Autoantibodies are detectable in the serum of more than 90% of SSc patients, which are directed against well identified ubiquitous nuclear proteins without evidence of a pathogenic role. Other autoantibodies bind to endothelial cells and/or fibroblasts and may exert a pathogenic role.

It has been proposed, by analogy to chronic graft versus host disease, that fetal cells might play a role in the pathogenesis of SSc [7]. Thus, although histologic and immunologic parameters differ between chronic graft versus host disease and SSc [8], it has been postulated that SSc might be understood as a type of chronic graft versus host disease resulting from transplacental transfer of cells between mother and fetus [9]. This hypothesis was further supported by the identification of fetal Y DNA and cells in skin lesions from women with SSc and a past history of delivery of male children [7]. Although a higher incidence of Y microchimerism (the persistence of foetal cells in the mother after delivery) has been reported in females with scleroderma who gave birth of child of male sex, than in healthy control females [10], these data remain controversial since not confirmed in other studies, particularly because of a higher incidence of detection of Y microchimerism in healthy control females than in the initial publications. Thus, if microchimerism has been suspected to play a role in the pathogenesis of SSc [11, 12], this postulate is actually controversial.

4. Influence of SSc on pregnancy

4.1 Fertility

Infertility is defined by difficulty in conception and the failure to achieve a successful pregnancy by the age of 35. Reports are contradictory in females with SSc. Silman and Black [13] reported a significantly higher spontaneous abortion rate in cases than in controls, with 33 (28.7%) vs 20 (17.4%), corresponding to a relative risk of 2.1 ($p=0.05$). In addition, multiple abortions were more frequently reported in women with SSc. In a Swedish national population-based registry [14], nulliparity was associated with increased risk of SSc (odds ratio = 1.37, 95% confidence interval: 1.22-1.55). Another study reported that both delay in conception and infertility were more common in patients who subsequently developed SSc. Women with SSc were more likely than women in the whole population to have had a delay in conception (> or = 12 months): OR 2.6 (1.1, 5.7) or be infertile: OR 2.3 (0.7, 7.2). These differences were not apparent when the group of patients with SSc was compared to the group of women with Raynaud's phenomenon, with OR's of 0.7 and 1.1, respectively [15]. In an Italian case-control study, the risk of SSc was found to be 70 percent lower for women with a past history of pregnancy (odds ratio = 0.3, 95% confidence interval: 0.1, 0.8) and the risk decreased with increasing parity [16]. It has been also reported that infertility was 3 times higher than in healthy controls in SSc patients before the diagnosis was made [6]. Similar findings were reported by Englert et al [15]. An alternative explanation might be that women, who develop SSc early in life, cannot or may not want to get pregnant.

In recent studies, the frequency of miscarriage and neonatal survival rate did not differ in patients with SSc as compared to healthy controls. Thus, Giordano et al did not find significant level of infertility among a series of 86 women with SSc when compared with matched healthy controls [17], although they observed a significantly increased frequency of miscarriages per pregnancy (50 of 299 pregnancies in patients with SSc versus 32 of 322 pregnancies in controls; $p<0.05$). Steen and Medsger reported that fertility in SSc patients did not differ significantly from that observed in either of the control groups [18]. In addition, the proportion of nulliparous women did not differ significantly between SSc and control patients.

4.2 Spontaneous abortion

Rates of early pregnancy loss of 14%-15% are somewhat increased from the estimated 10% in the general population. Late pregnancy losses occurred scarcely, generally in women with severe diffuse SSc [18]. The anti-Ro/SSA antibody might be associated with spontaneous abortion [19]. A retrospective study of Silman did not find increased risk of fetal loss in SSc patients [13].

4.3 Preterm delivery and fetal outcomes

Reported preterm delivery rates ranged from 8% to 40% in patients with SSc [18, 20, 21], most of them being observed on or after gestational age 34.

The frequency of small full-term babies was slightly increased among SSc patients [18]. Low birth weight infants (<10th% tile for gestational age) ranged from 0% to 50%.

4.4 Delivery

The optimal mode of delivery in patients with SSc remains controversial. Vaginal delivery is associated with fewer shifts in blood volume but has a prolonged second stage of labor and issues regarding increased pressure with contractions. Cesarean delivery reduces the second stage of labor and may be necessary in cases of extreme maternal or fetal distress but increases risks of infection and thrombosis [22]. Among women who had an elective termination, 87.5% had diffuse SSc whereas 12.5% had limited SSc ($p<0.0001$) [6]. Cases of preeclampsia were isolated [18]. Labor and delivery represent a very vulnerable period in this setting, and extended observation in the hospital following delivery may be required, particularly in patients with PAH, although PAH is a contra-indication to pregnancy [23].

4.5 Placenta

The placenta, which embodies the maternal-fetal interface, may be involved in women with SSc, with vascular abnormalities inducing placental ischemia [22, 23]. The higher rates of prematurity and low birth weight infants encountered in SSc may be the direct consequence of placental vascular insufficiency [23]. In a large study, 13 placentas from women with SSc were examined and correlations were made with perinatal outcomes. In 5/13 placentas, marked decidual vasculopathy was noted, in association with intrauterine fetal demise between week 16 and 30 in 4 cases [24]. These findings are similar to those observed in eclampsia. In 1986, Labarrere and colleagues investigated 18 placentas of 15 mothers with various autoimmune diseases including idiopathic thrombocytopenic purpura, autoimmune thyroid diseases, and multiple sclerosis. Interestingly, the group of patients with autoimmune diseases had significantly more maternal vascular lesions and chronic villitis of unknown etiology than the control group. Investigators failed to identify lesions that could be attributed to any of the diseases in particular. Placental vascular damage with deposits of IgM, C3, and C1q was more prominent in a patient with SSc. In both of these diseases, these lesions were related to poor fetal outcome. Placental vascular damage with deposits of IgM, C3, and C1q was more prominent in a patient with SSc and these lesions were related to poor fetal outcome [25]. Thus, we are convinced that systematic placental examination might help to identify the role of placental vasculopathy in pregnancy outcome [23].

5. Influence of pregnancy on the course of SSc

For years, SSc has been considered as a strict contraindication for pregnancy because of physiologic changes observed during gestation, including blood volume, vascular resistance, cardiac output and oxygen consumption, with a peak at the end of the second trimester of pregnancy. Recent studies demonstrated that women with SSc have acceptable pregnancy outcomes. More provocatively, it has been proposed that pregnancy might be protective against SSc [2, 12, 20]. Artlett at al suggested in a retrospective study that pregnancy was protective, since diffuse disease and worsening interstitial lung disease were more common in nulliparous women with SSc. Alternatively, it has been reported that pregnancy-related phenomena may contribute to SSc development [26, 27], and Cockrill at al. [28] proposed in a large cohort of women with SSc and sibling controls that immune responses associated with early childhood infections might predispose to the occurrence of SSc. In this study, it was observed that the risk of SSc increased with increasing birth order, and that a history of one or more pregnancy losses without any live births had the strongest association with SSc development.
Visceral involvement represents the major hurdle to pregnancy outcome in women with SSc, particularly in patients with pulmonary arterial hypertension (PAH), advanced pulmonary fibrosis and/or scleroderma renal crisis (SRC). Thus, a past history and/or de novo severe visceral involvement in a woman with SSc during pregnancy represent major risk factors for the occurrence of complications and/or materno-foetal mortality. Overall, during pregnancy, SSc remains clinically stable in 40-60% of patients, deteriorates in 20%, and improves in 20%. The variation probably relates to the heterogeneous nature of SSc [2, 29].

5.1 Vasculopathy

Vasculopathy is a prominent feature of SSc which may influence pregnancy outcome in women with preexisting SSc [23]. Thus, 22.9% of pregnant women with SSc develop hypertensive disorders including preeclampsia, corresponding to a four-fold increased as compared to the general population (85% CI, 2.4-6.6) [29]. Similarly, a nearly four-fold increased rate of intrauterine growth restriction was observed in the same study.

5.2 Scleroderma renal crisis

Scleroderma renal crisis (SRC) represent the worst complication that may occur in pregnant SSc patients. SRC is characterized by malignant hypertension, proteinuria, acute renal failure and in more than half of the cases thrombotic microangiopathy. SRC occur in patients with rapidly progressing diffuse skin disease of less than four years evolution. The frequency of maternal complications in SSc women with either diffuse or limited disease is not increased as compared with healthy controls, except for SRC [30]. This risk of SRC is lower if pregnancy is planned within 3-5 years from onset of symptoms [31]. Many of the perinatal deaths reported among SSc women are reported in those who develop SRC [32, 33]. Steen reported two cases of SRC in retrospective study of 86 pregnancies occurring after the diagnosis of SSc [34]. One woman developed end-stage renal disease, and the other died from status epilepticus. In a prospective study of 91 pregnancies, two cases of renal crisis were reported [20]. Both women required hemodialysis after delivery. Overall, it remains unclear if rates of SRC are increased in pregnant women compared to non pregnant women with severe diffuse disease [23]. Finally, SRC may be difficult to distinguish from preeclampsia in the pregnant SSc patient and renal biopsy may be indicated in case of difficulties to distinguish both disorders [35].

5.3 Pulmonary arterial hypertension

Pulmonary arterial hypertension is a major cause of morbidity and mortality in patients with SSc. In contrast to SRC, PAH can occur both in patients with limited or diffuse disease. Women with PAH identified by right heart catheterism are at extremely high risk of severe hemodynamic complications during pregnancy. Thus, the reserve in the pulmonary arterioles is markedly reduced and as a consequence vascular resistance cannot be reduced to accommodate the increased blood volume and cardiac output that occurs during pregnancy [23]. Reports estimated a 30%-56% maternal mortality rate in women with PAH . This maternal mortality rate is relevantly higher (56%) in women with secondary vascular pulmonary hypertension included connective tissues diseases, than in primary PAH and Eisenmenger's syndrome (30% and 36% respectively). The most vulnerable period occurring with delivery and the first two weeks postpartum [36]. Women with PAH should be strongly discouraged from becoming pregnant. All complaints of dyspnea in pregnant SSc women should prompt an immediate evaluation for the occurrence or worsening of PAH. Despite currently available treatments, a pregnancy is a principle-cons in pregnant women with PAH and a contraception is recommended for women of childbearing age.

5.4 Other complications

Gastro-oesophageal reflux increases during third trimester of pregnancy. Skin thickening has been reported to increase during post-partum in women with diffuse SSc.

Raynaud's phenomenon is characterized by vascular hyperactivity and vasospasm. Among all vascular complications of SSc, Raynaud's phenomenon and digital ulcers are the most likely to improve during pregnancy and worsen in postpartum [37]. Raynaud's phenomenon should not be considered a contraindication to pregnancy, even in patients with recurrent digital ulcers [23]. Reduction in skin fibrosis has been reported in SSc patients during pregnancy, with improvement lasting for up to one year post partum [38].

6. Management of pregnancy in patients with SSc

Women with SSc who become pregnant should be considered at high risk for complication related to the pregnancy. Multidisciplinary approach and aggressive prenatal monitoring are necessary for the management of women presenting with complications. PAH requires careful hemodynamic monitoring and specific management in collaboration with pneumologists. Women with SSc require extended observation in hospitalisation following delivery. Pregnancy must be planned when the disease is stable. Pregnancies should be avoided in women with SSc with significant cardio-pulmonary or renal disease because of the increased risk of maternal death. If women with SSc carefully consider the timing of pregnancy recomanded by their physician and are closely monitored, successful outcome can be obtained without excessive risk for the mother or the foetus [18].

7. Medications during pregnancy

At the time of diagnosis of pregnancy, drugs associated with an increased risk of fetal toxicity must be stopped. The treatment of severe hypertension during pregnancy in patients with SSc is difficult despite the use of multiple antihypertensive agents [39]. The routine use of ACE inhibitors is not recommended during pregnancy. An increased risk of fetal waste, teratogenic effects, fetal distress, and severe postpartum neonatal renal failure has been reported in the literature in this setting [40]. However, if the women has a history of SRC or is at high risk for developing SRC, an immediate initiation of Angiotensin conversing enzyme (ACE) inhibitors may be indicated. In cases of profound maternal or fetal distress, emergent delivery may be the most appropriate option followed by initiation of ACE inhibitor therapy. The severity of SRC during pregnancy and the benefits of ACE inhibitor treatment are highly likely to outweigh the risks of fetotoxicity [23].

Hydroxychloroquine in the setting of polyarthritis, intravenous immunoglobulin in the setting of documented myositis and low doses of steroids may be safely used during pregnancy. In case of pulmonary hypertension, successful use of epoprostenol and sildenafil has been reported in patients with PAH during pregnancy. Anticoagulation with low-molecular-weigth heparin is recommended to reduce risk of thromboembolism, since anti-vitamine K agents are teratogenic [41].

Calcium channel blockers are classically contra-indicated during pregnancy. However, Wilson and Kirby reported the successful conception and pregnancy in a woman with SSc while receiving continuous treatment with nifedipine 30 mg/day, after a previously poor obstetric record and involuntary secondary infertility. They speculated that nifedipine might have had a beneficial effect on conceiving and maintaining the pregnancy in this patient [42]. In addition, calcium channel blockers might prevent hypertension and premature labour. Thus, nifedipine is regularly prescribed in women with SSc during pregnancy. Finally, Basso and Ghio reported the first case of successful pregnancy in a woman with SSc treated with cyclosporine [43].

A Japan team reported the case of a woman with SSc who experienced two spontaneous abortions before delivering a healthy baby after administration of vitamin E. Vitamin E is known to have properties of antioxidants and anti-platelet aggregation agents and may prevent placental ischemia induced by decidual vasculopathy [19].

Among immunosuppressive treatments prescribed in patients with SSc, azathioprine is the only one which can be prescribed during pregnancy. Thus, the drug does not seem to be teratogenic in humans [44], whereas cyclophosphamide, methotrexate and mycophenolate mofetyl are teratogenic. Because of the potential for carcinogenesis and the unknown long-term effects of fetal immunosuppression, the use of azathioprine should be reserved for pregnant women whose diseases are severe or life-threatening. Reduction of the azathioprine dose at 32 weeks' gestation may prevent serious neonatal leukopenia and thrombocytopenia. Close prenatal monitoring for growth and long-term evaluation of the offspring are essential [45].

8. Conclusion

Pregnancies in patients with SSc are infrequent. There is no increase in the frequency of miscarriages but an increased premature births and small full-term babies in patients with SSc. Vascular manifestations including SRC and PAH should be considered as contraindications for pregnancy due to the increased risk of both maternal and fetal morbidity and mortality. The use of ACE inhibitors is recommended in pregnant women with SRC despite the risk of teratogenicity. In order to minimize risks, a multidisciplinary approach is necessary to suggest the best timing for pregnancy and provide adequate supportive treatment to patients with SSc during pregnancy.

SSc : Systemic sclerosis

SRC : Scleroderma renal crisis

PAH : Pulmonary arterial hypertension

ACE : Angiotensin conversing enzyme

9. References

[1] Ranque B, Mouthon L. Geoepidemiology of systemic sclerosis. Autoimmun Rev 2010;9(5):A311-8.

[2] Weiner ES, Brinkman CR, Paulus HE. Scleroderma CREST syndrome and pregnancy [abstract]. Arthritis Rheum 1986;29(suppl):S51.

[3] Johnson TR, Banner EA, Winkelmann RK. Scleroderma and pregnancy. Obstet Gynecol 1964;23:467-9.

[4] Artlett CM, Rasheed M, Russo-Stieglitz KE, Sawaya HH, Jimenez SA. Influence of prior pregnancies on disease course and cause of death in systemic sclerosis. Ann Rheum Dis. 2002 Apr;61(4):346-50.

[5] Silman AJ. Pregnancy and scleroderma. Am J Reprod Immunol. 1992 Oct-Dec;28(3-4):238-40.

[6] Silman AJ, Black C. Increased incidence of spontaneous abortion and infertility in women with scleroderma before disease onset: a controlled study. Ann Rheum Dis. 1988 Jun;47(6):441-4.

[7] Bianchi DW, Zickwolf GK, Weil GJ, Sylvester S, DeMaria MA. Male fetal progenitor cells persist in maternal blood for as long as 27 years postpartum. Proc Natl Acad Sci U S A. 1996 Jan 23;93(2):705-8.

[8] Chosidow O, Bagot M, Vernant JP, Roujeau JC, Cordonnier C, Kuentz M, Wechsler J, André C, Touraine R, Revuz J. Sclerodermatous chronic graft-versus-host disease. Analysis of seven cases. J Am Acad Dermatol. 1992 Jan;26(1):49-55.

[9] Black CM, Stevens WM. Scleroderma. Rheum Dis Clin North Am. 1989 May;15(2):193-212.

[10] Artlett CM, Smith JB, Jimenez SA. Identification of fetal DNA and cells in skin lesions from women with systemic sclerosis. N Engl J Med. 1998 Apr 23;338(17):1186-91.

[11] Adams KM, Nelson JL. Microchimerism: an investigative frontier in autoimmunity and transplantation. JAMA. 2004 Mar 3;291(9):1127-31.

[12] Nelson JL, Furst DE, Maloney S, Gooley T, Evans PC, Smith A, Bean MA, Ober C, Bianchi DW. Microchimerism and HLA-compatible relationships of pregnancy in scleroderma. Lancet. 1998 Feb 21;351(9102):559-62.

[13] Silman AJ, Black C. Increased incidence of spontaneous abortion and infertility in women with scleroderma before disease onset: a controlled study. Ann Rheum Dis. 1988 Jun;47(6):441-4.

[14] Lambe M, Björnådal L, Neregård P, Nyren O, Cooper GS. Childbearing and the risk of scleroderma: a population-based study in Sweden. Am J Epidemiol. 2004 Jan 15;159(2):162-6.

[15] Englert H, Brennan P, McNeil D, Black C, Silman AJ. Reproductive function prior to disease onset in women with scleroderma. J Rheumatol. 1992 Oct;19(10):1575-9.

[16] Pisa FE, Bovenzi M, Romeo L, Tonello A, Biasi D, Bambara LM, Betta A, Barbone F. Reproductive factors and the risk of scleroderma: an Italian case-control study. Arthritis Rheum. 2002 Feb;46(2):451-6.

[17] Giordano M, Valentini G, Lupoli S, Giordano A. Pregnancy and systemic sclerosis. Arthritis Rheum. 1985 Feb;28(2):237-8.

[18] Steen VD, Medsger TA Jr. Fertility and pregnancy outcome in women with systemic sclerosis. Arthritis Rheum. 1999 Apr;42(4):763-8.

[19] Harada M, Kumemura H, Harada R, Komai K, Sata M. Scleroderma and repeated spontaneous abortions treated with vitamin E-a case report-Kurume Med J. 2005;52(3):93-5.

[20] Steen VD, Conte C, Day N, Ramsey-Goldman R, Medsger TA Jr. Pregnancy in women with systemic sclerosis. Arthritis Rheum. 1989 Feb;32(2):151-7.

[21] Chung L, Flyckt RL, Colón I, Shah AA, Druzin M, Chakravarty EF. Outcome of pregnancies complicated by systemic sclerosis and mixed connective tissue disease. Lupus. 2006;15(9):595-9.

[22] Bédard E, Dimopoulos K, Gatzoulis MA. Has there been any progress made on pregnancy outcomes among women with pulmonary arterial hypertension? Eur Heart J. 2009 Feb;30(3):256-65. Epub 2009 Jan 15.

[23] Chakravarty EF. Vascular Complications of Systemic Sclerosis during Pregnancy. Int J Rheumatol. 2010;2010. pii: 287248. Epub 2010 Aug 11.

[24] Doss BJ, Jacques SM, Mayes MD, Qureshi F. Maternal scleroderma: placental findings and perinatal outcome. Hum Pathol. 1998 Dec;29(12):1524-30.

[25] Labarrere CA, Catoggio LJ, Mullen EG, Althabe OH. Placental lesions in maternal autoimmune diseases.Am J Reprod Immunol Microbiol. 1986 Nov;12(3):78-86.

[26] Bernatsky S, Hudson M, Pope J, Vinet E, Markland J, Robinson D, Jones N, Docherty P, Abu-Hakima M, Leclercq S, Dunne J, Smith D, Mathieu JP, Khalidi N, Sutton E,

Baron M. Assessment of reproductive history in systemic sclerosis. Arthritis Rheum. 2008 Nov 15;59(11):1661-4.

[27] Launay D, Hebbar M, Hatron PY, Michon-Pasturel U, Queyrel V, Hachulla E, Devulder B. Relationship between parity and clinical and biological features in patients with systemic sclerosis. J Rheumatol. 2001 Mar;28(3):509-13.

[28] Cockrill T, del Junco DJ, Arnett FC, Assassi S, Tan FK, McNearney T, Fischbach M, Perry M, Mayes MD. Separate influences of birth order and gravidity/parity on the development of systemic sclerosis. Arthritis Care Res (Hoboken). 2010 Mar;62(3):418-24.

[29] Chakravarty EF, Khanna D, Chung L. Pregnancy outcomes in systemic sclerosis, primary pulmonary hypertension, and sickle cell disease. Obstet Gynecol. 2008 Apr;111(4):927-34.

[30] Steen VD. Pregnancy in women with systemic sclerosis. Obstet Gynecol. 1999 Jul;94(1):15-20.

[31] Steen VD. Scleroderma and pregnancy. Rheum Dis Clin North Am. 1997 Feb;23(1):133-47.

[32] Ramsay B, De Belder A, Campbell S, Moncada S, Martin JF. A nitric oxide donor improves uterine artery diastolic blood flow in normal early pregnancy and in women at high risk of pre-eclampsia. Eur J Clin Invest. 1994 Jan;24(1):76-8.

[33] Younker D, Harrison B. Scleroderma and pregnancy. Anaesthetic considerations. Br J Anaesth. 1985 Nov;57(11):1136-9.

[34] Steen VD, Mayes MD, Merkel PA. Assessment of kidney involvement. Clin Exp Rheumatol. 2003;21(3 Suppl 29):S29-31.

[35] Mok CC, Kwan TH, Chow L. Scleroderma renal crisis sine scleroderma during pregnancy. Scand J Rheumatol. 2003;32(1):55-7.

[36] Weiss BM, Zemp L, Seifert B, Hess OM. Outcome of pulmonary vascular disease in pregnancy: a systemic overview from 17978 through 1996. J Am Coll Cardiol.1998 Jun;31(7):1650-7.

[37] Steen VD. Pregnancy in scleroderma. Rheum Dis Clin North Am. 2007 May;33(2):345-58, vii.

[38] Goplerud CP. Scleroderma. Clin Obstet Gynecol. 1983 Sep;26(3):587-91.

[39] Scarpinato L, Mackenzie AH. Pregnancy and progressive systemic sclerosis. Case report and review of the literature. Cleve Clin Q. 1985 Summer;52(2):207-11.

[40] Broughton Pipkin F, Turner SR, Symonds EM. Possible risk with captopril in pregnancy: some animal data. Lancet. 1980 Jun 7;1(8180):1256.

[41] Madden BP. Pulmonary hypertension and pregnancy. Int J Obstet Anesth. 2009 Apr;18(2):156-64. Epub 2009 Feb 14.

[42] Wilson AG, Kirby JD. Successful pregnancy in a woman with systemic sclerosis while taking nifedipine. Ann Rheum Dis. 1990 Jan;49(1):51-2.

[43] Basso M, Ghio M, Filaci G, Setti M, Indiveri F. A case of successful pregnancy in a woman with systemic sclerosis treated with cyclosporin. Rheumatology (Oxford). 2004 Oct;43(10):1310-1.

[44] Rudolph J, Schweizer R, Bartus S. Pregnancy in renal transplant patients. Transplantation. 1979;27:26-29.

[45] Janssen NM, Genta MS. The effects of immunosuppressive and anti-inflammatory medications on fertility, pregnancy, and lactation. Arch Intern Med. 2000 Mar 13;160(5):610-9.